REFERENCE
GUIDE TO THE
OCCUPATIONAL
THERAPY

CODE OF
ETHICS & ETHICS
STANDARDS

2010 EDITION

Deborah Yarett Slater,
MS, OT/L, FAOTA
Editor

Foreword by
Florence Clark,
PhD, OTR/L, FAOTA

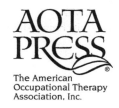

AOTA
PRESS
The American
Occupational Therapy
Association, Inc.

AOTA Centennial Vision
We envision that occupational therapy is a powerful, widely recognized, science-driven, and evidence-based profession with a globally connected and diverse workforce meeting society's occupational needs.

Mission Statement
The American Occupational Therapy Association advances the quality, availability, use, and support of occupational therapy through standard-setting, advocacy, education, and research on behalf of its members and the public.

AOTA Staff
Frederick P. Somers, *Executive Director*
Christopher M. Bluhm, *Chief Operating Officer*

Chris Davis, *Director, AOTA Press*
K. Hyde Loomis, *Production Consultant*
Ashley Hofmann, *Development/Production Editor*
Victoria Davis, *Production Editor/Editorial Assistant*

Beth Ledford, *Director, Marketing*
Emily Zhang, *Technology Marketing Specialist*
Jennifer Folden, *Marketing Specialist*

American Occupational Therapy Association, Inc.
4720 Montgomery Lane
Bethesda, MD 20814
Phone: 301-652-AOTA (2682)
TDD: 800-377-8555
Fax: 301-652-7711
www.aota.org
To order: http://store.aota.org

Disclaimers
This publication is designed to provide accurate and authoritative information in regard to the subject matter covered. It is sold or distributed with the understanding that the publisher is not engaged in rendering legal, accounting, or other professional service. If legal advice or other expert assistance is required, the services of a competent professional person should be sought.
—*From the Declaration of Principles jointly adopted by the American Bar Association and a Committee of Publishers and Associations*

It is the objective of the American Occupational Therapy Association to be a forum for free expression and interchange of ideas. The opinions expressed by the contributors to this work are their own and not necessarily those of the American Occupational Therapy Association.

ISBN 10: 1-56900-310-6
ISBN 13: 978-1-56900-310-7

Library of Congress Control Number: 2011925107

Cover Design by Sarah Ely and Jennifer Farr
Composition by Maryland Composition, Laurel, MD
Printed by Automated Graphic Systems, Inc., White Plains, MD

Contents

Foreword

Radical changes in the health care environment have led to challenges in the diverse roles that occupational therapists and occupational therapy assistants fulfill. Although perhaps most evident in the practice arena, these changes also influence the way students of the profession are educated and the way research related to the field is carried out.

The focus of occupational therapy practice, professional education, and research typically revolves around competency. In fact, the *Occupational Therapy Code of Ethics and Ethics Standards (2010)* (referred to as the "Code and Ethics Standards"; American Occupational Therapy Association [AOTA], 2010b) contains significant language related directly and indirectly to competency in all three areas under Principle 1 (Beneficence):

1. *Practice:* The Code and Ethics Standards refer to the use of appropriate and current assessment tools, provision of services that "are within each practitioner's level of competence and scope of practice" (Principle 1E), use of evidence-based techniques and equipment where possible (Principle 1F), and the obligation to "take responsible steps (e.g., continuing education, research, supervision, training) and use careful judgment to ensure their own competence and weigh potential for client harm when generally recognized standards do not exist in emerging technology or areas of practice" (Principle 1G).

2. *Professional education:* Educators, too, are mandated to "provide occupational therapy education, continuing education, instruction, and training that are within the instructor's subject area of expertise and level of competence" while also providing students with education related to the Code and Ethics Standards and resolving or reporting ethical conflict (Principles 1J and 1K).

3. *Research:* Finally, researchers must "ensure that occupational therapy research is conducted in accordance with currently accepted ethical guidelines and standards for the protection of research participants and the dissemination of results" (Principle 1L).

Regardless of their specific role, all occupational therapy personnel are expected to "report to appropriate authorities any acts in practice, education, and research that appear unethical or illegal" (Principle 1M). Principle 5 (Procedural Justice), particularly 5F, also contains important language about our responsibility "for maintaining high standards and continuing competence in practice, education, and research." So by virtue of inclusion in this Code and Ethics Standards document, practical competency to perform our work-related responsibilities, regardless of the venue, is clearly an important ethical mandate.

However, performing our work-related responsibilities to meet professional and other standards involves more than practical competency alone. Along with critical, procedural, and interactive reasoning, ethical reasoning is a core competency and must inform not only professional conduct but also daily decisions in the workplace. The public grants professionals greater autonomy when the profession establishes a code of ethics to set standards of behavior and guide actions and has in place an enforcement process to ensure compliance. It is the responsibility of educators to provide students with knowledge and skills related to ethical reasoning that can be further developed and applied as they move into clinical practice, education, or research. These qualifications are invaluable in addressing the inevitable challenges of providing services that meet the primary goal of benefiting our clients, particularly in these times of limited health care resources and administrative and reimbursement constraints. The Code and Ethics Standards, along with additional ethics-related educational materials, provide a foundation for ethical actions and decisions, whether they occur in the clinic, at the university, or while conducting research.

The purpose of this *Reference Guide to the Occupational Therapy Code of Ethics and Ethics Standards* is to support and guide members of the occupational therapy profession in the area of ethics. Situations in which ethical dilemmas or questions arise have become remarkably common in today's world. They are part of everyday practice (including education and research) and, as witnessed by the volume of inquiries to AOTA, can appear with surprising frequency and considerable complexity. With increased awareness of and reflection on ethics, occupational therapists, occupational therapy assistants, and students may be challenged to rethink their usual responses to situations in their daily work. Resolution of ethical issues and dilemmas can cause significant angst, even to experienced professionals in the field. This *Reference Guide* aims to address these challenges by linking aspirational principles, factual case descriptions, and a framework for analysis and decision making to assist readers in resolving these conflicts.

In addition to the new Code and Ethics Standards and most recent *Enforcement Procedures for the Occupational Therapy Code of Ethics and Ethics Standards* (AOTA, 2010a), this book contains new content, including new advisory opinions, ethics-related articles, and advice about suggested learning activities for educators using content from the *Reference Guide*. The 2010 edition of the Code and Ethics Standards has expanded language to broaden its relevance not only to educators and researchers (in addition to clinical practitioners, the traditional audience) but also to those in roles such as consultant, administrator or manager, business owner, emerging technology developer or user, and elected or appointed volunteer. Like other AOTA ethics and continuing education resources, this *Reference Guide* uses real-life situations to illustrate the analysis and application of ethical concepts to promote the resolution of ethical dilemmas. The goal is to illustrate, as readers approach and reason through complicated and challenging situations, the relevance of ethics to the practical world of everyday life and work. This knowledge ultimately promotes better client care, competency, and professional satisfaction.

—*Florence Clark, PhD, OTR/L, FAOTA*
President
American Occupational Therapy Association

REFERENCES

American Occupational Therapy Association. (2010a). Enforcement procedures for the *Occupational Therapy Code of Ethics and Ethics Standards. American Journal of Occupational Therapy, 64*(Suppl.), S4–S16. doi:10.5014/ajot.2010.64S4

American Occupational Therapy Association. (2010b). Occupational therapy code of ethics and ethics standards (2010). *American Journal of Occupational Therapy, 64*(Suppl.), S17–S26. doi:10.5014/ajot.2010.64S17

Acknowledgments

This edition of the *Reference Guide to the Occupational Therapy Code of Ethics and Ethics Standards* was updated by the members of the AOTA Ethics Commission:

Barbara Hemphill, DMin, OTR, FAOTA, FMOTA, *Chairperson*

Kathlyn L. Reed, PhD, OTR, FAOTA, MLIS, *Past Chairperson*

Lea Cheyney Brandt, OTD, MA, OTR/L, *Member at Large*

Ann Moodey Ashe, MHS, OTR/L, *Practice Representative*

Loretta Jean Foster, MS, COTA/L, *OTA Representative*

Joanne Estes, MS, OTR/L, *Education Representative*

Donna F. Homenko, PhD, RHD, *Public Member*

Craig R. Jackson, JD, MSW, *Public Member*

Deborah Yarett Slater, MS, OT/L, FAOTA, *AOTA Staff Liaison*

The Ethics Commission refined, organized, and made additions to the contents of this new edition to enhance its functionality and relevance as a fundamental resource for members of the occupational therapy profession and those they serve.

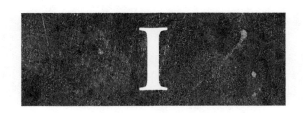

OCCUPATIONAL THERAPY CODE OF ETHICS AND ETHICS STANDARDS (2010)

CHAPTER 1

Reference Guide to the Occupational Therapy Code of Ethics and Ethics Standards

AOTA Ethics Commission

The Ethics Commission (EC) of the American Occupational Therapy Association (AOTA) was established in 1975 by the AOTA Representative Assembly with the passage of Resolution 461–75. As stated in the AOTA Bylaws (AOTA, 2009b), the purpose of the EC is "to serve the Association members and public through the identification, development, review, interpretation, and education of the AOTA *Occupational Therapy Code of Ethics and Ethics Standards* and to provide the process whereby the ethics of the Association are enforced" (Art. 7, §7).

AOTA has developed the *Occupational Therapy Code of Ethics and Ethics Standards (2010)* (referred to as the "Code and Ethics Standards"; AOTA, 2010b) and *Standards of Practice for Occupational Therapy* (AOTA, 2010e) to promote quality care and professional conduct. The EC is responsible for reviewing and enforcing ethics standards related to practice, education, and research. The contents of this edition of the *Reference Guide to the Occupational Therapy Code of Ethics and Ethics Standards* have an increased focus on all aspects of professional conduct and its application to the many roles in which occupational therapists, occupational therapy assistants, or students may find themselves. These roles go beyond traditional practice, education, and research and include elected and volunteer leadership roles in the profession.

The EC has no jurisdiction over certification or accreditation standards. Initial certification is the responsibility of the National Board for Certification in Occupational Therapy (NBCOT), formed in 1986. Compliance with accreditation standards for occupational therapy educational programs is the responsibility of the Accreditation Council for Occupational Therapy Education. Note that violations of the Code and Ethics Standards also may be reported to state regulatory boards (SRBs) or the NBCOT for consideration. Similarly, SRBs or the NBCOT may refer cases of violation of professional conduct, licensure, or certification standards to the EC for their information and action as deemed appropriate.

Relationship to State Regulatory Boards

States with regulatory laws governing occupational therapy personnel have the responsibility to investigate alleged violations that have caused or have the potential to cause harm to the public in that state and to take disciplinary action as defined within those state laws and regulations. Disciplinary language in state regulations may reflect or reference AOTA documents on standards of practice and ethical conduct. When informed of disciplinary action by SRBs, the EC may take further action or may take independent action if the individual is a member of AOTA.

AOTA Standards of Practice

AOTA, through the Commission on Practice and the Commission on Continuing Competence and Professional Development, has developed practice standards and related documents for occupational therapy practitioners. The AOTA Representative Assembly recently adopted revisions to the following standards:

- *Standards of Practice for Occupational Therapy* (AOTA, 2010e)
- *Guidelines for Supervision, Roles, and Responsibilities During the Delivery of Occupational Therapy Services* (AOTA, 2009a)
- *Standards for Continuing Competence* (AOTA, 2010d)
- *Scope of Practice* (AOTA, 2010c).

Code and Ethics Standards

The *Occupational Therapy Code of Ethics* was initially adopted in 1977 and was revised in 1979, 1988, 1994, 2000, 2005, and 2010. It is reviewed for potential revision, at a minimum, every 5 years. The Representative Assembly adopted the current Code and Ethics Standards in April 2010; this document replaces the 2005 *Occupational Therapy Code of Ethics* (AOTA, 2005) and integrates two other previous AOTA documents: the *Guidelines to the Occupational Therapy Code of Ethics* (AOTA, 2006), and the *Core Values and Attitudes of Occupational Therapy Practice* (AOTA, 1993). The three documents were merged to make it easier for AOTA constituents to locate and apply information about the core concepts and standards that guide the profession.

The Code and Ethics Standards apply to AOTA members at all levels in professional roles such as practitioner, educator, fieldwork educator or coordinator, clinical supervisor, manager, administrator, consultant, faculty, program director, researcher or scholar, private practice owner, entrepreneur, student, and others, including elective and appointed volunteer roles within AOTA. The Code and Ethics Standards are available to AOTA members and the public on AOTA's Web site (www.aota.org) and through AOTA's Ethics Office. They were also published in Volume 64 of the *American Journal of Occupational Therapy* (AOTA, 2010b).

Enforcement Procedures

To ensure maintenance of the Code and Ethics Standards and compliance by AOTA members, *Enforcement Procedures for the Occupational Therapy Code of Ethics and Ethics Standards* (AOTA, 2010a) have been developed for the investigation and adjudication of alleged violations. These procedures, initially approved by the 1996 Representative Assembly and most recently updated in 2009, enable the Association to act fairly in the performance of its responsibilities as a professional membership organization. Their purpose also is to safeguard the rights of individuals against whom complaints have been made. The most current Enforcement Procedures are included in this *Reference Guide*.

References

American Occupational Therapy Association. (1993). Core values and attitudes of occupational therapy practice. *American Journal of Occupational Therapy, 47,* 1085–1086.

American Occupational Therapy Association. (2005). Occupational therapy code of ethics. *American Journal of Occupational Therapy, 59,* 639–642.

American Occupational Therapy Association. (2006). Guidelines to the occupational therapy code of ethics. *American Journal of Occupational Therapy, 60,* 652–658.

American Occupational Therapy Association. (2009a). Guidelines for supervision, roles and responsibilities during the delivery of occupational therapy services. *American Journal of Occupational Therapy, 63,* 797–803. doi:10.5014/ajot.63.6.797

American Occupational Therapy Association. (2009b). *The official bylaws of the American Occupational Therapy Association, Inc.* Retrieved

November 17, 2010, from www.aota.org/Governance/bylaws.aspx

American Occupational Therapy Association. (2010a). Enforcement procedures for the *Occupational Therapy Code of Ethics and Ethics Standards*. *American Journal of Occupational Therapy, 64*(6 Suppl.), S4–S16. doi:10.5014/ajot.2010.64S4

American Occupational Therapy Association. (2010b). Occupational therapy code of ethics and ethics standards (2010). *American Journal of Occupational Therapy, 64*(6 Suppl.), S17–S26. doi:10.5014/ajot.2010.64S17

American Occupational Therapy Association. (2010c). Scope of practice. *American Journal of Occupational Therapy, 64*(6 Suppl.), S70–S77. doi:10.5014/ajot.2010.64S70

American Occupational Therapy Association. (2010d). Standards for continuing competence. *American Journal of Occupational Therapy,* 64(6 Suppl.), S103–S105. doi:10.5014/ajot.2010.64S103

American Occupational Therapy Association. (2010e). Standards of practice for occupational therapy. *American Journal of Occupational Therapy,* 64(6 Suppl.), S106–S111. doi:10.5014/ajot.2010.64S106

Penny Kyler, MA, OTR/L, FAOTA

AOTA Staff Liaison to the Ethics Commission

Deborah Yarett Slater, MS, OT/L, FAOTA

AOTA Staff Liaison to the Ethics Commission

This chapter was originally published in the 2006 edition of the *Reference Guide to the Occupational Therapy Code of Ethics*. It has been revised to reflect updated AOTA official documents, Web sites, AOTA style, and additional resources.

Occupational Therapy Code of Ethics and Ethics Standards (2010)

PREAMBLE

The American Occupational Therapy Association (AOTA) *Occupational Therapy Code of Ethics and Ethics Standards (2010)* ("Code and Ethics Standards") is a public statement of principles used to promote and maintain high standards of conduct within the profession. Members of AOTA are committed to promoting inclusion, diversity, independence, and safety for all recipients in various stages of life, health, and illness and to empower all beneficiaries of occupational therapy. This commitment extends beyond service recipients to include professional colleagues, students, educators, businesses, and the community.

Fundamental to the mission of the occupational therapy profession is the therapeutic use of everyday life activities (occupations) with individuals or groups for the purpose of participation in roles and situations in home, school, workplace, community, and other settings. "Occupational therapy addresses the physical, cognitive, psychosocial, sensory, and other aspects of performance in a variety of contexts to support engagement in everyday life activities that affect health, well-being, and quality of life" (AOTA, 2004, p. 694). Occupational therapy personnel have an ethical responsibility primarily to recipients of service and secondarily to society.

The *Occupational Therapy Code of Ethics and Ethics Standards (2010)* was tailored to address the most prevalent ethical concerns of the profession in education, research, and practice. The concerns of stakeholders including the public, consumers, students, colleagues, employers, research participants, researchers, educators, and practitioners were addressed in the creation of this document. A review of issues raised in ethics cases, member questions related to ethics, and content of other professional codes of ethics were utilized to ensure that the revised document is applicable to occupational therapists, occupational therapy assistants, and students in all roles.

The historical foundation of this Code and Ethics Standards is based on ethical reasoning surrounding practice and professional issues, as well as on empathic reflection regarding these interactions with others (see e.g., AOTA, 2005, 2006). This reflection resulted in the establishment of principles that guide ethical action, which goes beyond rote following of rules or application of principles. Rather, *ethical action* is a manifestation of moral character and mindful reflection. It is a commitment to benefit others, to virtuous practice of artistry and science, to genuinely good behaviors, and to noble acts of courage.

While much has changed over the course of the profession's history, more has remained the same. The profession of occupational therapy remains grounded in seven core concepts, as identified in the *Core Values and Attitudes of Occupational Therapy Practice* (AOTA, 1993): *altruism, equality, freedom, justice, dignity, truth,* and *prudence. Altruism* is the individual's ability to place the needs of others before their own. *Equality* refers to the desire to promote fairness in interactions with others. The concept of *freedom* and personal choice is paramount in a profession in which the desires of the client must guide our interventions. Occupational therapy practitioners, educators, and researchers relate in a fair and impartial manner to individuals with whom they interact and respect and adhere to the applicable laws and standards regarding their area of practice, be it direct care, education, or research *(justice).* Inherent in the practice of occupational therapy is the promotion and preservation of the individuality and *dignity* of the client, by assisting him or her to engage in occupations that are meaningful to him or her regardless of level of disability. In all situations, occupational therapists, occupational therapy assistants, and students must provide accurate information, both in oral and written form *(truth).* Occupational therapy personnel use their clinical and ethical reasoning skills, sound judgment, and reflection to make decisions to direct them in their area(s) of practice *(prudence).* These seven core values provide a foundation by which occupational therapy personnel guide their interactions with others, be they students, clients, colleagues, research participants, or communities. These values also define the ethical principles to which the profession is committed and which the public can expect.

The *Occupational Therapy Code of Ethics and Ethics Standards (2010)* is a guide to professional conduct when ethical issues arise. Ethical decision making is a process that includes awareness of how the outcome will impact occupational therapy clients in all spheres. Applications of Code and Ethics Standards Principles are considered situation-specific, and where a conflict exists, occupational therapy personnel will pursue responsible efforts for resolution. These Principles apply to occupational therapy personnel engaged in any professional role, including elected and volunteer leadership positions.

The specific purposes of the *Occupational Therapy Code of Ethics and Ethics Standards (2010)* are to

1. Identify and describe the principles supported by the occupational therapy profession.
2. Educate the general public and members regarding established principles to which occupational therapy personnel are accountable.
3. Socialize occupational therapy personnel to expected standards of conduct.
4. Assist occupational therapy personnel in recognition and resolution of ethical dilemmas.

The *Occupational Therapy Code of Ethics and Ethics Standards (2010)* define the set of principles that apply to occupational therapy personnel at all levels:

Definitions

Recipient of service: Individuals or groups receiving occupational therapy.

Student: A person who is enrolled in an accredited occupational therapy education program.

Research participant: A prospective participant or one who has agreed to participate in an approved research project.

Employee: A person who is hired by a business (facility or organization) to provide occupational therapy services.

Colleague: A person who provides services in the same or different business (facility or organization) to which a professional relationship exists or may exist.

Public: The community of people at large.

BENEFICENCE

Principle 1. Occupational therapy personnel shall demonstrate a concern for the well-being and safety of the recipients of their services.

Beneficence includes all forms of action intended to benefit other persons. The term *beneficence* connotes acts of mercy, kindness, and charity (Beauchamp & Childress, 2009). Forms of beneficence typically include altruism, love, and humanity. Beneficence requires taking action by helping others, in other words, by promoting good, by preventing harm, and by removing harm. Examples of beneficence include protecting and defending the rights of others, preventing harm from occurring to others, removing conditions that will cause harm to others, helping persons with disabilities, and rescuing persons in danger (Beauchamp & Childress, 2009).

Occupational therapy personnel shall

A. Respond to requests for occupational therapy services (e.g., a referral) in a timely manner as determined by law, regulation, or policy.

B. Provide appropriate evaluation and a plan of intervention for all recipients of occupational therapy services specific to their needs.

C. Reevaluate and reassess recipients of service in a timely manner to determine if goals are being achieved and whether intervention plans should be revised.

D. Avoid the inappropriate use of outdated or obsolete tests/assessments or data obtained from such tests in making intervention decisions or recommendations.

E. Provide occupational therapy services that are within each practitioner's level of competence and scope of practice (e.g., qualifications, experience, the law).

F. Use, to the extent possible, evaluation, planning, intervention techniques, and therapeutic equipment that are evidence-based and within the recognized scope of occupational therapy practice.

G. Take responsible steps (e.g., continuing education, research, supervision, training) and use careful judgment to ensure their own competence and weigh potential for client harm when generally recognized standards do not exist in emerging technology or areas of practice.

H. Terminate occupational therapy services in collaboration with the service recipient or responsible party when the needs and goals of the recipient have been met or when services no longer produce a measurable change or outcome.

I. Refer to other health care specialists solely on the basis of the needs of the client.

J. Provide occupational therapy education, continuing education, instruction, and training that are within the instructor's subject area of expertise and level of competence.

K. Provide students and employees with information about the Code and Ethics Standards, opportunities to discuss ethical conflicts, and procedures for reporting unresolved ethical conflicts.

L. Ensure that occupational therapy research is conducted in accordance with currently accepted ethical guidelines and standards for the protection of research participants and the dissemination of results.

M. Report to appropriate authorities any acts in practice, education, and research that appear unethical or illegal.

N. Take responsibility for promoting and practicing occupational therapy on the basis of current knowledge and research and for further developing the profession's body of knowledge.

NONMALEFICENCE

Principle 2. Occupational therapy personnel shall intentionally refrain from actions that cause harm.

Nonmaleficence imparts an obligation to refrain from harming others (Beauchamp & Childress,

2009). The principle of nonmaleficence is grounded in the practitioner's responsibility to refrain from causing harm, inflicting injury, or wronging others. While beneficence requires action to incur benefit, nonmaleficence requires non-action to avoid harm (Beauchamp & Childress, 2009). Nonmaleficence also includes an obligation to not impose risks of harm even if the potential risk is without malicious or harmful intent. This principle often is examined under the context of *due care*. If the standard of due care outweighs the benefit of treatment, then refraining from treatment provision would be ethically indicated (Beauchamp & Childress, 2009).

Occupational therapy personnel shall

A. Avoid inflicting harm or injury to recipients of occupational therapy services, students, research participants, or employees.

B. Make every effort to ensure continuity of services or options for transition to appropriate services to avoid abandoning the service recipient if the current provider is unavailable due to medical or other absence or loss of employment.

C. Avoid relationships that exploit the recipient of services, students, research participants, or employees physically, emotionally, psychologically, financially, socially, or in any other manner that conflicts or interferes with professional judgment and objectivity.

D. Avoid engaging in any sexual relationship or activity, whether consensual or nonconsensual, with any recipient of service, including family or significant other, student, research participant, or employee, while a relationship exists as an occupational therapy practitioner, educator, researcher, supervisor, or employer.

E. Recognize and take appropriate action to remedy personal problems and limitations that might cause harm to recipients of service, colleagues, students, research participants, or others.

F. Avoid any undue influences, such as alcohol or drugs, that may compromise the provision of occupational therapy services, education, or research.

G. Avoid situations in which a practitioner, educator, researcher, or employer is unable to maintain clear professional boundaries or objectivity to ensure the safety and well-being of recipients of service, students, research participants, and employees.

H. Maintain awareness of and adherence to the Code and Ethics Standards when participating in volunteer roles.

I. Avoid compromising client rights or well-being based on arbitrary administrative directives by exercising professional judgment and critical analysis.

J. Avoid exploiting any relationship established as an occupational therapist or occupational therapy assistant to further one's own physical, emotional, financial, political, or business interests at the expense of the best interests of recipients of services, students, research participants, employees, or colleagues.

K. Avoid participating in bartering for services because of the potential for exploitation and conflict of interest unless there are clearly no contraindications or bartering is a culturally appropriate custom.

L. Determine the proportion of risk to benefit for participants in research prior to implementing a study.

AUTONOMY, CONFIDENTIALITY

Principle 3. Occupational therapy personnel shall respect the right of the individual to self-determination.

The principle of autonomy and confidentiality expresses the concept that practitioners have a duty to treat the client according to the client's desires, within the bounds of accepted standards of care and to protect the client's confidential information. Often *autonomy* is referred to as the *self-determination* principle. However, respect for autonomy goes beyond acknowledging an individual as a mere agent and also acknowledges a "person's right to hold views, to make choices, and to take actions based on personal values and beliefs" (Beauchamp & Childress, 2009, p. 103). Autonomy has become a prominent principle in health care ethics; the right to make a determination regarding care decisions that directly impact the life of the service recipient should reside with that individual. The principle of autonomy and confidentiality also applies to students in an educational program, to participants in research studies, and to the public who seek information about occupational therapy services.

Occupational therapy personnel shall

A. Establish a collaborative relationship with recipients of service, including families, significant others, and caregivers in setting goals and priorities throughout the intervention process. This includes full disclosure of the benefits, risks, and potential outcomes of any intervention; the personnel who will be providing the intervention(s); and/or any reasonable alternatives to the proposed intervention.
B. Obtain consent before administering any occupational therapy service, including evaluation, and ensure that recipients of service (or their legal representatives) are kept informed of the progress in meeting goals specified in the plan of intervention/care. If the service recipient cannot give consent, the practitioner must be sure that consent has been obtained from the person who is legally responsible for that recipient.
C. Respect the recipient of service's right to refuse occupational therapy services temporarily or permanently without negative consequences.
D. Provide students with access to accurate information regarding educational requirements and academic policies and procedures relative to the occupational therapy program/educational institution.
E. Obtain informed consent from participants involved in research activities, and

ensure that they understand the benefits, risks, and potential outcomes as a result of their participation as research subjects.
F. Respect research participants' right to withdraw from a research study without consequences.
G. Ensure that confidentiality and the right to privacy are respected and maintained regarding all information obtained about recipients of service, students, research participants, colleagues, or employees. The only exceptions are when a practitioner or staff member believes that an individual is in serious foreseeable or imminent harm. Laws and regulations may require disclosure to appropriate authorities without consent.
H. Maintain the confidentiality of all verbal, written, electronic, augmentative, and nonverbal communications, including compliance with HIPAA regulations.
I. Take appropriate steps to facilitate meaningful communication and comprehension in cases in which the recipient of service, student, or research participant has limited ability to communicate (e.g., aphasia or differences in language, literacy, culture).
J. Make every effort to facilitate open and collaborative dialogue with clients and/or responsible parties to facilitate comprehension of services and their potential risks/benefits.

SOCIAL JUSTICE

Principle 4. Occupational therapy personnel shall provide services in a fair and equitable manner.

Social justice, also called *distributive justice,* refers to the fair, equitable, and appropriate distribution of resources. The principle of social justice refers broadly to the distribution of all rights and responsibilities in society (Beauchamp & Childress, 2009). In general, the principle of social justice supports the concept of achieving justice in every aspect of society rather than merely the administration of law. The general idea is that individuals and groups should receive fair treatment and an impartial share of the benefits of society. Occupational therapy personnel have a vested interest in addressing unjust inequities that limit opportunities for participation in society (Braveman & Bass-Haugen, 2009). While opinions differ regarding the most ethical approach to addressing distribution of health care resources and reduction of health disparities, the issue of social justice continues to focus on limiting the impact of social inequality on health outcomes.

Occupational therapy personnel shall

A. Uphold the profession's altruistic responsibilities to help ensure the common good.

B. Take responsibility for educating the public and society about the value of occupational therapy services in promoting health and wellness and reducing the impact of disease and disability.

C. Make every effort to promote activities that benefit the health status of the community.

D. Advocate for just and fair treatment for all patients, clients, employees, and colleagues, and encourage employers and colleagues to abide by the highest standards of social justice and the ethical standards set forth by the occupational therapy profession.

E. Make efforts to advocate for recipients of occupational therapy services to obtain needed services through available means.

F. Provide services that reflect an understanding of how occupational therapy service delivery can be affected by factors such as economic status, age, ethnicity, race, geography, disability, marital status, sexual orientation, gender, gender identity, religion, culture, and political affiliation.

G. Consider offering *pro bono* ("for the good") or reduced-fee occupational therapy services for selected individuals when consistent with guidelines of the employer, third-party payer, and/or government agency.

PROCEDURAL JUSTICE

Principle 5. Occupational therapy personnel shall comply with institutional rules, local, state, federal, and international laws and AOTA documents applicable to the profession of occupational therapy.

Procedural justice is concerned with making and implementing decisions according to fair processes that ensure "fair treatment" (Maiese, 2004). Rules must be impartially followed and consistently applied to generate an unbiased decision. The principle of procedural justice is based on the concept that procedures and processes are organized in a fair manner and that policies, regulations, and laws are followed. While *the law* and *ethics* are not synonymous terms, occupational therapy personnel have an ethical responsibility to uphold current reimbursement regulations and state/territorial laws governing the profession. In addition, occupational therapy personnel are ethically bound to be aware of organizational policies and practice guidelines set forth by regulatory agencies established to protect recipients of service, research participants, and the public.

Occupational therapy personnel shall

A. Be familiar with and apply the Code and Ethics Standards to the work setting, and share them with employers, other employees, colleagues, students, and researchers.

B. Be familiar with and seek to understand and abide by institutional rules, and when those rules conflict with ethical practice, take steps to resolve the conflict.

C. Be familiar with revisions in those laws and AOTA policies that apply to the profession of occupational therapy and inform employers, employees, colleagues, students, and researchers of those changes.

D. Be familiar with established policies and procedures for handling concerns about the Code and Ethics Standards, including familiarity with national, state, local, district, and territorial procedures for handling ethics complaints as well as policies and procedures created by AOTA and certification, licensing, and regulatory agencies.

E. Hold appropriate national, state, or other requisite credentials for the occupational therapy services they provide.

F. Take responsibility for maintaining high standards and continuing competence in practice, education, and research by participating in professional development and educational activities to improve and update knowledge and skills.

G. Ensure that all duties assumed by or assigned to other occupational therapy personnel match credentials, qualifications, experience, and scope of practice.

H. Provide appropriate supervision to individuals for whom they have supervisory responsibility in accordance with AOTA official documents and local, state, and federal or national laws, rules, regulations, policies, procedures, standards, and guidelines.

I. Obtain all necessary approvals prior to initiating research activities.

J. Report all gifts and remuneration from individuals, agencies, or companies in accordance with employer policies as well as state and federal guidelines.

K. Use funds for intended purposes, and avoid misappropriation of funds.

L. Take reasonable steps to ensure that employers are aware of occupational therapy's ethical obligations as set forth in this Code and Ethics Standards and of the implications of those obligations for occupational therapy practice, education, and research.

M. Actively work with employers to prevent discrimination and unfair labor practices, and advocate for employees with disabilities to ensure the provision of reasonable accommodations.

N. Actively participate with employers in the formulation of policies and procedures

to ensure legal, regulatory, and ethical compliance.

O. Collect fees legally. Fees shall be fair, reasonable, and commensurate with services delivered. Fee schedules must be available and equitable regardless of actual payer reimbursements/contracts.

P. Maintain the ethical principles and standards of the profession when participating in a business arrangement as owner, stockholder, partner, or employee, and refrain from working for or doing business with organizations that engage in illegal or unethical business practices (e.g., fraudulent billing, providing occupational therapy services beyond the scope of occupational therapy practice).

VERACITY

Principle 6. Occupational therapy personnel shall provide comprehensive, accurate, and objective information when representing the profession.

Veracity is based on the virtues of truthfulness, candor, and honesty. The principle of *veracity* in health care refers to comprehensive, accurate, and objective transmission of information and includes fostering the client's understanding of such information (Beauchamp & Childress, 2009). Veracity is based on respect owed to others. In communicating with others, occupational therapy personnel implicitly promise to speak truthfully and not deceive the listener. By entering into a relationship in care or research, the recipient of service or research participant enters into a contract that includes a right to truthful information (Beauchamp & Childress, 2009). In addition, transmission of information is incomplete without also ensuring that the recipient or participant understands the information provided. Concepts of veracity must be carefully balanced with other potentially competing ethical principles, cultural beliefs, and organizational policies. Veracity ultimately is valued as a means to establish trust and strengthen professional relationships. Therefore, adherence to the Principle also requires thoughtful analysis of how full disclosure of information may impact outcomes.

Occupational therapy personnel shall

A. Represent the credentials, qualifications, education, experience, training, roles, duties, competence, views, contributions, and findings accurately in all forms of communication about recipients of service, students, employees, research participants, and colleagues.

B. Refrain from using or participating in the use of any form of communication that contains false, fraudulent, deceptive, misleading, or unfair statements or claims.

C. Record and report in an accurate and timely manner, and in accordance with applicable regulations, all information related to professional activities.

D. Ensure that documentation for reimbursement purposes is done in accordance with applicable laws, guidelines, and regulations.

E. Accept responsibility for any action that reduces the public's trust in occupational therapy.

F. Ensure that all marketing and advertising are truthful, accurate, and carefully presented to avoid misleading recipients of service, students, research participants, or the public.

G. Describe the type and duration of occupational therapy services accurately in professional contracts, including the duties and responsibilities of all involved parties.

H. Be honest, fair, accurate, respectful, and timely in gathering and reporting fact-based information regarding employee job performance and student performance.

I. Give credit and recognition when using the work of others in written, oral, or electronic media.

J. Not plagiarize the work of others.

FIDELITY

Principle 7. Occupational therapy personnel shall treat colleagues and other professionals with respect, fairness, discretion, and integrity.

The principle of fidelity comes from the Latin root *fidelis* meaning loyal. *Fidelity* refers to being faithful, which includes obligations of loyalty and the keeping of promises and commitments (Veatch & Flack, 1997). In the health professions, fidelity refers to maintaining good-faith relationships between various service providers and recipients. While respecting fidelity requires occupational therapy personnel to meet the client's reasonable expectations (Purtillo, 2005), Principle 7 specifically addresses fidelity as it relates to maintaining collegial and organizational relationships. Professional relationships are greatly influenced by the complexity of the environment in which occupational therapy personnel work. Practitioners, educators, and researchers alike must consistently balance their duties to service recipients, students, research participants, and other professionals as well as to organizations that may influence decision making and professional practice.

Occupational therapy personnel shall

A. Respect the traditions, practices, competencies, and responsibilities of their own and other professions, as well as those of the institutions and agencies that constitute the working environment.

B. Preserve, respect, and safeguard private information about employees, colleagues, and students unless otherwise mandated by national, state, or local laws or permission to disclose is given by the individual.

C. Take adequate measures to discourage, prevent, expose, and correct any breaches of the Code and Ethics Standards, and report any breaches of the former to the appropriate authorities.

D. Attempt to resolve perceived institutional violations of the Code and Ethics Standards by utilizing internal resources first.

E. Avoid conflicts of interest or conflicts of commitment in employment, volunteer roles, or research.

F. Avoid using one's position (employee or volunteer) or knowledge gained from that position in such a manner that gives rise to real or perceived conflict of interest among the person, the employer, other Association members, and/or other organizations.

G. Use conflict resolution and/or alternative dispute resolution resources to resolve organizational and interpersonal conflicts.

H. Be diligent stewards of human, financial, and material resources of their employers, and refrain from exploiting these resources for personal gain.

REFERENCES

American Occupational Therapy Association. (1993). Core values and attitudes of occupational therapy practice. *American Journal of Occupational Therapy, 47,* 1085–1086.

American Occupational Therapy Association. (2004). Policy 5.3.1: Definition of occupational therapy practice for state regulation. *American Journal of Occupational Therapy, 58,* 694–695.

American Occupational Therapy Association. (2005). Occupational therapy code of ethics (2005). *American Journal of Occupational Therapy, 59,* 639–642.

American Occupational Therapy Association. (2006). Guidelines to the occupational therapy code of ethics. *American Journal of Occupational Therapy, 60,* 652–658.

Beauchamp, T. L., & Childress, J. F. (2009). *Principles of biomedical ethics* (6th ed.). New York: Oxford University Press.

Braveman, B., & Bass-Haugen, J. D. (2009). Social justice and health disparities: An evolving discourse in occupational therapy research and intervention. *American Journal of Occupational Therapy, 63,* 7–12.

Maiese, M. (2004). *Procedural justice.* Retrieved July 29, 2009, from http://www.beyondintractability.org/essay/procedural_justice/

Purtillo, R. (2005). *Ethical dimensions in the health professions* (4th ed.). Philadelphia: Elsevier/Saunders.

Veatch, R. M., & Flack, H. E. (1997). *Case studies in allied health ethics.* Upper Saddle River, NJ: Prentice Hall.

Authors

Ethics Commission (EC):

Kathlyn Reed, PhD, OTR, FAOTA, MLIS, *Chairperson*

Barbara Hemphill, DMin, OTR, FAOTA, FMOTA, *Chair-Elect*

Ann Moodey Ashe, MHS, OTR/L

Lea C. Brandt, OTD, MA, OTR/L

Joanne Estes, MS, OTR/L

Loretta Jean Foster, MS, COTA/L

Donna F. Homenko, PhD, RDH

Craig R. Jackson, JD, MSW

Deborah Yarett Slater, MS, OT/L, FAOTA, *AOTA Staff Liaison*

Adopted by the Representative Assembly 2010CApr17.

Note. This document replaces the following rescinded Ethics documents 2010CApril18: the *Occupational Therapy Code of Ethics (2005) (American Journal of Occupational Therapy, 59,* 639–642); the *Guidelines to the Occupational Therapy Code of Ethics (American Journal of Occupational Therapy, 60,* 652–658); and the *Core Values and Attitudes of Occupational Therapy Practice (American Journal of Occupational Therapy, 47,* 1085–1086).

Citation. American Occupational Therapy Association. (2010). Occupational therapy code of ethics and ethics standards (2010). *American Journal of Occupational Therapy, 64*(6 Suppl.), S17–S26. doi: 10.5014/ajot.2010.64S17

This chapter was originally published in the *American Journal of Occupational Therapy, 64*(6 Suppl.), S17–S26.

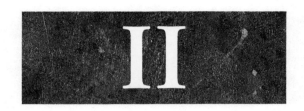

II

ENFORCEMENT

Overview of the Enforcement Procedures for the Occupational Therapy Code of Ethics and Ethics Standards

The *Enforcement Procedures for the Occupational Therapy Code of Ethics and Ethics Standards,* revised most recently in 2009 (American Occupational Therapy Association [AOTA], 2010a), articulate the procedures that AOTA's Ethics Commission (EC) follows as it carries out its duties to enforce the *Occupational Therapy Code of Ethics and Ethics Standards (2010)* (referred to as the "Code and Ethics Standards"; AOTA, 2010b). A major goal of these procedures is to ensure objectivity and fundamental fairness to all individuals who may be parties in an ethics complaint.

The Code and Ethics Standards are a public statement of the values and principles used as a guide in promoting and maintaining high standards of professional conduct in occupational therapy. The Code and Ethics Standards apply to occupational therapy personnel at all levels and in the diverse roles they may occupy, not only as clinicians, educators, researchers, and students, but also in elected and voluntary leadership roles, whether within AOTA or in the community, where the occupational therapy perspective can provide a valuable benefit. The Enforcement Procedures are used to help ensure compliance with the values and principles that members of the profession have identified as important.

Several revisions have been made to this document since the Enforcement Procedures were last published in the 2008 edition of the *Reference Guide to the Occupational Therapy Ethics Standards:* Procedures for regular versus sua sponte complaints are more clearly delineated, and the organizational flow has been improved to aid readers in following the enforcement process. The disciplinary actions enforceable by the EC and its jurisdiction, however, remain unchanged.

The Enforcement Procedures begin with an "Introduction," which discusses the jurisdiction of the Code and Ethics Standards, disciplinary actions, the circumstances under which complaints may be dismissed, and educational options such as advisory opinions or educative letters. Section 2, "Complaints," identifies the different types of complaints (interested party vs. sua sponte), how they may be received, and how correspondence is handled to ensure confidentiality and receipt.

Section 3, "EC Review and Investigations," establishes the procedures used by AOTA's Ethics Office and the EC to evaluate and investigate cases, as well as criteria for dismissal. This section also includes the investigation timeline and the circumstances under which a complaint may be referred to another jurisdiction or stayed. Section 3.4, "Investigation," outlines circumstances under which a complaint may be dismissed and the investigation process should evidence be deemed sufficient to open a case for further review. Section 4, "EC Review and Decision," is now divided to describe this process in detail for both regular and de jure complaints. The presentation of the procedures for each type of complaint has been reorganized to make the process easier to follow.

Section 5 discusses the role of the Disciplinary Council and outlines a procedure for selecting members and convening a hearing in which the respondent can refute the decision of a formal charge or sanction by the EC. The hearing is also held to allow the EC, represented by its chairperson, to present evidence to support the charge or sanction. The timelines for the Council's hearing and decision also are presented. If the respondent chooses to appeal the Council's decision, the final step is to request an Appeal Panel. The process for this is described in Section 6, "Appeal Process." As with other procedures delineated in this document, this section presents the timelines and process for selecting and convening the panel, handling the case review, and issuing a decision. The final sections of the Enforcement Procedures address Notifications (Section 7), Records and Reports (Section 8), Publication (Section 9), and Modification (Section 10).

The EC and AOTA's Ethics Office make the *Enforcement Procedures for the Occupational Therapy Code of Ethics and Ethics Standards* public and available to members of the profession, state regulatory boards, consumers, and others for their use. When questions arise concerning the AOTA Code and Ethics Standards and their Enforcement Procedures, the Ethics Office at AOTA is available for assistance.

REFERENCES

American Occupational Therapy Association. (2010a). Enforcement procedures for the *Occupational Therapy Code of Ethics and Ethics Standards*. *American Journal of Occupational Therapy, 64*(6 Suppl.), S4–S16. doi:10.5014/ajot.2010.64S4

American Occupational Therapy Association. (2010b). Occupational therapy code of ethics and ethics standards (2010). *American Journal of Occupational Therapy, 64*(6 Suppl.), S17–S26. doi:10.5014/ajot.2010.64S17

Deborah Yarett Slater, MS, OT/L, FAOTA
AOTA Staff Liaison to the Ethics Commission

This chapter was originally published in the 2006 edition of the *Reference Guide to the Occupational Therapy Code of Ethics*. It has been revised to reflect updated AOTA official documents, Web sites, AOTA style, and additional resources.

Enforcement Procedures *for the* Occupational Therapy Code of Ethics and Ethics Standards

1. INTRODUCTION

The principal purposes of the *Occupational Therapy Code of Ethics and Ethics Standards* (hereinafter referred to as the "Code and Ethics Standards") are to help protect the public and to reinforce its confidence in the occupational therapy profession rather than to resolve private business, legal, or other disputes for which there are other more appropriate forums for resolution. The Code and Ethics Standards also is an aspirational document to guide occupational therapists, occupational therapy assistants, and occupational therapy students toward appropriate professional conduct in all aspects of their diverse roles. It applies to any conduct that may affect the performance of occupational therapy as well as to behavior that an individual may do in another capacity that reflects negatively on the reputation of occupational therapy.

The *Enforcement Procedures for the Occupational Therapy Code of Ethics and Ethics Standards* (formerly the *Enforcement Procedures for the Occupational Therapy Code of Ethics*) have undergone a series of revisions by the American Occupational Therapy Association's (AOTA's) Ethics Commission (hereinafter referred to as the *EC*) since their initial adoption. The most recent update was in 2009. This public document articulates the procedures that are followed by the EC as it carries out its duties to enforce the Code and Ethics Standards. A major goal of these Enforcement Procedures is

to ensure objectivity and fundamental fairness to all individuals who may be parties in an ethics complaint.

The Enforcement Procedures are used to help ensure compliance with the Code and Ethics Standards, which represent the values and principles that members of the profession have identified as important. Acceptance of AOTA membership commits individuals to adherence to the Code and Ethics Standards and cooperation with its Enforcement Procedures. These are established and maintained by the EC: The EC and AOTA's Ethics Office make the Enforcement Procedures public and available to members of the profession, state regulatory boards, consumers, and others for their use.

The EC urges particular attention to the following issues:

1.1. Professional Responsibility, Other Processes—All occupational therapy personnel have an obligation to maintain the Code and Ethics Standards of their profession and to promote and support these Standards among their colleagues. Each AOTA member must be alert to practices that undermine these Standards and is obligated to take action that is appropriate in the circumstances. At the same time, members must carefully weigh their judgments as to potentially unethical practice to ensure that they are based on objective evaluation and not on personal bias or prejudice, inadequate information, or simply differences of professional viewpoint. It is recognized that individual occupational therapy personnel may not have the authority or ability to address or correct all situations of concern. Whenever feasible and appropriate, members should first pursue other corrective steps within the relevant institution or setting and discuss ethical concerns directly with the potential Respondent before resorting to AOTA's ethics complaint process.

1.2. Jurisdiction—The Code and Ethics Standards apply to persons who are or were AOTA members at the time of the conduct in question. Later nonrenewal or relinquishment of membership does not affect Association jurisdiction. The Enforcement Procedures that shall be utilized in any complaint shall be those in effect at the time the complaint is initiated.

1.3. Disciplinary Actions/Sanctions (Pursuing a Complaint)—If the EC determines that unethical conduct has occurred, it may impose sanctions, including reprimand, censure, probation (with terms), suspension, or permanent revocation of AOTA membership. In all cases, except those involving only reprimand, the Association will report the conclusions and sanctions in its official publications and also will communicate to any appropriate persons or entities. The potential sanctions are defined as follows:

1.3.1. Reprimand—A formal expression of disapproval of conduct communicated privately by letter from the EC Chairperson that is nondisclosable and noncommunicative to other bodies (e.g., state regulatory boards [SRBs], National Board for Certification in Occupational Therapy® [NBCOT®]).
1.3.2. Censure—A formal expression of disapproval that is public.

1.3.3. Probation of Membership Subject to Terms—Failure to meet terms will subject an AOTA member to any of the disciplinary actions or sanctions.
1.3.4. Suspension—Removal of AOTA membership for a specified period of time.
1.3.5. Revocation—Permanent denial of AOTA membership.
    1.3.5.1. If an individual is on either the Roster of Fellows (ROF) or the Roster of Honor (ROH), the EC Chairperson (via the EC Staff Liaison) shall notify the Recognitions Committee Chairperson (and AOTA Executive Director) of their membership revocation. That individual shall have their name removed from either the ROF or the ROH and no longer has the right to use the designated credential of FAOTA or ROH.

1.4. Educative Letters—If the EC determines that the alleged conduct may or may not be a true breach of the Code and Ethics Standards but in any event does not warrant any of the sanctions set forth in Section 1.3 or is not completely in keeping with the aspirational nature of the Code and Ethics Standards or within the prevailing standards of practice or good professionalism, the EC may send a letter to educate the Respondent about relevant standards of practice and/or appropriate professional behavior. In addition, a different educative letter, if appropriate, may be sent to the Complainant.

1.5. Advisory Opinions—The EC may issue general advisory opinions on ethical issues to inform and educate the AOTA membership. These opinions shall be publicized to the membership and are available in the *Reference Guide to the Occupational Therapy Code of Ethics and Ethics Standards* as well as in other locations.

1.6. Rules of Evidence—The EC proceedings shall be conducted in accordance with fundamental fairness. However, formal rules of evidence that are used in legal proceedings do not apply to these Enforcement Procedures. The Disciplinary Council (see Section 5) and the Appeal Panel (see Section 6) can consider any evidence that they deem appropriate and pertinent.

1.7. Confidentiality and Disclosure—The EC develops and adheres to strict rules of confidentiality in every aspect of its work. This requires that participants in the process refrain from any communication relating to the existence and subject matter of the complaint other than with those directly involved in the enforcement process. Maintaining confidentiality throughout the investigation and enforcement process of a formal ethics complaint is essential in order to ensure fairness to all parties involved. These rules of confidentiality pertain not only to the EC but also apply to others involved in the complaint process. Beginning with the EC Staff Liaison and support staff, strict rules of confidentiality are followed. These same rules of confidentiality apply to Complainants, Respondents and their attorneys, and witnesses involved with the EC's investigatory process. Due diligence must be exercised by everyone involved in the investigation to avoid compromising the confidential nature of the process. Any AOTA member who breaches these rules of confidentiality may become subject to an ethics complaint/investigatory process himself or herself. Non–AOTA members may lodge an ethics complaint against an Association member, and these individuals are still expected to adhere to the Association's confidentiality rules. The Association reserves the right to take appropriate action against non–AOTA members who violate confidentiality rules, including notification of their appropriate licensure boards.

1.7.1. Disclosure—When the EC investigates a complaint, it may request information from a variety of sources. The process of obtaining additional information is carefully executed in order to maintain confidentiality. The EC may request information from a variety of sources, including state licensing agencies, academic councils, courts, employers, and other persons and entities. It is within the EC's purview to determine what disclosures are appropriate for particular parties in order to effectively implement its investigatory obligations. Public sanctions by the EC, Disciplinary Council, or Appeal Panel will be publicized as provided in these Enforcement Procedures. Normally, the EC does not disclose information or documentation reviewed in the course of an investigation unless the EC determines that disclosure is necessary to obtain additional, relevant evidence or to administer the ethics process or is legally required.

Individuals who file a complaint (i.e., *Complainant*) and those who are the subject of one (i.e., *Respondent*) must not disclose to anyone outside of those involved in the complaint process their role in an ethics complaint. Disclosing this information in and of itself may jeopardize the ethics process and violate the rules of fundamental fairness by which all parties are protected. Disclosure of information related to any case under investigation by the EC is prohibited and, if done, will lead to repercussions as outlined in these Enforcement Procedures (see Section 2.2.3).

2. COMPLAINTS

2.1. Interested Party Complaints

2.1.1. Complaints stating an alleged violation of the Code and Ethics Standards may originate from any individual, group, or entity within or outside AOTA. All complaints must be in writing, signed by the Complainant(s), and submitted to the EC Chairperson at the address of the AOTA

Headquarters. Complainants must complete the Formal Statement of Complaint Form at the end of this document. All complaints shall identify the person against whom the complaint is directed (the Respondent), the ethical principles that the Complainant believes have been violated, and the key facts and date(s) of the alleged ethical violations. If lawfully available, supporting documentation should be attached.

2.1.2. Within 90 days of receipt of a complaint, the EC shall make a preliminary assessment of the complaint and decide whether it presents sufficient questions as to a potential ethics violation that an investigation is warranted in accordance with Section 3. Commencing an investigation does not imply a conclusion that an ethical violation has in fact occurred or any judgment as to the ultimate sanction, if any, that may be appropriate. In the event the EC determines at the completion of an investigation that the complaint does rise to the level of an ethical violation, the EC may initiate a charge as set forth in Section 4 below. In the event the EC determines that the complaint does not rise to the level of an ethical violation, the EC may direct the parties to utilize *Roberts Rules* and/or other conflict resolution resources via an educative letter. This applies to all complaints, including those involving AOTA elected/volunteer leadership related to their official roles.

2.2. Complaints Initiated by the EC

2.2.1. The EC itself may initiate a complaint (a *sua sponte complaint*) when it receives information from a governmental body, certification or similar body, public media, or other source indicating that a person subject to its jurisdiction may have committed acts that violate the Code and Ethics Standards. The Association will ordinarily act promptly after learning of the basis of a sua sponte complaint, but there is no specified time limit.

If the EC passes a motion to initiate a sua sponte complaint, the AOTA Staff Liaison to the EC will complete the Formal Statement of Complaint Form (at the end of this document) and will describe the nature of the factual allegations that led to the complaint and the manner in which the EC learned of the matter. The Complaint Form will be signed by the EC Chairperson on behalf of the EC. The form will be filed with the case material in the Association's Ethics Office.

2.2.2. De Jure Complaints—Where the source of a sua sponte complaint is the findings and conclusions of another official body, the EC classifies such sua sponte complaints as *de jure*. The procedure in such cases is addressed in Section 4.2.

2.2.3. The EC shall have the jurisdiction to investigate, charge, or sanction any matter or person for violations based on information learned in the course of investigating a complaint under Section 2.2.2.

2.3. Continuation of Complaint Process—

If an AOTA member relinquishes membership, fails to renew membership, or fails to cooperate with the ethics investigation, the EC shall nevertheless continue to process the complaint, noting in its report the circumstances of the Respondent's action. Such actions shall not deprive the EC of jurisdiction. All correspondence related to the EC complaint process is in writing and sent by certified mail, return receipt requested. In the event that any written correspondence does not have delivery confirmation, the AOTA Ethics Office will make an attempt to search for an alternate address or make a second attempt to send to the original address. If Respondent does not claim correspondence after two attempts to deliver, delivery cannot be confirmed, or correspondence is returned to the Association as undeliverable, the EC shall consider that it has made good-faith effort and shall proceed with the ethics enforcement process.

3. EC Review and Investigations

3.1. Initial Action
—The purpose of the preliminary review is to decide whether or not the information submitted with the complaint warrants opening the case. If in its preliminary review of the complaint the EC determines that an investigation is not warranted, the Complainant will be so notified.

3.2. Dismissal of Complaints
—The EC may at any time dismiss a complaint for any of the following reasons:

3.2.1. Lack of Jurisdiction
—The EC determines that it has no jurisdiction over the Respondent (e.g., a complaint against a person who is or was not an AOTA member at the time of the alleged incident or who has never been a member).

3.2.2. Absolute Time Limit/Not Timely Filed
—The EC determines that the violation of the Code and Ethics Standards is alleged to have occurred more than 7 years prior to the filing of the complaint.

3.2.3. Subject to Jurisdiction of Another Authority
—The EC determines that the complaint is based on matters that are within the authority of and are more properly dealt with by another governmental or nongovernmental body, such as an SRB, NBCOT, an Association component other than the EC, an employer, or a court (e.g., accusing a superior of sexual harassment at work, accusing someone of anti-competitive practices subject to the antitrust laws).

3.2.4. No Ethics Violation
—The EC finds that the complaint, even if proven, does not state a basis for action under the Code and Ethics Standards (e.g., simply accusing someone of being unpleasant or rude on an occasion).

3.2.5. Insufficient Evidence
—The EC determines that there clearly would not be sufficient factual evidence to support a finding of an ethics violation.

3.2.6. Corrected Violation
—The EC determines that any violation it might find already has been or is being corrected and that this is an adequate result in the given case.

3.2.7. Other Good Cause.

3.3. Investigator (Avoidance of Conflict of Interest)
—The investigator chosen shall not have a conflict of interest (i.e., shall never have had a substantial professional, personal, financial, business, or volunteer relationship with either the Complainant or the Respondent). In the event that the EC Staff Liaison has such a conflict, the EC Chairperson shall appoint an alternate investigator who has no conflict of interest.

3.4. Investigation
—If an investigation is deemed warranted, the EC Chairperson shall do the following within thirty (30) days: Appoint the EC Staff Liaison at the AOTA Headquarters to investigate the complaint and notify the Respondent (by certified, return-receipt mail) that a complaint has been received and an investigation is being conducted. A copy of the complaint and supporting documentation shall be enclosed with this notification. The Complainant also will receive notification by certified, return-receipt mail that the complaint is being investigated.

3.4.1.
Ordinarily, the Investigator will send questions formulated by the EC to be answered by the Complainant and/or the Respondent.

3.4.2.
The Complainant shall be given thirty (30) days from receipt of the questions to respond in writing to the Investigator.

3.4.3.
The Respondent shall be given thirty (30) days from receipt of the questions to respond in writing to the Investigator.

3.4.4.
The EC ordinarily will notify the Complainant of any substantive new evidence adverse to the Complainant's initial complaint that is discovered in the course of the ethics investigation and allow the Complainant to respond to such adverse

evidence. In such cases, the Complainant will be given a copy of such evidence and will have fourteen (14) days in which to submit a written response. If the new evidence clearly shows that there has been no ethics violation, the EC may terminate the proceeding. In addition, if the investigation includes questions for both the Respondent and the Complainant, the evidence submitted by each party in response to the investigatory questions shall be provided to the Respondent and available to the Complainant on request. The EC may request reasonable payment for copying expenses depending on the volume of material to be sent.

3.4.5. The Investigator, in consultation with the EC, may obtain evidence directly from third parties without permission from the Complainant or Respondent.

3.5. Investigation Timeline—The investigation will be completed within ninety (90) days after receipt of notification by the Respondent or his or her designee that an investigation is being conducted, unless the EC determines that special circumstances warrant additional time for the investigation. All timelines noted here can be extended for good cause at the discretion of the EC, including the EC's schedule and additional requests of the Respondent. The Respondent and the Complainant shall be notified in writing if a delay occurs or if the investigational process requires more time.

3.6. Case Files—The investigative files shall include the complaint and any documentation on which the EC relied in initiating the investigation.

3.7. Cooperation by Member—Every AOTA member has a duty to cooperate reasonably with enforcement processes for the Code and Ethics Standards. Failure of the Respondent to participate and/or cooperate with the investigative process of the EC shall

not prevent continuation of the ethics process, and this behavior itself may constitute a violation of the Code and Ethics Standards.

3.8. Referral of Complaint—The EC may at any time refer a matter to NBCOT, the SRB, or other recognized authorities for appropriate action. Despite such referral to an appropriate authority, the EC shall retain jurisdiction. EC action may be stayed for a reasonable period pending notification of a decision by that authority, at the discretion of the EC (and such delays will extend the time periods under these Procedures). A stay in conducting an investigation shall not constitute a waiver by the EC of jurisdiction over the matters. The EC shall provide written notice by mail (requiring signature and proof of date of receipt) to the Respondent and the Complainant of any such stay of action.

4. EC REVIEW AND DECISION

4.1. Regular Complaint Process

4.1.1. Charges—The EC shall review the relevant materials resulting from the investigation and shall render a decision on whether a charge by the EC is warranted within 90 days of receipt. The EC may, in the conduct of its review, take whatever further investigatory actions it deems necessary. If the EC determines that an ethics complaint warrants a charge, the EC shall proceed with a disciplinary proceeding by promptly sending a notice of the charge(s) to the Respondent and Complainant by mail with signature and proof of date received. The notice of the charge(s) shall describe the alleged conduct that, if proven in accordance with these Enforcement Procedures, would constitute a violation of the Code and Ethics Standards. The notice of charge(s) shall describe the conduct in sufficient detail to inform the Respondent of the nature of the unethical behavior that is alleged. The EC may indicate in the notice its preliminary

view (absent contrary facts or mitigating circumstances) as to what sanction would be warranted if the violation is proven in accordance with these Enforcement Procedures.

4.1.2. Respondent's Response—Within 30 days of notification of the EC's decision to charge, and proposed sanction, if any, the Respondent shall

4.1.2.1. Advise the EC Chairperson in writing that he or she accepts the EC's charge of an ethics violation and the proposed sanction and waives any right to a Disciplinary Council hearing, or

4.1.2.2. Advise the EC Chairperson in writing that he or she accepts the EC's charge of an ethics violation but believes the sanction is not justified or should be reduced with a rationale to support a reduced sanction.

4.1.2.3. Advise the EC Chairperson in writing that he or she contests the EC's charge and the proposed sanction and requests a hearing before the Disciplinary Council.

Failure of the Respondent to take one of these actions within the time specified will be deemed to constitute acceptance of the charge and proposed sanction. If the Respondent requests a Disciplinary Council hearing, it will be scheduled. If the Respondent does not request a Disciplinary Council hearing but accepts the decision, the EC will notify all relevant parties and implement the sanction.

4.2. De Jure Complaint Process

4.2.1. The EC Staff Liaison will present to the EC any findings from external sources (as described above) that come to his or her attention and that may warrant sua sponte complaints pertaining to individuals who are or were AOTA members at the time of the alleged incident.

4.2.2. Because *de jure complaints* are based on the findings of fact or conclusions of another official body, the EC will decide whether or not to act based on such findings or conclusions and will not ordinarily initiate another investigation, absent clear and convincing evidence that such findings and conclusions were erroneous or not supported by substantial evidence. Based on the information presented by the EC Staff Liaison, the EC will determine whether the findings of the public body also are sufficient to demonstrate an egregious violation of the Code and Ethics Standards and therefore warrant an ethics charge.

4.2.3. If the EC decides that a formal charge is warranted, the EC Chairperson will notify the Respondent in writing of the formal charge and the proposed education and/or disciplinary action. In response to the de jure sua sponte charge by the EC, the Respondent may

4.2.3.1. Accept the decision of the EC (as to both the ethics violation and the sanction) based solely on the findings of fact and conclusions of the EC or the public body, or

4.2.3.2. Accept the charge that the Respondent committed unethical conduct but within thirty (30) days submit to the EC a statement setting forth the reasons why any sanction should not be imposed or reasons why the sanction should be mitigated or reduced.

4.2.3.3. Within thirty (30) days, present information showing the findings of fact of the official body relied on by the EC to initiate the charge are clearly erroneous and request reconsideration by the EC. The EC may have the option of opening an investigation or modifying the sanction in the event they find clear and convincing evidence that the findings and the conclusions of the other body are erroneous.

4.2.4. In cases of de jure complaints, a Disciplinary Council hearing can later be requested (pursuant to Section 5 below) only if the Respondent has first exercised Options 4.2.3.2 or 4.2.3.3.

4.2.5. Respondents in an ethics case may utilize Options 4.2.3.2 or 4.2.3.3 (reconsideration) once in responding to the EC. Following one review of the additional information submitted by the Respondent, if the EC reaffirms its original sanction, the Respondent has the option of accepting the violation and proposed sanction or requesting a Disciplinary Council hearing. Repeated requests for reconsideration will not be accepted by the EC.

5. THE DISCIPLINARY COUNCIL

5.1. Purpose—The purpose of the Disciplinary Council (hereinafter to be known as *the Council*) hearing is to provide the Respondent an opportunity to present evidence and witnesses to answer and refute the charge and/or the proposed sanction and to permit the EC Chairperson or designee to present evidence and witnesses in support of his or her charge. The Council shall consider the matters alleged in the complaint; the matters raised in defense as well as other relevant facts, ethical principles, and federal or state law, if applicable. The Council may question the parties concerned and determine ethical issues arising from the factual matters in the case even if those specific ethical issues were not raised by the Complainant. The Council also may choose to apply Principles or other language from the AOTA Code and Ethics Standards not originally identified by the EC. The Council may affirm the decision of the EC or reverse or modify it if it finds that the decision was clearly erroneous or a material departure from its written procedure.

5.2. Parties—The parties to a Council Hearing are the Respondent and the EC Chairperson.

5.3. Criteria and Process for Selection of Council Chairperson

5.3.1. Criteria
5.3.1.1. Must have experience in analyzing/reviewing cases.

5.3.1.2. May be selected from the pool of candidates for the Council or a former EC member who has been off the EC for at least three (3) years.

5.3.1.3. The EC Chairperson shall not serve as the Council Chairperson.

5.3.2. Process
5.3.2.1. The Representative Assembly (RA) Speaker (in consultation with EC Staff Liaison) will select the Council Chairperson.

5.3.2.2. If the RA Speaker needs to be recused from this duty, the RA Vice Speaker will select the Council Chairperson.

5.4. Criteria and Process for Selection of Council Members

5.4.1. Criteria
5.4.1.1. AOTA Administrative SOP guidelines in Policy 2.6 shall be considered in the selection of qualified potential candidates for the Council, which shall be composed of qualified individuals and AOTA members drawn from a pool of candidates who meet the criteria outlined below. In the interest of financial prudence and efficiency, every effort will be made to assemble Council members who meet the criteria below but also who are within geographic proximity to the AOTA Headquarters.

5.4.1.2. Members ideally will have some knowledge or experience in the areas of activity that are at issue in the case. They also will have experience in disciplinary hearings and/or general knowledge about ethics as demonstrated by education, presentations, and/or publications.

5.4.1.3. No conflict of interest may exist with either the Complainant or the Respondent (refer to Association Policy 1.22—Conflict of Interest for guidance).

5.4.1.4. No individual may serve on the Council who is currently a member of the EC or the AOTA Board of Directors.

5.4.1.5. No individual may serve on the Council who has previously been the subject of an ethics complaint that resulted in a specific EC disciplinary action.

5.4.1.6. The public member on the Council shall have knowledge of the profession and ethical issues.

5.4.1.7. The public member shall not be an occupational therapy practitioner, educator, or researcher.

5.4.2. Process

5.4.2.1. Potential candidates for the Council pool will be recruited through public postings in AOTA publications and via the electronic forums. Association leadership will be encouraged to recruit qualified candidates. Potential members of the Council shall be interviewed to ascertain the following:

a. Willingness to serve on the Council and availability for a period of three (3) years and

b. Qualifications per criteria outlined in Section 5.3.1.

5.4.2.2. The AOTA President and EC Staff Liaison will maintain a pool of no less than six (6) and no more than twelve (12) qualified individuals.

5.4.2.3. The President, with input from the EC Staff Liaison, will select from the pool the members of each Council within thirty (30) days of notification by a Respondent that a Council is being requested.

5.4.2.4. Each Council shall be composed of three (3) AOTA members in good standing and a public member.

5.4.2.5. The EC Staff Liaison will remove anyone with a potential conflict of interest in a particular case from the potential Council pool.

5.5. Notification of Parties (EC Chairperson, Complainant, Respondent, Council Members)

5.5.1. The EC Staff Liaison shall schedule a hearing date in coordination with the Council Chairperson.

5.5.2. The Council (via the EC Staff Liaison) shall notify all parties at least forty-five (45) days prior to the hearing of the date, time, and place.

5.5.3. Case material will be sent to all parties and the Council members by national delivery service or mail with signature required and proof of date received with return receipt.

5.6. Hearing Witnesses, Materials, and Evidence

5.6.1. Within thirty (30) days of notification of the hearing, the Respondent shall submit to the Council a written response to the charges, including a detailed statement as to the reasons that he or she is appealing the decision and a list of potential witnesses (if any) with a statement indicating the subject matter they will be addressing.

5.6.2. The Complainant before the Council also will submit a list of potential witnesses (if any) to the Council with a statement indicating the subject matter they will be addressing. Only under limited circumstances may the Council consider additional material evidence from the Respondent or the Complainant not presented or available prior to the issuance of their proposed sanction. Such new or additional evidence may be considered by the Council if the Council is satisfied that the Respondent or the Complainant has demonstrated the new evidence was previously unavailable and provided it is submitted to all parties in writing no later than fifteen (15) days prior to the hearing.

5.6.3. The Council Chairperson may permit testimony by conference call (at no expense to the participant), limit participation of witnesses in order to curtail repetitive testimony, or prescribe other reasonable arrangements or limitations. The Respondent may elect to appear (at Respondent's own expense) and present testimony. If alternative technology options are available for the hearing, the Respondent, Council members, and EC Chairperson shall be so informed when the hearing arrangements are sent.

5.7. Counsel—The Respondent may be represented by legal counsel at his or her own expense. AOTA's Legal Counsel shall advise and represent the Association at the hearing. AOTA's Legal Counsel also may advise the Council regarding procedural matters to ensure fairness to all parties. All parties and the AOTA Legal Counsel (at the request of the EC or the Council) shall have the opportunity to question witnesses.

5.8. Hearing

5.8.1. The Council hearing shall be recorded by a professional transcription service or telephone recording transcribed for Council members and shall be limited to two (2) hours.

5.8.2. The Council Chairperson will conduct the hearing and does not vote except in the case of a tie.

5.8.3. Each person present shall be identified for the record, and the Council Chairperson will describe the procedures for the Council hearing. An oral affirmation of truthfulness will be requested from each participant who gives factual testimony in the Council hearing.

5.8.4. The Council Chairperson shall allow for questions.

5.8.5. The EC Chairperson shall present the ethics charge, a summary of the evidence resulting from the investigation, and the EC-proposed disciplinary action against the Respondent.

5.8.6. The Respondent may present a defense to the charge(s) after the EC presents its case.

5.8.7. Each party and/or his or her legal representative shall have the opportunity to call witnesses to present testimony and to question any witnesses including the EC Chairperson or his or her designee. The Council Chairperson shall be entitled to provide reasonable limits on the extent of any witnesses' testimony or any questioning.

5.8.8. The Council Chairperson may recess the hearing at any time.

5.8.9. The Council Chairperson shall call for final statements from each party before concluding the hearing.

5.8.10. Decisions of the Council will be by majority vote.

5.9. Disciplinary Council Decision

5.9.1. An official copy of the transcript shall be sent to each Council member, the EC Chairperson, the AOTA Legal Counsel, the EC Staff Liaison, and the Respondent and his or her counsel as soon as it is available from the transcription company.

5.9.2. The Council Chairperson shall work with the EC Staff Liaison and the AOTA Legal Counsel in preparing the text of the final decision.

5.9.3. The Council shall issue a decision in writing to the AOTA Executive Director within thirty (30) days of receiving the written transcription of the hearing (unless special circumstances warrant additional time). The Council decision shall be based on the record and evidence presented and may affirm, modify, or reverse the decision of the EC, including increasing or decreasing the level of sanction or determining that no disciplinary action is warranted.

5.10. Action, Notification, and Timeline Adjustments

5.10.1. A copy of the Council's official decision and appeal process (Section 6) is sent to the Respondent, the EC Chairperson, and other appropriate parties within fifteen (15) business days via mail (with signature and proof of date received) after notification of the AOTA Executive Director.

5.10.2. The time limits specified in the *Enforcement Procedures for the Occupational Therapy Code of Ethics and Ethics Standards* may be extended by mutual consent of the Respondent, Complainant, and Council Chairperson for good cause by the Chairperson.

5.10.3. Other features of the preceding Enforcement Procedures may be adjusted in particular cases in light of extraordinary circumstances, consistent with fundamental fairness.

5.11. Appeal—Within thirty (30) days after notification of the Council's decision, a Respondent upon whom a sanction was imposed may appeal the decision as provided in Section 6. Within thirty (30) days after notification of the Council's decision, the EC also may appeal the decision as provided in Section 6. If no appeal is filed within that time, the AOTA Executive Director or EC Staff Liaison shall publish the decision in accordance with these procedures and make any other notifications deemed necessary.

6. APPEAL PROCESS

6.1. Appeals—Either the EC or the Respondent may appeal. Appeals shall be written, signed by the appealing party, and sent by certified mail to the AOTA Executive Director in care of the AOTA Ethics Office. The grounds for the appeal shall be fully explained in this document. When an appeal is requested, the other party will be notified.

6.2. Grounds for Appeal—Appeals shall generally address only the issues, procedures, or sanctions that are part of the record before the Council. However, in the interest of fairness, the Appeal Panel may consider newly available evidence relating to the original charge only under extraordinary circumstances.

6.3. Composition and Leadership of Appeal Panel—The AOTA Vice President, Secretary, and Treasurer shall constitute the Appeal Panel. In the event of vacancies in these positions or the existence of a conflict of interest, the Vice President shall appoint replacements drawn from among the other AOTA Board of Directors members. If the entire Board has a conflict of interest (e.g., the Complainant or Respondent is or was recently a member of the Board), the Board Appeal process shall be followed. The President shall not serve on the Appeal Panel. No individual may serve on the Council who has previously been the subject of an ethics complaint that resulted in a specific EC disciplinary action.

The Appeal Panel Chairperson will be selected by its members from among themselves.

6.4. Appeal Process—The AOTA Executive Director shall forward any letter of appeal to the Appeal Panel within fifteen (15) business days of receipt. Within thirty (30) days after the Appeal Panel receives the appeal, the Panel shall determine whether a hearing is warranted. If the Panel decides that a hearing is warranted, timely notice for such hearing shall be given to the parties. Participants at the hearing shall be limited to the Respondent and legal counsel (if so desired), the EC Chairperson, the Council Chairperson, the AOTA Legal Counsel, or others approved in advance by the Appeal Panel as necessary to the proceedings.

6.5. Decision

6.5.1. The Appeal Panel shall have the power to (a) affirm the decision; or (b) modify the decision; or (c) reverse or remand to the EC, but only if there were procedural errors materially prejudicial to the outcome of the proceeding or if the Council decision was against the clear weight of the evidence.

6.5.2. Within thirty (30) days after receipt of the appeal if no hearing was granted, or within thirty (30) days after receipt of the transcript if a hearing was held, the Appeal

Panel shall notify the AOTA Executive Director of its decision. The AOTA Executive Director shall promptly notify the Respondent, the original Complainant, appropriate Association bodies, and any other parties deemed appropriate (e.g., SRB, NBCOT). For Association purposes, the decision of the Appeal Panel shall be final.

7. NOTIFICATIONS

All notifications referred to in these Enforcement Procedures shall be in writing and shall be delivered by national delivery service or mail with signature and proof of date of receipt required.

8. RECORDS AND REPORTS

At the completion of the enforcement process, the written records and reports that state the initial basis for the complaint, material evidence, and the disposition of the complaint shall be retained in the AOTA Ethics Office for a period of five (5) years.

9. PUBLICATION

Final decisions will be publicized only after any Appeal Panel process has been completed.

10. MODIFICATION

AOTA reserves the right to (a) modify the time periods, procedures, or application of these Enforcement Procedures for good cause consistent with fundamental fairness in a given case and (b) modify its Code and Ethics Standards and/or these Enforcement Procedures, with such modifications to be applied only prospectively.

Adopted by the Representative Assembly 2009CONov146 as Attachment A of the Standard Operating Procedures (SOP) of the Ethics Commission.

Reviewed by BPPC 1/04, 1/05, 9/06, 1/07, 9/09

Adopted by RA 4/96, 5/04, 5/05, 11/06, 4/07, 11/09

Revised by SEC 4/98, 4/00, 1/02, 1/04, 12/04, 9/06

Revised by EC 12/06, 2/07, 8/09

Note. The Commission on Standards and Ethics (SEC) changed to Ethics Commission (EC) in September 2005 as per Association Bylaws.

Citation. American Occupational Therapy Association. (2010). Enforcement procedures for the *Occupational Therapy Code of Ethics and Ethics Standards. American Journal of Occupational Therapy, 64*(6 Suppl.), S4–S16. doi: 10.5014/ajot.2010.64S4

This chapter was originally published in the *American Journal of Occupational Therapy, 64*(6 Suppl.), S4–S16.

AMERICAN OCCUPATIONAL THERAPY ASSOCIATION
ETHICS COMMISSION

Formal Complaint of Alleged Violation of the *Occupational Therapy*
Code of Ethics and Ethics Standards

If an investigation is deemed necessary, a copy of this form will be provided to the individual against whom the complaint is filed.

Date _____

Complainant: (Information regarding individual filing the complaint)

Name _____   Phone _____

Address _____   Email _____

City _____ State _____ Zip Code _____

Respondent: (Information regarding individual against whom the complaint is directed)

Name _____   Phone _____

Address _____   Email _____

City _____ State _____ Zip Code _____

1. **Summarize** in a written attachment the **facts and circumstances, including dates and events**, which support a violation of the *Code of Ethics and Ethics Standards* and this complaint. Include steps, if any, that have been taken to resolve this complaint before filing.
2. **Please sign and date all documents you have written and are submitting**. *Do not include confidential documents such as patient or employment records.*
3. **If you have filed a complaint about this same matter with any other agency (e.g., NBCOT; SRB; academic institution; any federal, state, or local official), indicate to whom it was submitted, the approximate date(s), and resolution if known.**

I certify that the statements/information within this complaint are correct and truthful to the best of my knowledge and are submitted in good faith, not for resolution of private business, legal, or other disputes for which other appropriate forums exist.

_____
Signature

Send completed form, with accompanying documentation, **IN AN ENVELOPE MARKED** *CONFIDENTIAL* **to:**

Ethics Commission
American Occupational Therapy Association, Inc.
Attn: Staff Liaison to the EC/Ethics Office
4720 Montgomery Lane, PO Box 31220
Bethesda, MD 20824-1220

Office Use Only:
Membership Dates:_____
Verified by:_____

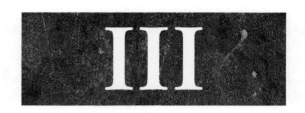

III

JURISDICTION

CHAPTER 5

Disciplinary Action: Whose Responsibility?

JURISDICTION

- **National Board for Certification in Occupational Therapy (NBCOT)**—All certified individuals (occupational therapists and occupational therapy assistants) and persons who are currently applicants to sit for the occupational therapist and occupational therapy assistant examinations.
- **State regulatory boards (SRBs)**—All individuals regulated in that state (varies from state to state)—for example, occupational therapists and occupational therapy assistants.
- **American Occupational Therapy Association (AOTA)**—All members of AOTA, including all membership categories (i.e., occupational therapists, occupational therapy assistants, students, and associates).

Ruth A. Hansen, PhD, OTR, FAOTA
Chairperson, Commission on Standards and Ethics (1988–1994)

This chapter was originally published in the 2006 version of the *Reference Guide to the Occupational Therapy Code of Ethics*. It has been revised to reflect updated AOTA official documents, Web sites, AOTA style, and additional resources.

| | JURISDICTION | | |
QUESTION	NBCOT	SRB	AOTA
1. Who should I call if I have questions about the following?			
a. Ethical violations that could cause harm or have potential to cause harm to a consumer or the public	X	X	X
b. Violations that do not cause harm or have a limited potential for causing harm to a consumer or the public			X
c. Violations of professional values that do not relate directly to potential harm to the public			X
2. Where did the alleged violation occur, and who was involved in the alleged incident?			
a. Took place in a state with rules, regulations, and disciplinary procedures in place	X	X	X
b. Took place in an unregulated state	X		X
c. Was committed by an AOTA member	X	X	X
d. Was committed by a person who is not an AOTA member	X	X	
3. What is the disciplinary action that you wish as a consequence of filing a complaint?			
a. Restrict or revoke licensure		X	
b. Restrict or revoke certification	X		
c. Restrict or prohibit membership in AOTA			X

FIGURE 5.1. Disciplinary Responsibility

REFERENCE GUIDE TO THE OCCUPATIONAL THERAPY CODE OF ETHICS AND ETHICS STANDARDS

Overview of the Ethical Jurisdictions of AOTA, NBCOT, and State Regulatory Boards

Three entities have jurisdiction over and concerns about the ethical and professional conduct of occupational therapy personnel: the American Occupational Therapy Association (AOTA), the National Certification Board for Occupational Therapy (NBCOT), and state regulatory boards (SRBs).

AOTA

AOTA is a voluntary membership organization that represents and promotes the profession and the interests of individuals who choose to become members. Because membership is voluntary, AOTA has no direct authority over occupational therapists and occupational therapy assistants who are not members. AOTA also has no direct legal mechanism for preventing nonmembers who are incompetent, unethical, or unqualified from practicing. That role is the responsibility of SRBs.

It is important to remember that AOTA is concerned about ethical conduct across the multiple roles that occupational therapists and occupational therapy assistants can play—student, researcher, educator, manager, practitioner, entrepreneur, elected or appointed volunteer leader, and so forth. The Ethics Commission (EC) is the volunteer-sector component of AOTA that is responsible for writing, revising, and enforcing the *Occupational Therapy Code of Ethics and Ethics Standards (2010)* (referred to as the "Code and Ethics Standards"; AOTA, 2010b). The EC is also responsible for informing and educating members about current ethical trends and issues and for reviewing allegations of unethical conduct by AOTA members.

There are five types of potential disciplinary action:

1. *Reprimand* is a formal expression of disapproval of conduct communicated privately by letter from the chairperson of the EC.
2. *Censure* is a formal expression of disapproval that is public (e.g., published in *OT Practice,* in the *American Journal of Occupational Therapy,* and at www.aota.org).
3. *Probation* of membership subject to certain terms—membership is conditional depending on compliance with specific requirements (e.g., continuing education). Failure to meet these terms will subject a member to any of the disciplinary actions or sanctions.
4. *Suspension* is removal of membership for a specified time.
5. *Revocation* prohibits a person from being a member of AOTA indefinitely (AOTA, 2010a).

NBCOT

NBCOT is a private, not-for-profit, nongovernmental credentialing organization that oversees and administers the entry-level certification examination for occupational therapists and occupational therapy assistants. This examination is what the SRBs use as one of the criteria for licensure (or other forms of regulation). NBCOT uses the examination as one of the criteria for initial NBCOT certification.

NBCOT certifies eligible individuals as Occupational Therapist Registered OTR® (OTR) or Certified Occupational Therapy Assistant COTA® (COTA). The "R" (registered) and "C" (certified) credentials are registered trademarks owned by NBCOT. Certification by NBCOT indicates to the public that the OTR or the COTA has met all of NBCOT's educational, fieldwork, and examination requirements (NBCOT, cited in Smith & Willmarth, 2003). Maintaining NBCOT certification entitles individuals to the continued use of NBCOT's registered certification marks OTR® or COTA®. Individuals who choose not to renew this certification are not permitted by NBCOT to use its certification marks.

States or jurisdictions commonly require occupational therapists and occupational therapy assistants to be initially certified (i.e., pass the NBCOT entry-level certification exam) before they can qualify for a license. Most states or jurisdictions, however, do not require practitioners to renew this certification to maintain their licenses to practice. There are a few exceptions. Occupational therapy assistants are not regulated in Hawaii or Colorado, and those in New York are not required to take the exam. Occupational therapists and occupational therapy assistants in Puerto Rico are not required to take the exam for licensure and may instead take a test developed by the Puerto Rico Occupational Therapy Board. South Carolina is the only state at this time requiring current certification for licensure renewal.

NBCOT does not use AOTA's Code and Ethics Standards as its guide in reviewing complaints about incompetent or impaired practitioners but has its own set of procedures for disciplinary action. NBCOT takes action when there is a clear violation of its Candidate/Certificant Code of Conduct (NBCOT, 2010a). The three main categories of violations that warrant disciplinary action are incompetence, unethical behavior, and impairment.

When NBCOT receives a complaint, it initiates an intensive, confidential review process to determine whether the allegations are warranted. If so, the Qualifications and Compliance Review Committee may recommend one of six types of disciplinary action, depending on the seriousness of the misconduct; all but reprimand and ineligibility are made public (NBCOT, 2010a):

1. *Ineligibility for certification:* An individual is barred from certification by NBCOT, either indefinitely or for a certain duration.
2. *Reprimand:* A formal expression of disapproval is retained in the certificant's file but is not publicly announced.
3. *Censure:* A formal expression of disapproval is publicly announced.
4. *Probation:* Continued certification is subject to fulfillment of specified conditions (e.g., monitoring, education, supervision, counseling).
5. *Suspension:* An individual loses certification for a certain duration, after which he or she may be required to apply for reinstatement.
6. *Revocation:* Loss of certification is permanent (NBCOT, 2010b).

STATE REGULATORY BOARDS

Occupational therapy SRBs are public bodies created by state legislatures to ensure the health and safety of the citizens of that state and to enforce the state's occupational therapy practice act. These bodies are sometimes known as *councils* or *advisory committees*, and in some states the state agency is solely responsible for enforcement of the practice act. Their responsibility is to protect the public in that state from potential harm caused by incompetent or unqualified practitioners, and there is a process for reviewing and handling any complaint against a practitioner that may be filed with the board.

State regulation may be in the form of licensure, registration, certification, or title protection. Only those states with licensure, registration, or certification laws have regulatory boards (or advisory councils or committees) to enforce the law. States with title protection (or trademark law) do not have SRBs; laws that protect consumers are usually enforced by the state's consumer protection agency or attorney general. The legal guidelines of states with licensure define the scope of practice for the profession and the qualifications that professionals must meet to practice.

In several states, SRBs have adopted AOTA's Code and Ethics Standards for this purpose. The majority of those states use the Code and Ethics Standards as their template for reviewing complaints about harm to the public by a practitioner who is licensed in that state. States often adopt the Code and Ethics Standards at a point in time and update regulations infrequently, which means that the adopted Code and Ethics Standards may become outdated in a particular state. Other states have language describing professional conduct as a standard.

Each SRB has direct jurisdiction over practitioners who are licensed or regulated in that state. By nature of this limited jurisdiction, each state can monitor the practitioners in that state more closely than can national organizations such as AOTA and NBCOT. In addition, an SRB has the authority by state law to discipline members of a profession practicing in that state if they have caused harm to residents of that state. This authority gives the SRB legal authority to conduct investigations, including the subpoena of witnesses, as well as impose fines or recommend imprisonment. Violations of the law at the level of criminal activity may be referred to the attorney general's office for potential prosecution. By virtue of their authority to suspend or revoke a license, SRBs control individual practitioners' ability to practice occupational therapy. SRBs also can intervene in situations in which they are made aware of actions through the judicial system that may affect professional practice (e.g.,

misappropriation of funds through false billing practices) or in which behaviors were not directly related to practice but demonstrated potential harm to the consumer in some way (e.g., poor decision making as evidenced by multiple drunk driving convictions).

When an SRB determines that an individual has violated the law, it can mandate one or more sanctions as a disciplinary measure. Examples of disciplinary actions are public censure, temporary or permanent suspension of a license to practice in that state, probationary license with conditions, and monetary fine.

WHERE TO GO FIRST

As one can see, AOTA, NBCOT, and SRBs have specific jurisdictions over occupational therapy practitioners (see Figure 5.1). Some areas of concern overlap among the three entities; others are separate and distinct. Individuals who need information or want to file a complaint must know which of the three is the most appropriate to contact. The following questions may assist in clarifying where to file:

1. In what state did the alleged violation take place, and what level of regulation does that state have for occupational therapy?
2. Is the individual a member of AOTA, or was he or she a member at the time of the alleged incident? Is the individual currently certified by NBCOT?
3. What consequences are considered appropriate if the complaint is determined to be justified?

In some instances, an individual may feel that it is appropriate to file a complaint with any or all of the three entities. For example, all three have concerns if there has been harm or potential harm to a consumer. But ethical violations of professional values that have no potential to cause harm would likely be of interest only to AOTA. For example, AOTA would be concerned about plagiarism of a colleague's professional work, but NBCOT and the SRB would not.

Individuals should also consider what disciplinary action they would consider appropriate for a particular violation: revoking or restricting the person's state license to practice? suspending or revoking the individual's certification? restricting or prohibiting the person's ability to be a member of AOTA? An individual considering an action should seek advice before filing a complaint to be sure that he or she has selected the agency with the jurisdiction to achieve the consequences commensurate to the violation (see Chapter 5).

CONCLUSION

Three primary organizations have ethical oversight of the occupational therapy profession. In some cases, their jurisdictions may overlap, but each focuses on particular areas of ethical behavior and has procedures for enforcing appropriate professional conduct. Occupational therapists and occupational therapy assistants have a responsibility to be aware of and comply with the policies and procedures of these organizations.

REFERENCES

American Occupational Therapy Association. (2010a). Enforcement procedures for the *Occupational Therapy Code of Ethics and Ethics Standards. American Journal of Occupational Therapy, 64*(6 Suppl.), S4–S16. doi:10.5014/ajot.2010.64S4

American Occupational Therapy Association. (2010b). Occupational therapy code of ethics and ethics standards (2010). *American Journal of Occupational Therapy, 64*(6 Suppl.), S17–S26. doi:10.5014/ajot.2010.64S17

National Board for Certification in Occupational Therapy. (2010a). *NBCOT candidate/certificant code of conduct.* Retrieved June 24, 2010, from http://www.nbcot.org/pdf/Candidate-Certificant-Code-of-Conduct.pdf

National Board for Certification in Occupational Therapy. (2010b). *Procedures for the enforcement of the NBCOT® candidate/certificant code of conduct.* Retrieved June 24, 2010, from http://www.nbcot.org/pdf/Enforcement_Procedures.pdf

Smith, K. C., & Willmarth, C. (2003). State regulation of occupational therapists and occupational therapy assistants. In G. L. McCormack, E. G. Jaffe, & M. Goodman-Lavey (Eds.), *The occupational therapy manager* (4th ed., pp. 439–459). Bethesda, MD: AOTA Press.

Ruth A. Hansen, PhD, OTR, FAOTA
Western Michigan University

Deborah Yarett Slater, MS, OT/L, FAOTA
AOTA Staff Liaison to the Ethics Commission

This chapter, originally published in the 2000 edition of the *Reference Guide to the Occupational Therapy Code of Ethics,* was adapted from Hansen, R. A. (1998). Ethics in occupational therapy. In M. E. Neistadt & E. B. Crepeau (Eds.), *Willard and Spackman's occupational therapy* (9th ed., pp. 819–827). Philadelphia: Lippincott. It has been revised to reflect updated AOTA official documents, Web sites, AOTA style, and additional resources.

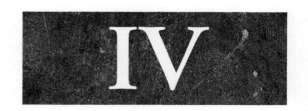

EDUCATIONAL
AND RESEARCH
RESOURCES

CHAPTER 7

Introduction: Educational and Research Resources

The Ethics Commission has two roles: enforcement and education. This section of the *Reference Guide to the Occupational Therapy Code of Ethics and Ethics Standards (2010)* (referred to as the "Code and Ethics Standards"; AOTA, 2010) provides tools to help members understand and apply ethics in their professional and volunteer work. Professional ethics applies to all licensed (or otherwise regulated) occupational therapists and occupational therapy assistants, including those who work in practice, education, and research, as well as to students and individuals who work in other paid or volunteer positions related to occupational therapy.

The chapters in this section provide foundational information about the role of ethics in the occupational therapy profession and additional resources to assist with practical application of the Code and Ethics Standards in a variety of situations. One overarching theme, both explicitly and implicitly, is the importance of conduct that positively reflects the behavior and values of the occupational therapy profession. This type of conduct is critically important not only among colleagues within a work setting but also in relationships and collaborative activities with outside organizations and the public.

To enhance the value of this section of the *Reference Guide,* a new chapter entitled "How to Use This *Reference Guide:* For Educators" is included with suggested learning activities and applications of content to the classroom. Additional new content in this edition of the *Reference Guide* includes "Occupational Therapy Values and Beliefs: A New View of Occupation and the Profession, 1950–1969," which describes the underpinnings of AOTA's ethics documents, and an article on "Combating Moral Distress," which appeared in *OT Practice,* that identifies workplace factors that can lead to moral or ethical distress and describes strategies to address them. This and other articles discuss the personal obligations practitioners have to maintain ethical standards in the face of increasing pressure to maximize productivity and reimbursement, often at the expense of appropriate clinical judgment and the client's best interests. Additional content in this section focuses on specific areas in which member queries have shown that there is greater need for ethical awareness and assistance with resolving issues.

Finally, as more occupational therapists and occupational therapy assistants pursue research and publication, there is a greater need for guidance related to the responsible conduct of research, plagiarism and authorship, human subjects, and intellectual property. An annotated bibliography with resources for online training and education in these areas is a new addition to this section.

REFERENCE

American Occupational Therapy Association. (2010). Occupational therapy code of ethics and ethics standards (2010). *American Journal of Occupational Therapy, 64*(6 Suppl.), S17–S26. doi:10.5014/ajot.2010.64S17

Deborah Yarett Slater, MS, OT/L, FAOTA
AOTA Staff Liaison to the Ethics Commission

CHAPTER 8

How to Use This Reference Guide: For Educators

The *Reference Guide to the Occupational Therapy Code of Ethics and Ethics Standards* is a rich resource for educators and students in academic settings that can help guide students on their journey toward becoming competent and ethical in their future professional roles. Students can purchase a copy of the book when they enter the occupational therapy program and review it during orientation to begin integrating ethical awareness into their thinking and reasoning processes. Educators can use the book as a resource throughout the curriculum, assigning specific chapters to coincide with course topics. The *Reference Guide* can also serve as a textbook for an occupational therapy ethics course. Chapter readings are especially helpful in explaining the specific principles to students learning the *Occupational Therapy Code of Ethics and Ethics Standards (2010)* (referred to as the "Code and Ethics Standards"; American Occupational Therapy Association [AOTA], 2010b).

Specific content of the *Reference Guide* can serve as a springboard for classroom learning activities. Many of the chapters include real-life case vignettes that students can explore in whole-class or small-group discussion, role-playing, debate, mock ethics committee proceedings, or "Theater of the Oppressed"

(see Brown & Gillespie, 1997). Chapter 13, "Is It Possible to Be Ethical?" includes a model for ethical decision making that students can apply in seeking a resolution to one of the case studies in a group discussion or written paper. A case study can also serve as the basis for learning the *Enforcement Procedures for the Occupational Therapy Code of Ethics and Ethics Standards* (AOTA, 2010a), which are used to process complaints filed with AOTA's Ethics Commission; students can simulate the process and recommend a course of action. To promote integration of ethics terminology, students can be encouraged to apply terms included in Appendix A, Glossary of Ethics Terms, during all these activities. Finally, student ethical reflection (Tillich, 1965) during and following these activities is an important part of the learning process.

The *Reference Guide* offers comprehensive information important to ethical occupational therapy practice. Students benefit from the wide scope of knowledge included in the book, and educators benefit from the up-to-date information and resources, allowing them to better prepare students to be competent and ethical occupational therapists or occupational therapy assistants.

REFERENCES

American Occupational Therapy Association. (2010a). Enforcement procedures for the *Occupational Therapy Code of Ethics and Ethics Standards. American Journal of Occupational Therapy, 64*(6 Suppl.), S4–S16. doi:10.5014/ajot.2010.64S4

American Occupational Therapy Association. (2010b). Occupational therapy code of ethics and ethics standards (2010). *American Journal of Occupational Therapy, 64*(6 Suppl.), S17–S26. doi:10.5014/ajot.2010.64S17

Brown, K. H., & Gillespie, D. (1997). "We become brave by doing brave acts": Teaching moral courage through the Theater of the Oppressed. *Literature and Medicine, 16*(1), 108–120.

Tillich, P. (1965). *Systematic theology* (Vol. 3). Chicago: University of Chicago Press.

Joanne Estes, MS, OTR/L
Education Representative, Ethics Commission (2009–2012)

Barbara Hemphill, DMin, OTR/L, FAOTA, FMOTA
Chairperson, Ethics Commission (2010–2013)

CHAPTER 9

The Function of
Professional Ethics

A profession organizes its ethics code based on the activities of its members. Professionals are expected to uphold a higher degree of ethical behavior than the general public. In turn, the public grants rights or privileges to professionals beyond those normally granted to all citizens. This arrangement is designed to protect the public and the recipients of professional services.

The American Occupational Therapy Association (AOTA) has adopted eight ethical concepts, which have been organized into seven statements. These statements are the *Occupational Therapy Code of Ethics and Ethics Standards (2010)* (referred to as the "Code and Ethics Standards"; AOTA, 2010b). Four of the concepts are considered moral principles: beneficence, nonmaleficence, autonomy, and procedural justice (Principles 1, 2, 3, and 5). Four concepts are viewed as rules that service providers must follow: confidentiality, social justice, veracity, and fidelity (Principles 3, 4, 6, and 7). These concepts are further illustrated in the following summary of the seven ethical statements in the Code and Ethics Standards:

- *Beneficence* includes all forms of action intended to benefit recipients of services that occupational therapy personnel are expected to provide, including protecting and defending the rights of others, preventing harm from occurring to others, removing conditions that will cause harm to others,

helping persons with disabilities, and rescuing persons in danger (Principle 1).
- *Nonmaleficence* imparts an obligation by occupational therapy personnel to avoid or refrain from harming others, to not inflict injury or wrong others, and to not impose risks of harm even if the potential risk is without malicious or harmful intent (Principle 2).
- *Autonomy* and *confidentiality* express the concept that occupational therapy personnel have a duty to treat recipients of service according to each person's desire for self-determination within the bounds of accepted standards of care and to not reveal or disclose confidential information to unauthorized persons or groups (Principle 3).
- *Social justice,* also called "distributive justice," refers to a vested interest occupational therapy personnel have to advocate for the distribution of health care resources in a fair, equitable, and appropriate manner that will provide opportunities for recipients of service to participate in society (Principle 4).
- *Procedural justice* is concerned with making and implementing decisions according to fair processes that ensure the fair treatment of all individuals and that form the foundation for policies, regulations, and laws that occupational therapy personnel are expected to follow (Principle 5).
- *Veracity* is based on the virtues of truthfulness, candor, and honesty, and occupational therapy personnel fulfill their obligation of

veracity by ensuring that information or data about recipients of service is comprehensive, accurate, and objective and is presented in a manner that service recipients understand (Principle 6).

- *Fidelity* refers to maintaining good-faith relationships between service providers, such as occupational therapy personnel, and service recipients and includes an obligation to treat colleagues and other professionals with respect, fairness, discretion, and integrity (Principle 7).

Professionals usually develop their concepts of moral ideals and accepted rules of ethical conduct by developing and implementing a written code of ethics through a professional association or organization. Three types of ethical codes can be adopted: aspirational, educational, or regulatory. *Aspirational codes* encourage competent and moral behavior but do not provide guidelines for ethical conduct or sanctions for failure to follow the intent of the code. *Educational codes* state what constitutes ethical behavior and may provide case examples as illustrations but do not provide sanctions for failure to follow the code. *Regulatory codes* spell out the expected behavior, state guidelines for expected conduct, and give specific descriptions of sanctions for failures to follow the code.

AOTA's Ethics Commission (EC) has described the *Occupational Therapy Code of Ethics and Ethics Standards (2010)* as aspirational. The Code and Ethics Standards are complemented by the *Enforcement Procedures for the Occupational Therapy Code of Ethics and Ethics Standards* (AOTA, 2010a), which offer members and the public the regulatory component to support the Code and Ethics Standards and ensure compliance.

The EC's approach is advantageous in that collective thinking is used to develop and update the Code and Ethics Standards, and peers are encouraged to monitor the behavior of their colleagues. The disadvantage is that the Code

and Ethics Standards can be applied only to members of the professional association. Occupational therapists and occupational therapy assistants who are not AOTA members are not under the jurisdiction of the Code and Ethics Standards, nor can they be held accountable to the conduct that it embraces. However, the public's access to the Code and Ethics Standards and the Enforcement Procedures may result in their expectation that all members of the profession adhere to the ethical standards approved by the professional association. Many state regulatory boards (SRBs), over time, have adopted the Code and Ethics Standards in whole or in part or have used similar language related to professional conduct; subsequently, many of the ethical concepts articulated by AOTA have been incorporated to varying degrees throughout the profession.

Although the Enforcement Procedures are regulatory, primary reliance on regulatory action to enforce the Code and Ethics Standards does not meet the EC's intent and spirit. Ethical behavior is a learned process that is best enforced through daily practice. Thus, voluntary compliance is both encouraged and endorsed. That is, members are encouraged to educate themselves and to help other members conform to the behavior stated in the Code and Ethics Standards before any sanctions are considered or applied. This approach of identifying and supporting desired behavior contrasts with standards that require certain behavior and have specific sanctions for noncompliance, even for a first offense.

Finally, ethics involves a dynamic process. As society changes, so do ideas about ethical behavior. AOTA has recognized the changing concepts of ethics by adopting a (minimum) 5-year review cycle to consider revisions of the Code and Ethics Standards. The process begins with members of the EC conducting an internal review of the document and then drafting revisions for review by the AOTA membership. Once the review process is complete, the revised Code and Ethics Standards are sent to the Representative Assembly for action. The final version is published in the *American Journal of Occupational Therapy* as part of the Association's official documents. The Code and Ethics Standards are also posted on AOTA's Web site (www.aota.org) in both the consumer and members-only sections.

In the past, the chairperson of the EC has received a variety of complaints concerning alleged violations of the Code and Ethics Standards that indicate that members may not understand clearly the criteria to which professional ethics can be applied. The misconceptions can be organized into 10 major areas:

1. The Code and Ethics Standards

    apply to persons who are or were members of the AOTA at the time of the conduct in question. Later nonrenewal or relinquishment of membership does not affect Association jurisdiction. The Enforcement Procedures that shall be utilized in any complaint shall be those in effect at the time the complaint is initiated. (AOTA, 2010a, pp. S4–S5)

    If the alleged violator was not a member at the time of the incident, other language related to professional conduct, such as that stated in a state licensure law, may apply.

2. The Code and Ethics Standards apply to those behaviors that occupational therapists and occupational therapy assistants have agreed are important. Other professions and professionals may have different ideas about ethical and unethical behavior. To determine the ethics that apply to another professional, occupational therapists must read the code of ethics adopted by that professional's organization or the state's licensure law. Most, if not all, professional codes of ethics are publicly available on the professional organization's Web site. If an occupational therapist or occupational therapy assistant feels that a member of another profession has violated

an ethics principle, he or she must review that profession's code of ethics for instructions or procedures to follow in reporting alleged violations.

3. When AOTA members or members of the public suspect that an occupational therapist or occupational therapy assistant has violated a regulation governing occupational therapy practice, an established code of conduct, or the Code and Ethics Standards, the alleged violation should be reported to the appropriate body. It is permissible to report alleged violations to more than one agency, organization, or association (e.g., SRB and AOTA, the National Certification Board for Occupational Therapy [NBCOT] and AOTA). Occupational therapy professionals can refer to "Overview of the Ethical Jurisdictions of AOTA, NBCOT, and State Regulatory Boards" (Chapter 6 in this book) for additional information. Any alleged breach of ethical conduct by an AOTA member should be reported to the EC.

4. The Code and Ethics Standards are a set of desired behaviors. A code does not take the place of disciplinary procedures that may be applied for failure to perform according to one's position description or employee policy manual. Managers should take action to ensure that an occupational therapy practitioner performs duties stated in the position description or apply the remedy as stated in the manual of the employing organization. Institutional rules and guidelines articulated in student handbooks should be considered for those in academia (e.g., students, faculty).

5. The Code and Ethics Standards delineate expected ethical behaviors, but they cannot substitute for a position description or contract. Occupational therapists and occupational therapy assistants need to know what their position description or contract states. Questions about job duties should be addressed to the manager in charge of occupational therapy. If the manager is

unable or unwilling to address the problem or question, the occupational therapist or occupational therapy assistant should follow the procedures outlined in the employee policy manual for addressing grievances. The advice of a lawyer specializing in employment law and/or business and contracts may be useful. Examples of problems related to job duties include productivity requirements, inappropriate referrals, lack of equipment or supplies, disagreements about the use of various therapy interventions, disputes about the number of therapy sessions to be provided, and termination procedures to end therapy. In some cases, fraud also may be involved (see Item 7 below).

6. If an AOTA member is convicted of an offense or a violation of federal, state, or local laws and regulations, the EC will review the charges. The member will be afforded due process. Only after careful review of the details of the charge will the EC determine if disciplinary action is indicated and the nature and extent of such action.

7. EC and AOTA officials cannot resolve disputes about billing procedures, record keeping, and documentation. False billing for services not rendered, double billing, or overcharging are examples of fraud. Deviations from accepted record keeping and documentation procedures done for financial gain also are examples of fraud. All states have mechanisms to oversee and review reported cases of suspected fraud through the state attorney general or similar state official or office. In addition, questionable business practices can be reported to the Better Business Bureau. Accrediting agencies for health and educational organizations may be notified, as fraud convictions can adversely affect accreditation. Insurance companies are usually quick to respond to reported cases of alleged fraud, because fraud usually increases the cost of doing business, may increase premiums, or

diverts funds that could be used to provide additional services. If federal funds are involved, fraud is a misappropriation of tax money, which is a federal offense. If an AOTA member is cited or convicted of fraudulent behavior, the EC and the Association may subject that member to disciplinary action.

8. EC or AOTA officials cannot resolve complaints about unsafe working conditions, such as electrical equipment improperly maintained, exposure to hazardous chemicals or waste, unsanitary conditions, improper storage of dangerous substances, structural weaknesses, or other alleged safety violations. Local building inspectors or fire departments often are charged with making local inspections. The federal Occupational Safety and Health Administration maintains offices in all states. If a member is convicted of or fined for violations related to health and safety, that person may be subjected to disciplinary action by the EC and the Association.

9. EC and AOTA officials cannot intervene on behalf of a student who alleges unfair grading procedures, lack of opportunity to take specific courses or obtain a desired fieldwork placement, or problems with other educational activity. Such complaints must be handled through college or university grievance procedures or civil courts. In some cases, notification of educational accrediting agencies may be in order. However, if an educational institution determines that an AOTA member has engaged in unfair or discriminatory practices against a student or colleague, that member may be subjected to disciplinary action by the EC and the Association.

10. The ultimate sanction that AOTA can apply to a member is permanent revocation of membership. AOTA cannot remove an occupational therapist's or occupational therapy assistant's right to practice. Removal of occupational therapy certification

is the responsibility of NBCOT. Only a court of law or government agency (state or federal) with legal authority (e.g., state licensure board) can take away or suspend a person's ability to practice occupational therapy. AOTA may, however, be called to testify about actions that it has taken against the member. If the member loses certification as an occupational therapy practitioner or is convicted of a crime by a legal authority related to services provided by that person in the capacity of an occupational therapist or occupational therapy assistant, disciplinary action may be initiated by the EC and the Association.

SUMMARY

A professional code of ethics contains statements of desired behaviors that members are encouraged to follow. Peers should support members' efforts to adopt the desired behavior. When a violation of the Code and Ethics Standards is thought to have taken place, enforcement of appropriate ethical behavior should begin as an educational process between the individuals directly involved. If the resolution cannot occur on the "local" level, a complaint should be filed with one or more of the most appropriate agencies or bodies, depending on the level of infraction and desired outcome (Figure 5.1 contains a chart outlining this information). The AOTA Ethics Office also can provide guidance with this decision. If an AOTA member is allegedly involved in a violation of the Code and Ethics Standards, the allegation should be reported to the EC, even if complaints have been filed with other regulatory authorities. The ultimate sanction that the AOTA can supply, revocation of membership or a permanent denial of membership, should be applied only on sound evidence of failure or unwillingness to comply with appropriate conduct.

REFERENCES

American Occupational Therapy Association. (2010a). Enforcement procedures for the *Occupational Therapy Code of Ethics and Ethics Standards. American Journal of Occupational Therapy, 64*(6 Suppl.), S4–S16. doi:10.5014/ajot.2010.64S4

American Occupational Therapy Association. (2010b). Occupational therapy code of ethics and ethics standards (2010). *American Journal of Occupational Therapy, 64*(6 Suppl.), S17–S26. doi:10.5014/ajot.2010.64S17

Kathlyn L. Reed, PhD, OTR, FAOTA, MLIS, AHIP
Associate Professor, Texas Woman's University–Houston Center
Chairperson, Ethics Commission (2006–2010)

Deborah Yarett Slater, MS, OT/L, FAOTA
AOTA Staff Liaison to the Ethics Commission

This chapter was originally published in the 2008 edition of the *Reference Guide to the Occupational Therapy Ethics Standards*. It has been revised to reflect updated AOTA official documents, Web sites, AOTA style, and additional resources.

CHAPTER 10

Scope of the AOTA Ethics Commission

The Ethics Commission (EC) is a body of the Representative Assembly (RA) of the American Occupational Therapy Association (AOTA). The purpose of the EC is "to serve the Association members and public through the identification, development, review, interpretation, and education of the AOTA *Occupational Therapy Code of Ethics and Ethics Standards (2010)* and to provide the process whereby the ethics of the Association are enforced" (AOTA Bylaws; AOTA, 2009, Art. 7, §7). The EC promotes and maintains professional conduct in all occupational therapy roles and supports the delivery of high-quality services and contributions to society's health and well-being.

The AOTA *Occupational Therapy Code of Ethics and Ethics Standards (2010)* (referred to as the "Code and Ethics Standards"; AOTA, 2010b) is a public statement of the values and principles that guide the behavior of members of the profession and to which they should aspire. The EC is responsible for the development and oversight of the Code and Ethics Standards, which apply to occupational therapy personnel at all levels and to all professional roles, including those of practitioner, educator, fieldwork educator or coordinator, clinical supervisor, manager, administrator, consultant, faculty, program director, researcher or scholar, private practice owner, entrepreneur, student, and elected and appointed volunteer within AOTA.

To ensure that AOTA members adhere to the Code and Ethics Standards, the EC has developed procedures for the investigation and adjudication of alleged violations. The *Enforcement Procedures for the Occupational Therapy Code of Ethics and Ethics Standards* (AOTA, 2010a) define the scope of disciplinary action for violations of the Code and Ethics Standards. These procedures are intended to enable AOTA to implement its responsibilities in a fair and equitable manner to best serve its members and society.

ROLE OF THE EC

The EC has two roles: education and enforcement. The EC's jurisdiction for enforcement is limited to individuals who are members of the Association (or were members at the time of the alleged incident), including occupational therapists, occupational therapy assistants, associates, and students.

FUNCTIONS OF THE EC

The functions of the EC include the following:

- To develop and revise AOTA's occupational therapy ethics documents and submit revisions to the RA for approval
- To provide a process for reviewing and monitoring existing and proposed documents from an ethical perspective for consistency with the Code and Ethics Standards
- To inform and educate Association members and consumers regarding the Code and Ethics Standards

- To establish and maintain procedures for considering and reviewing allegations of nonconformance with the Code and Ethics Standards
- To serve as a resource for any Association body requiring interpretation of the Code and Ethics Standards
- To issue Advisory Opinions on the interpretation and application of the Code and Ethics Standards and ethical trends
- To clarify for members and Association bodies the roles of the regulatory or associated agencies or bodies (e.g., National Board for Certification in Occupational Therapy, state regulatory boards) that oversee the delivery of occupational therapy services and educational programs (AOTA, 2009).

MEMBERS OF THE EC

The EC chairperson, elected by the AOTA membership, serves 1 year in the role of chairperson-elect and 3 years as chairperson. The chairperson appoints AOTA member volunteers and public members to serve on the EC. The EC is made up of an occupational therapist, an occupational therapy assistant, an educator, a practitioner, a member at large, and two public members (a total of seven members, including the chairperson). The chairperson and appointed volunteers serve 3-year terms. The chairperson serves one term, but EC members have the possibility of serving a maximum of two consecutive terms.

AOTA's National Office staff liaison and legal counsel support the work of the EC. Specifically, the liaison provides administrative and procedural support, and the legal counsel provides legal expertise as needed.

OVERVIEW OF THE EC

One of the primary roles of the EC is ethics education. Accordingly, the EC periodically issues Advisory Opinions; provides an "Everyday Ethics" workshop at the AOTA Annual Conference & Expo; and develops and provides other educational materials in response to member needs, inquiries, and ethical trends.

The EC reviews and investigates ethics complaints filed against AOTA members. The EC may recommend disciplinary actions that include reprimand, censure, probation, suspension, and revocation. For specific information about the disciplinary process used by the EC, see the *Enforcement Procedures for the Occupational Therapy Code of Ethics and Ethics Standards* in this *Reference Guide*. The EC meets monthly by conference call.

Along with the EC, other agencies that have oversight over the occupational therapy profession include state regulatory boards (SRBs) and the National Board for Certification in Occupational Therapy (NBCOT). Each has a defined jurisdiction and areas of specific concern. More information on the ethical jurisdictions of AOTA, NBCOT, and SRBs is available in Chapter 6 of this *Reference Guide*.

REFERENCES

American Occupational Therapy Association. (2009). *The official bylaws of the American Occupational Therapy Association, Inc.* Retrieved November 17, 2010, from www.aota.org/Governance/bylaws.aspx

American Occupational Therapy Association. (2010a). Enforcement procedures for the *Occupational Therapy Code of Ethics and Ethics Standards*. *American Journal of Occupational Therapy, 64*(6 Suppl.), S4–S16. doi:10.5014/ajot.2010.64S4

American Occupational Therapy Association. (2010b). Occupational therapy code of ethics and ethics standards (2010). *American Journal of Occupational Therapy, 64*(6 Suppl.), S17–S26. doi:10.5014/ajot.2010.64S17

Deborah Yarett Slater, MS, OT/L, FAOTA
AOTA Staff Liaison to the Ethics Commission

This chapter was originally published in the 2006 edition of the *Reference Guide to the Occupational Therapy Code of Ethics*. It has been revised to reflect updated AOTA official documents, Web sites, AOTA style, and additional resources.

CHAPTER 11

Occupational Therapy Values and Beliefs: The Formative Years, 1904–1929

"The social values of a professional group are its basic and fundamental beliefs, the unquestioned premises upon which its very existence rests. Foremost among these values is the essential worth of the service which the professional group extends to the community" (Greenwood, 1957, p. 52). "One of the major differences between the professions and other occupations is that the professions are assumed to be concerned with the fulfillment of certain intrinsic values . . ." (Lipset & Schwartz, 1966, p. 307).

Occupational therapy values and beliefs were shaped by the times and events of the 19th and early 20th centuries, during which the profession was created. The Progressive Era (1890–1914) was at its height of influence as occupational therapy was being formally organized. The United States was being transformed by political, social, and economic reform (Gould, 2001). There was a "revolution in manners and morals" (Lear, 1981, p. xvi) that "was part of a broader shift from a Protestant ethos of salvation through self-denial to a therapeutic ideal of self-fulfillment in this world through exuberant health and intense experience" (Lear, 1981, p. xvi).

As Elizabeth Greene Upham said in 1918,

Occupational therapy is neither a new movement nor one which has suddenly come into prominence through a spectacular publicity campaign. It is, rather, a movement which has gradually developed by justifying itself over a long period of years. It was initiated by the doctors in insane hospitals who first dared the experiment of putting their patients to work; and by those other doctors who were groping after something which might give to their neurasthenic patients a healthy interest and a new grip on life. The healing value of occupation is so well established that occupational therapy is no longer confined to the insane or neurasthenic but has been found equally beneficent in tuberculosis, in long orthopedic treatments, and in extensive convalescences in a general hospital. (Upham, 1918, pp. 48–49)

As the profession approaches its 100th year of formal organization, a review of the values and beliefs that formed the basic premises is in order.

In the Beginning

The development of occupational therapy as a profession is unique. According to Maxwell and Maxwell (1984),

The development appeared to reflect not so much the emergence of a new technology or scientific advance, such as the development of the occupational role of X-ray technician following the invention of X-rays by Roentgen, but rather the organizing of existing knowledge into a new occupational role. . . . Since the knowledge base was not specific, occupational therapists faced from the beginning the problem of identity. (p. 339)

In other words, the development of occupational therapy did not fit the existing pattern recognized in sociology for a new profession—that is, as a consequence of a new technology or an advance in scientific knowledge. Instead, occupational therapy was created by selecting among knowledge already established from a variety of sources, including educators, artists, craftsmen and craftswomen, religious and spiritual leaders, engineers, nurses, physicians, social services workers, women's social groups, civic leaders and reformers, attendants, aides, and the patients or clients themselves. Such a variety of sources provided many values and beliefs, and even the early leaders were aware of the need to organize them into a set of principles.

The first set of principles proposed to the professional organization was published in 1919 in the January issue of the *Maryland Psychiatric Quarterly* (Dunton, 1919b) and in a book by William R. Dunton, Jr., MD (Dunton, 1919a). They were reprinted in 1923 (American Occupational Therapy Association [AOTA], 1923), 1925 (AOTA, 1925), and 1940 (AOTA, 1940; see Figure 11.1). The last two printings appeared in *Occupational Therapy and Rehabilitation,* the organization's official journal before the *American Journal of Occupational Therapy.* The principles were written by Eleanor Clarke Slagle, William L. Russell, and Norman L. Burnette (from Canada). Dunton had already published a shorter set of principles in 1918 (Dunton, 1918; see Figure 11.2). After the early efforts, the idea of documenting the values and beliefs of occupational therapy was not revisited for many years.

WHY LOOK BACK?

The current project grew from a concern expressed by members of the Representative Assembly Coordinating Committee in 2003 that the historical and philosophical roots of occupational therapy were not known to all current members of the profession. Responding to this concern, the 2003 Representative Assembly adopted a motion to form an ad hoc committee to identify those roots. The committee consists of myself as the chair, along with Suzanne Peloquin, PhD, OTR, FAOTA, and Christine Peters, MA, OTR.

The project began by identifying a time frame, 1904 to 1929, that represents a significant period of formation for the profession, based on an analysis of historical patterns in occupational therapy. We identified several subject areas that emerged during that time and that had an influence on the development or application of occupational therapy. The subject areas relate to social, educational, and philosophical movements; to the national government; to the application of therapeutic techniques; and to important contributions by particular individuals. By 1930 only Slagle, Kidner, and Dunton remained active; the other founders and early leaders had died or were inactive. In addition, no new textbooks were published from 1928 until the 1940s.

To assemble information from the subject areas, we created an outline for data collection that included a description of the subject area; dates when the subject began and ended; names and places associated with the subject; the purpose(s) of the subject; where, when, and how the subject interacted with occupational therapy; names and places associated with occupational therapy interaction; and the beliefs and values relevant to occupational therapy based on its involvement with the subject area.

As might be expected, some outlines were more complete than others because of the availability of more source material. Cross-references to other subjects were listed because many were interrelated. All references identified from the occupational literature about each subject were listed. However, a

FIGURE 11.1. Basic Principles of Occupational Therapy, 1919

To the members of the National Society for the Promotion of Occupational Therapy: Your Committee on Principles has agreed upon the following as representing the basic principles of occupational therapy:

1. Occupational therapy is a method of treating the sick or injured by means of instruction and employment of productive occupation.
2. The objects sought are to arouse interest, courage, and confidence; to exercise mind and body in healthy activity; to overcome functional disability; and to re-establish capacity for industrial and social usefulness.
3. In applying occupational therapy, system and precision are as important as in other forms of treatment.
4. The treatment should be administered under constant medical advice and supervision, and correlated with the other treatment of the patient.
5. The treatment should, in each case, be specifically directed to the individual's needs.
6. Though some patients do best alone, employment in groups is usually advisable because it provides exercise in social adaptation and the stimulating influence of example and comment.
7. The occupation selected should be within the range of the patient's estimated interests and capability.
8. As the patient's strength and capability increase, the type and extent of occupation should be regulated and graded accordingly.
9. The only reliable measure of the value of the treatment is the effect on the patient.
10. Inferior workmanship, or employment in an occupation which would be trivial for the healthy, may be attended with the greatest benefit to the sick or injured. Standards worthy of entirely normal persons must be maintained for proper mental stimulation.
11. The production of well-made, useful, and attractive articles, or the accomplishment of a useful task, requires healthy exercise of mind and body, gives the greatest satisfaction, and thus produces the most beneficial effects.
12. Novelty, variety, individuality, and utility of the products enhance the value of an occupation as a treatment measure.
13. Quality, quantity, and salability of the products may prove beneficial by satisfying and stimulating the patient but should never be permitted to obscure the main purpose.
14. Good craftsmanship, and ability to instruct, are essential qualifications in the occupational therapist; understanding, sincere interest in the patient, and an optimistic, cheerful outlook and manner are equally essential.
15. Patients under treatment by means of occupational therapy should also engage in recreational or play activities. It is advisable that gymnastics and calisthenics, which may be given for habit training, should be regarded as work. Social dancing and all recreational and play activities should be under the definite head of recreations.

Committee members: Eleanor Clarke Slagle, Dr. William L. Russell, and Mr. Norman L. Burnette (Canada)

Source: Dunton, W. R. (1919b). N.S.P.O.T. *Maryland Psychiatry Quarterly, 13*(3), 68–73. Reprinted in Dunton, W. R. (1919a). Appendix. In *Reconstruction therapy* (pp. 229). Philadelphia: W. B. Saunders.

separate literature search on each subject area was not done, such as searching several data sources for all articles and books on the Arts and Crafts movement or all articles published about humanism.

Of the 42 subject areas identified, developmental psychology, play as a skill for children, and progressive education did not produce useful literature or references. The remaining 39 subject areas are listed in Figure 11.3.

Reference sources included textbooks on the treatment of war injuries (during World War I), vocational reeducation and training, and occupational therapy literature published from 1904 to 1929. Journal articles came from four primary sources: *Maryland Psychiatric*

FIGURE 11.2. Principles Written by Dr. William R. Dunton, Jr., 1918

1. That work should be carried on with cure as the main object.
2. The work must be interesting.
3. The patient should be carefully studied.
4. The one form of occupation should not be carried to the point of fatigue.
5. That it should have some useful end.
6. That it preferably should lead to an increase in the patient's knowledge.
7. That it should be carried on with others.
8. That all possible encouragement should be given the worker.
9. The work resulting in a poor or useless product is better than idleness.

Source: Dunton, W. R. (1919a). Appendix. In *Reconstruction therapy* (pp. 229). Philadelphia: W. B. Saunders. *Original source:* Dunton, W. R. (1918). The principles of occupational therapy. *Public Health Nurse, 18,* 316–321. *Committee members:* Eleanor Clarke Slagle, Dr. William L. Russell, and Mr. Norman L. Burnette (Canada).

Quarterly (1914–1923), *Archives of Occupational Therapy* (1922–1924), *Occupational Therapy and Rehabilitation* (1925–1929), and *Modern Hospital* (1917–1929). Other relevant journals related mostly to psychiatry, mental hygiene, tuberculosis, orthopedics, surgery, and social welfare. Historical review articles were also identified to examine the values, beliefs, and ideas of the time. Approximately 40 books and 400 articles were scanned and screened for content. We used the Internet to identify some resources that were not readily available in the occupational therapy literature, such as major names and places associated with the manual training movement.

From these data we extracted values and beliefs, then organized them by principle (see Figure 11.4). McKenzie (1919) may have best summarized the uniqueness of occupational therapy as a therapeutic agent when he wrote that "treatment by occupation differs from all other forms . . . in that the remedy is given in increasing doses with its patient's improvement" (p. 105). Hall (1921), a past pres-

FIGURE 11.3. Subject Areas (in alphabetical order)

Arts and Crafts movement	Interest or interests	Progressive Era
Curative workshops	Manual training	Public health and welfare
Education of occupational therapists	Mechanism or mechanistic philosophy	Purposive psychology
Emmanuel movement	Mechano-therapy	Reconstruction aides
Federal Board of Vocational Education	Medical education	Reeducation of the disabled
Feminism	Mental hygiene	Settlement houses
Functional reeducation	Meyer and psychobiology	The simple life
Habit training	Moral treatment	Surgeon General's Office (including divisions and departments)
Holism and gestalt psychology	Motion study (Gilbreths)	
Humanism	Motivation	Therapeutic occupation
Humanitarianism	Neuropsychiatry	Treatment of tuberculosis
Idleness	Occupational therapy	Vocational reeducation and training
Industrial reeducation	Orthopedics	
	Pragmatism	Work and the work ethic

REFERENCE GUIDE TO THE OCCUPATIONAL THERAPY CODE OF ETHICS AND ETHICS STANDARDS

FIGURE 11.4. Summary of Principles Drawn From Values and Beliefs: 1904–1929

Note: The following cites only the occupational therapist, because the occupational therapy assistant position was not created until 1959.

Principles related to goals and outcomes

- The primary goal of occupational therapy is to return the person to active life and for the person to function in normal society as a whole person in body and soul.
- Additional goals may include attainment of self-control (of behavior), self-reliance and self-sufficiency (for attaining basic needs), manual skills (dexterity, strength, and coordination), and good work habits (accuracy, orderliness, neatness, patience, and perseverance).
- Where disease or injury has occurred, the goal of occupational therapy is to contribute to and hasten recovery.
- The outcome of occupational therapy is to enable the person to learn to develop better, easier, or more interesting methods of performing daily occupation.
- The purpose of occupational therapy may address physical, mental, and/or social occupations.
- Occupational therapy is the making of a man (individual) stronger physically, mentally, and spiritually than he was before.
- Occupational therapy makes the patient a creator, a doer (Crane, 1919).

Principles related to the process of occupational therapy

- All persons should be regarded as unique beings.
- All persons are capable of change and improvement regardless of diagnosis or situation.
- A person should not be excluded from intervention because his or her condition appears hopeless or unlikely to improve.
- The 24-hour cycle of time can be used successfully as a means of facilitating normal occupational behavior and organizing and structuring a person's daily occupations.
- The use of interest and motivation encourages a person to increase attention, to learn about the self and the environment, and to engage in occupations that promote self-realization.
- The person's interest in (or motivation for) occupation should always be considered and sustained.
- Interest and motivation may associate with physical, mental, or social activity.
- Appliances and assistive technology should meet the individual's needs for occupational performance and be kept to a minimum consistent with those needs.
- Appliances and assistive technology should be kept as simple as possible and still do the job.
- Occupations used in occupational therapy programs should be considered primarily for their therapeutic potential.
- Occupational therapists should focus on providing opportunities for people to practice the actual doing of occupation, not prescriptions focused on telling people which occupations to do.
- Occupational therapy should be provided in a pleasant (harmonious) environment in which useful occupations are provided and the occupational therapists act as role models.
- Occupation can be analyzed and graded along several continua including aptitude, ability, and interest. Therefore, occupation can be graded from simple and easy or complex and hard, require low or high level of skill, require little or extensive prior experience and education, and require a short or long time to complete.
- Occupation should be selected with the person's needs and abilities in mind.
- Occupational therapists need infinite patience, the ability to teach, and the power to inspire confidence in others.
- Occupational therapists need an optimistic temperament and a sense of humor.
- Occupational therapists must not become too paternal, killing personal responsibility (Crane, 1919).
- Occupational therapists should always praise the attempt and use constructive and suggestive criticism.
- Occupational therapy services can be designed to meet a variety of needs and purposes.
- It takes rare gifts and personalities to be pathfinders in this work (Meyer, 1922).
- It requires that one be true to one's nature and teach others to do the same (Meyer, 1922).
- Occupational therapy is an art and a science.
- Occupational therapy must lead somewhere, and the patient must want to follow (Cullimore, 1921).
- Occupational therapy requires understanding and give-and-take (Slagle, 1927).
- Occupational therapy requires spiritual vision of the end problem (Slagle, 1927).
- Visualizing results of therapy encourages the patient (Mock, 1919).
- The use of experimental, survey, case history, and analytical methodologies can be applied to the study of therapeutic occupation and its application to patients.

(continued)

- The use of systematic literature reviews can be applied to the study of therapeutic occupation and its application to patients.

Principles related to personal change through occupational therapy

- Occupational therapy is a method of treatment by means of instruction and employment of productive occupation (Dunton, 1919).
- Occupational therapists help the person to take control of his or her life situation.
- Occupational therapists encourage the person to learn to do things for himself or herself.
- Occupational therapists encourage the person to keep life simple and simplify life.
- Occupational therapists encourage the person to engage in wholesome (healthful and moral) occupations.
- Occupational therapists increase opportunities for the person to engage in social situations.
- Occupational therapy is the science of healing by occupation (Upham, 1918).

Principles related to the therapeutic application of occupation

- Focuses attention directly on the injury and uses occupation designed to promote and hasten return to function (direct approach).
- Focuses attention away from the pain of injury onto an absorbing occupation that promotes and hastens return of function through mental stimulation and doing/performing the actions required of the occupation (indirect approach).
- Keeps the mind occupied or absorbed with productive occupation and away from idleness, unreality, and self-absorbing thoughts (indirect approach).

- Keeps the mind and hands occupied so the body can rest.
- Uses a normal or familiar environment for doing/performing occupation.
- Can be graded along several criteria from bedside to workshop, diversional to work, individual to group, amusement to productive.
- Can be adjusted to fit individual needs as opposed to requiring the individual to adjust to it.
- Affords occasions for productivity and opportunity.
- Transforms environments and atmospheres.
- Aims to individualize with the temperament of each patient.
- Is a reeducation of faith and self-confidence.
- Is a scientific effort for the restoration to health of those mentally and physically ill.

Principles related to the therapeutic nature of occupation

- Occupation encourages doing and performing.
- Occupation can be goal directed.
- Occupation is important to good health.
- Occupation is natural and familiar to people.
- Occupation can arouse interest and motivation.
- Occupation can increase contact with the environment and reality.
- Occupation can be used to increase muscle power and strength.
- Occupation can be used to increase joint function.
- Occupation can be used to improve muscle tone (physical endurance, tolerance).
- Occupation can be used to improve sensation following nerve lesion.
- Occupation and health are linked.

- Occupation can be positive, purposeful, and controlled.
- Occupation can promote a healthier lifestyle.
- Occupation has recreational, educational, vocational, and therapeutic value.
- Occupation promotes the resumption of natural and healthy modes of thought.
- Occupation trains and engages attention.
- Occupation develops right habit formation.
- Occupation stimulates the mind and trains interest.
- Occupation fosters dignity, competence, and health.
- Occupation reduces despair and produces hope.
- The therapeutic value of occupation can be studied by recording the response (improved, much improved, or no relief) of clients to treatment.
- Occupations can be studied based on the type of effect various occupations have on recovery from different diagnoses or symptoms (e.g., calming or exciting the patient).
- Occupations can be studied for their potential as a therapeutic agent in various settings. Factors might include cost of supplies and equipment, number of tools needed, precautions to be observed, type of work area needed, and amount of training needed.

Principles related to philosophical assumptions

- Occupational therapy is based on the idea of helping others find their way toward health (Emmanuel movement).
- Occupational therapists assume the whole is different from and more than the sum of its parts and that the person should be

FIGURE 11.4. Summary of Principles Drawn From Values and Beliefs: 1904–1929 *(continued)*

treated as a whole (mind, body, and soul) (gestalt psychology). *Note:* Holism did not become a concept until 1926, but gestalt psychology existed prior to the First World War.

- Occupational therapists believe that man learns to organize time and does so through doing occupation (Meyer, 1922).
- Occupational therapists believe that time is a person's best asset and that validation of opportunity and performance is the best measure (Meyer, 1922).
- The occupation (of one's hands and muscles) enables a person to achieve and attain pleasure (Meyer, 1922).
- Illness, especially mental illness, may be conceptualized as problems of living rather than as diseases or disorders of the bodily constitution (Meyer, 1922).
- Man maintains and balances in contact with reality through active involvement in life and use of time in harmony with the self and the environment surrounding the self (Meyer, 1922).
- Occupational therapy involves more mental action than physical (Thorn & Singer, 1921).
- Every human being should have both physical and mental occupation (Dunton, 1919).

- Sick minds, bodies, and souls can be healed through occupation (Dunton, 1919).

Principles related to education: The occupational therapist should

- Learn by doing.
- Learn about functional abilities.
- Learn to care for others and see oneself as a caring person.
- Learn medical (biological) science and social science.
- Learn technical training in a variety of occupations and a variety of methods of presenting or teaching the occupations.

Principles related to sociocultural influences

- Individuals should be treated equally, regardless of political, economic, social status, or military rank (feminism and reconstruction aides).
- Occupational therapists who are women have the ability and capacity to work and interact in society.
- Occupational therapists should pay attention to urban, industrial, educational, social, and cultural issues in society.
- Occupational therapists who are women can participate in society outside the home.

- Occupational therapists facilitate the adjustment of immigrants to life and work in the new country.
- Occupational therapists can act as advocates for individuals in the neighborhood and in the nation.

References

Crane, B. T. (1919). Occupational therapy. *Boston Medical and Surgical Journal, 181*, 63–65.

Cullimore, A. R. (1921). Objectives and motivation in occupational therapy. *Modern Hospital, 17*, 537–538.

Dunton, W. R. (1919). *Reconstruction therapy*. Philadelphia: W. B. Saunders.

Meyer, A. (1922). The philosophy of occupation therapy. *Archives of Occupational Therapy, 1*(1), 1–10.

Mock, H. E. (1919). Curative work. *Carry On, 1*, 12–17.

Slagle, E. C. (1927). To organize an "OT" department. *Occupational Therapy and Rehabilitation, 6*, 125–130.

Thorn, D. A., & Singer, D. (1921). The care of neuro-psychiatric disabilities. *Public Health Reports, 36*, 2665–2677.

Upham, E. G. (1918). *Training of teachers for occupational therapy for the rehabilitation of disabled soldiers and sailors*. Washington, DC: Federal Board for Vocational Education.

ident of AOTA, reminded all practitioners that although the values and beliefs of a profession change little over the years, "the technic [sic] of the art, its practical application, is due for many changes, improvements, and readjustments" (p. 73). All occupational therapists and occupational therapy assistants should know and retain the inherent values and beliefs of the profession, even as societal and technological changes affect the technique.

Next Stage

The members of the Ad Hoc Committee on Historical Foundations are continuing to review professional values and beliefs during additional time periods. The second stage of our research covers the years from 1930 to 1949. Early data show that although we expect the original values and beliefs to remain intact, the profession continued its practice of drawing on knowledge from other fields. As this new knowledge was incorporated into practice, additional values and beliefs may have been added to the existing ones. Also, as changes occur in the politics, society, and economics of practice, some values and beliefs may be competing with others for the attention of occupational therapy practitioners. We look forward to sharing the report when it is completed. (*Editor's note:* This article, published in *OT Practice*, October 9, 2006, pp. 17–22, is not included in this volume.)

REFERENCES

American Occupational Therapy Association. (1923). *Bulletin No. 4.* Baltimore: Sheppard Hospital Press.

American Occupational Therapy Association. (1925). An outline of lectures on occupational therapy to medical students and physicians. *Occupational Therapy and Rehabilitation, 4,* 280–281.

American Occupational Therapy Association. (1940). Principles of occupational therapy. *Occupational Therapy and Rehabilitation, 19,* 19–20.

Dunton, W. R. (1918). The principles of occupational therapy. *Public Health Nurse, 18,* 316–321.

Dunton, W. R. (1919a). Appendix. In *Reconstruction therapy* (pp. 227–229). Philadelphia: W. B. Saunders.

Dunton, W. R. (1919b). N.S.P.O.T. *Maryland Psychiatry Quarterly, 13*(3), 68–73.

Gould, L. L. (2001). *America in the Progressive Era: 1890–1914.* Harlow, England: Pearson Education.

Greenwood, E. (1957). Attributes of a profession. *Social Work, 2*(1), 45–55.

Hall, H. J. (1921). Occupational therapy forecasts and suggestions. *Modern Hospital, 16,* 73.

Lear, T. J. (1981). *No place of grace: Antimodernism and the transformation of American culture, 1880–1920.* New York: Pantheon.

Lipset, S. M., & Schwartz, M. A. (1966). The politics of professionals. In H. M. Vollmer & D. L. Mills (Eds.), *Professionalization* (pp. 299–321). Englewood Cliffs, NJ: Prentice Hall.

Maxwell, J. D., & Maxwell, M. P. (1984). Inner fraternity and outer sorority: Social structure and the professionalization of occupational therapy. In A. Wipper (Ed.), *The sociology of work: Papers in honour of Oswald Hall* (pp. 330–358). Ottawa, Ontario, Canada: Carleton University Press.

McKenzie, R. T. (1919). *Reclaiming the maimed.* New York: Macmillan.

Upham, E. G. (1918). *Training of teachers for occupational therapy for the rehabilitation of disabled soldiers and sailors.* Washington, DC: Federal Board for Vocational Education.

Kathlyn L. Reed, PhD, OTR, FAOTA, MLIS
Associate Professor, Texas Woman's
University–Houston Center
Chairperson, Ethics Commission (2007–2010)

CHAPTER 12

Occupational Therapy Values and Beliefs: A New View of Occupation and the Profession, 1950–1969

I personally have little trust that we can continue to exist as an arts and crafts group which services muscle dysfunction or as an activity group which services the emotionally disabled. (Reilly, 1962, p. 4)

Mary Reilly (1962) stated a major theme leading to significant change in occupational therapy that evolved during the progressive movement of the 1960s. Inherent in her words is Reilly's futuristic view that occupational therapy was evolving as a science-based profession. At the same time, occupational therapy practitioners were increasingly concerned that arts and crafts, often viewed as diversional, did not fully explain the essence of occupation or occupational therapy. Arts and crafts projects seemed to be overemphasized, whereas the therapeutic value of occupation was being underemphasized (Murphy, 1951a, 1951b). Of importance to the profession is whether the values and beliefs inherent in the arts and crafts movement were still held within the profession when the teaching of arts and crafts was being deemphasized within the curriculum. A related question is whether the values and beliefs supported by the arts and crafts movement were broad enough to encompass an expanding view of occupation as a science-based concept within the profession.

The arts and crafts movement had advanced a number of ideas and ideals including design unity, joy in labor (work), individualism, regionalism, social responsibility, consistency and order, simplicity, and home and hearth (family and fireplace; E. Cummings & Kaplan, 1991; Kaplan, 1989). Many of these ideas focused on setting a tone and tempo of life in society through the organization of habits of work, play, rest, and sleep (Meyer, 1922). American social values had changed from conservative in the 1950s to progressive in the 1960s; in addition, the practice of medicine had changed after World War II (Starr, 1982). Physicians, with a focus on scientific methods, expanded their knowledge through working with former soldiers with physical and mental disabilities. For example, psychotropic medication introduced changes in mental health practice and hospitalization patterns, leading to community mental health and mental retardation legislation in 1963 (Mental Retardation Facilities and Community Mental Health Centers Construction Act, 1963). Given the changes in medical practice patterns and occupational therapy's predominant reliance on guidance from medicine, the ideas of the arts and crafts movement may have been a difficult fit. Medicine was developing a focus on short-term care, while the arts and crafts tradition fit better in a long-term-care approach.

Occupational therapy in physical medicine and mental health, or *neuropsychiatry* as it was referred to at the time, also had a new agenda. For example, Shields, Oelhafen, and Sheeham (1952) stated that the role of occupational therapy in physical medicine is to increase endurance, improve coordination and dexterity, improve muscle power and strength, improve joint range of motion, relieve tightness of fascial planes, and obtain the best functional results. The new focus was on the biomedical aspects of the body, not on the social or temporal life of the individual, which had been more conducive to the values of the arts and crafts movement. Similar views of the role of occupational therapy in physical medicine were expressed by V. Cummings (1968), Grove (1969), Helming (1964), and Huddleston (1956). Psychiatry, on the other hand, was focused on psychoanalytic psychotherapy, including the provision of the opportunity to satisfy the basic emotional need for security (e.g., the need to be loved, to be accepted, and to belong). Other occupational therapy objectives were to establish an atmosphere conducive to recovery, assist patients to undertake appropriate economic and social responsibilities, provide data for evaluation and diagnosis, and assist the patient to bridge the gap between hospital and community living (AOTA, 1958c). Again, the tone and tempo of the arts and crafts movement, which emphasized the practical, hands-on approach of crafts labor, were deemphasized.

CONTINUING THE DISCUSSION

This article is the third in a series and continues the process of identifying and organizing the beliefs, values, and ideas gleaned from the historical foundations of the profession. The first article, "Occupational Therapy Values and Beliefs: The Formative Years, 1904–1929," appeared in the April 17, 2006, issue of OT Practice (Reed, 2006). The second article, entitled "Occupational Therapy Values and Beliefs, Part II: The Great Depression and War Years: 1930–1949," appeared in the October 9, 2006, issue of OT Practice (Reed & Peters, 2006). The methods used and themes developed to guide the historical literature review project were discussed in the first two articles and included economics, education, health and medicine,

philosophy, politics and government, professions and professionals, psychology and psychological concepts, religion and spirituality, and social themes and movements. This article discusses some new categories that became evident in a literature search from 1950 to 1969. These categories will not follow the previous theme format. Rather, the topics represent a sampling of either concerns addressed by the American Occupational Therapy Association (AOTA) Board of Management or concerns external to the Association that shaped occupational therapy practice, education, or both.

THE GREATER PROFESSION
Defining Occupational Therapy

In 1969, for the first time, AOTA adopted the following formal definition of occupational therapy: "Occupational Therapy is the art and science of directing man's response to selected activity to promote and maintain health, to prevent disability, to evaluate behavior and to treat or train patients with physical or psychosocial dysfunction" (AOTA, 1969a, p. 185). This official definition replaced the commonly used definition that Pattison had developed in 1922 and expanded the description conveyed in AOTA's 1963 *A Statement of Basic Philosophy, Principle, and Policy* (see Figure 12.1). This definition, along with AOTA's 1958c definitions of function and 1961 *Statement of Policy* (see Figure 12.2), outlined the thought and direction of the occupational therapy profession and AOTA during the 1960s.

Responses From the Association

In response to changes in the profession during this time, the Association provided more direction and published more books. Of special interest are the previously mentioned documents *Statement of Policy* (AOTA, 1961) and *A Statement of Basic Philosophy, Principle, and Policy* (AOTA, 1963), along with two manuals: *The Objectives and Functions of Occupational Therapy* (AOTA, 1958c) and

FIGURE 12.1. A Statement of Basic Philosophy, Principle, and Policy

Occupational therapy is particularly concerned with man and his ability to meet the demands of his environment. The therapist administers treatment to the patient designed to (1) evaluate and increase his physical function in relation to activities of daily living, the needs of his family, and the requirements of his job, (2) improve his self-understanding and psychosocial function as a total human being. Treatment involves the scientific use of activity procedures and/or controlled social relationships to meet the specific needs of the individual patient (AOTA, 1963, p. 159).

Occupational Therapy Reference Manual for Physicians (AOTA, 1960). The two statements provided a description of the role of the Association and of occupational therapy. The two manuals outlined and detailed the services provided. The manuals and statements have been used as references in the preparation of this article. Perhaps of greatest value to the profession was the role of the Association in providing publications that were written by occupational therapists instead of relying on external publishing sources and physicians to advance the knowledge base and profession of occupational therapy.

Eleanor Clarke Slagle Lectureship and Award of Merit

To recognize the value of professional contributions, the Association established the Eleanor Clarke Slagle lectureship in 1953 (AOTA, 1954). The "honorary occupational therapy guest lectureship" was to be awarded "in recognition of meritorious service to the profession" (AOTA, 1954, p. 24):

> It perpetuates the memory of Mrs. Eleanor Clarke Slagle, one of the outstanding pioneers in the field (profession) of occupational therapy. The award is bestowed upon practicing therapists who are members of the AOTA and who have made or are making a significant contribution to the profession. (AOTA, 1960, p. 24)

Since its inception, the Slagle lectureship has been given to 44 individuals. The Award of Merit had already been established in 1950 to recognize distinguished service to the profession (AOTA, 1950).

CHANGES IN PRACTICE AREAS

Practice areas were also changing relative to advances in technology, medicine, and pharmacology. Occupational therapists had worked with clients who had tuberculosis from the

FIGURE 12.2. Statement of Policy

1. Maintain and control the voluntary registration of its practitioners.
2. Regulate, in conjunction with the Council on Medical Education and hospitals of the American Medical Association, the education of occupational therapists to prepare them for their treatment function.
3. Establish and maintain standards of clinical practice in occupational therapy which will improve patient treatment.
4. Foster continuing growth in the professional competence of occupational therapists.
5. Encourage and facilitate increase in the body of specific occupational therapy knowledge available to physicians.
6. Protect the standards of occupational therapy and the environment in which the occupational therapist functions.
7. Strongly oppose and protest any administrative policy or structure which ignores or weakens the treatment function of occupational therapy (AOTA, 1961, p. 24).

start of the profession, but sanatoriums treating tuberculosis were closing as drug therapy permitted outpatient care. The literature reflects the diminished practice area of tuberculosis, with the last article on this topic appearing in the *American Journal of Occupational Therapy* (*AJOT*) in 1960 (Appleby, Morton, Lawson, Loudon, & Brown, 1960). Similarly, the polio vaccination decreased rapidly the number of new cases of poliomyelitis in children and adults, and the last article on polio in *AJOT* appeared in 1957 (Halford, 1957). Curiously, vocational rehabilitation grants were still funding postprofessional education for occupational therapists in the areas of tuberculosis and polio, which kept them in both practice areas despite fewer patients (Peters, 2005).

During this time, as occupational therapists became more sophisticated in their education and their knowledge base grew, new areas of treatment appeared or were expanded on in the literature. For example, interest in neurology and perceptual motor dysfunction was increasing (Ayres, 1963, 1965), and articles on neurophysiology and facilitation techniques began to appear (Ayres, 1955; Rood, 1956).

Activities of Daily Living

A major new focus for occupational therapy was activities of daily living. The first form to assess activities of daily living appearing in the occupational therapy literature was the 1949 *Scale for Rating Functional Demands for Daily Living* (McLean, 1949). However, the term *activities of daily living* did not become popular in the occupational therapy literature until the 1950s. According to Isaac (1963), physician Howard Rusk, working with returning soldiers, established rehabilitation after World War II. Rusk defined activities of daily living as "all those little things a person does for himself, that make him miserable if he is unable to do them" (p. 58). Clinically, the initial work to develop the principles of activities of daily living was

done at the Institute for the Crippled and Disabled in New York City, but this work spread quickly across the country in all areas of occupational therapy practice.

The concepts of independence and independent living were closely associated with activities of daily living (Hightower, 1966). The independent living movement is closely aligned with the physical rehabilitation efforts of occupational therapy, but it is not as clearly defined in occupational therapy mental health history. Occupational therapists working in mental health were exposed to various ways of conceptualizing activities of daily living. For example, Maxwell Jones's 1953 *The Therapeutic Community* focused on role equality, with patients and staff members taking equal responsibility for daily housecleaning chores on a hospital unit or ward. In the 1950s, the community-based clubhouse models like Fountain House in New York created real-life situations for former patients to gather and share responsibility for the daily running and maintenance of their centers, from light cooking to administrative work (Flannery & Glickman, 1996).

Prescription Versus Referral

Although physicians continued to supervise occupational therapists, the nature of this relationship was changing. In 1958 Mazer and Goodrich suggested that the prescription for psychiatric occupational therapy services was an anachronistic procedure and should be discontinued. The argument was that occupational therapists did not need to have the details for treating a patient spelled out in a prescribed form because as professionals they could determine the needs for themselves. They needed the physician's permission to see the patient but could supply the expertise regarding treatment and intervention without physician assistance. Fidler (1963) concurred, and in 1964 the AOTA Board of Management recommended that the term *referral* be used in place of *prescription* (AOTA, 1964a). In 1969 the first statement on occupational therapy referral was adopted by the Association (AOTA, 1969c). Zamir (1966) expanded on the challenge to the relationship between medicine and occupational therapy by stating that history had shown that professional development almost always demands autonomy. She further stated that it was doubtful that any field could truly call itself a profession if it was merely a tool of another profession, working only under its direction and at its behest. Bockoven (1968) suggested that occupational therapy separate from medicine and focus on its concern for occupation.

Registration Versus Licensure

Although change was happening in some areas of occupational therapy, professional beliefs about the value of state licensure remained unchanged. In 1951 Wilma L. West, as executive director of AOTA, summarized the accepted view of state licensure as not necessary. Licensure was seen as a potential barrier to recruiting students (more costs), expensive to obtain because of legal fees, and having the potential to hinder the movement of occupational therapists across the country because states might have different requirements in their licensure regulations. The negative view of licensure was reinforced in 1969 when a position paper was adopted by the AOTA Delegate Assembly, stating that licensure had "done little to protect either the providers or consumers of specific services" and represented "an external attempt at imposing qualifications for entrance into the profession and to engage in practice" (AOTA, 1969b, p. 529). A more positive view of licensure would not occur for several years.

OCCUPATIONAL THERAPY EDUCATION

Occupational therapy curriculum design also began to change during this period. A new concern was expanded courses in medical conditions, activities analysis, and therapeutic application and a move away from a predominant arts and crafts curriculum. Nedra Gillette illustrated these shifts in 1965 when she summarized the recommendations of the AOTA Curriculum Study project as follows:

> . . . It was recommended that the traditional arts and crafts be deemphasized as treatment media with decreased time devoted to these in the curricula, decreased number of media taught, emphasis on *methods* of acquiring skills, and teaching of a core course in media. (p. 352)

Not only was curriculum content revamped, but occupational therapy levels of education became a topic of discussion. Given the 1963 adoption of a baccalaureate degree required for professional-level education, there was discussion about graduate education to promote scholarship.

Graduate Education

With a need for more research and for better-prepared occupational therapists in specialty areas of practice came a need for occupational therapists with postprofessional degrees. Academic leaders discussed two entrances to occupational therapy graduate education. The first was a master's degree in occupational therapy for baccalaureate-trained occupational therapists who were already practicing. The more controversial second option was a master's degree as the entry level to practice (AOTA, 1958a). The document *A Guide for the Development of Graduate Education Leading to Higher Degrees in Occupational Therapy* was adopted in 1958 (AOTA, 1958b). In 1964 the first proposed master's-level entry program, at the University of Southern California, was submitted and discussed in the Council on Education (AOTA, 1964b).

Certified Occupational Therapy Assistants

The lack of trained occupational therapists, particularly in large state hospitals, was also a focus of concern (Poole & Kassalow, 1968; Stattel, 1966). In 1957 the AOTA Board of Management voted to accept the title Certified Occupational Therapy Assistant (COTA) and to adopt the standards for organizing a training program for occupational therapy assistants (AOTA, 1958d). Educational programs for the occupational therapy assistant developed quickly throughout the country. Occupational therapy personnel were now recognized at two levels: professional and technical.

Summary

The years 1950 to 1969 witnessed change and growth of occupational therapy practice, education, and organization. Practice responded to the need for more organization of information into models to guide the development of theoretical knowledge and practice skills. Educational opportunities in occupational therapy expanded through the development of more schools at the professional level and the initiation of schools at the technical level. The professional organization recognized the need for assistants to provide more manpower in occupational therapy practice, changed the relationships with physicians from prescription to referral, and facilitated the publication of more manuals and textbooks on occupational therapy written by occupational therapists.

References

American Occupational Therapy Association. (1950). Meetings of the Board of Management. *American Journal of Occupational Therapy, 4,* 236.

American Occupational Therapy Association. (1954). Annual reports: Meetings of the House of Delegates. *American Journal of Occupational Therapy, 8,* 24.

American Occupational Therapy Association. (1958a). Committee on Graduate Study. *American Journal of Occupational Therapy, 12,* 109–110.

American Occupational Therapy Association. (1958b). A guide for the development of graduate education leading to higher degrees in occupational therapy. *American Journal of Occupational Therapy, 12,* 334–335.

American Occupational Therapy Association. (1958c). *The objectives and functions of occupational therapy.* Dubuque, IA: Wm. C. Brown.

American Occupational Therapy Association. (1958d). Report of the project committee on recognition of OT assistants. *American Journal of Occupational Therapy, 12,* 38–39.

American Occupational Therapy Association. (1960). *Occupational therapy reference manual for physicians.* New York: Author.

American Occupational Therapy Association. (1961). Statement of policy. *American Journal of Occupational Therapy, 15,* 24.

American Occupational Therapy Association. (1963). A statement of basic philosophy, principle, and policy. *American Journal of Occupational Therapy, 17,* 159.

American Occupational Therapy Association. (1964a). Board of Management minutes. *American Journal of Occupational Therapy, 18,* 165–170.

American Occupational Therapy Association. (1964b). Council on Education. *American Journal of Occupational Therapy, 18,* 266–269.

American Occupational Therapy Association. (1969a). Definition of occupational therapy. *American Journal of Occupational Therapy, 23,* 185.

American Occupational Therapy Association. (1969b). Licensing and standards of competency in occupational therapy. *American Journal of Occupational Therapy, 23,* 529–530.

American Occupational Therapy Association. (1969c). Statement on occupational therapy referral. *American Journal of Occupational Therapy, 23,* 530–531.

Appleby, L., Morton, J. E. C., Lawson, R. A., Loudon, R. G., & Brown, J. (1960). Toward a therapeutic community in a tuberculosis hospital. *American Journal of Occupational Therapy, 14,* 117–120.

Ayres, A. J. (1955). Proprioceptive facilitation elicited through the upper extremities: Part I. Background. *American Journal of Occupational Therapy, 9,* 1–9, 50.

Ayres, A. J. (1963). Eleanor Clarke Slagle Lecture—The development of perceptual–motor abilities: A theoretical basis for treatment of dysfunction. *American Journal of Occupational Therapy, 17,* 221–225.

Ayres, A. J. (1965). Patterns of perceptual–motor dysfunction in children: A factor analytic study. *Perceptual and Motor Skills, 20,* 335–368.

Bockoven, J. S. (1968). Challenge of the new clinical approaches. *American Journal of Occupational Therapy, 22,* 23–25.

Cummings, E., & Kaplan, W. (1991). *The arts and crafts movement.* London: Thames & Hudson.

Cummings, V. (1968). The occupational therapist. *Canadian Nurse, 64,* 38–39.

Fidler, G. S. (1963). Nationally Speaking—The prescription in occupational therapy. *American Journal of Occupational Therapy, 17,* 122–124.

Flannery, M., & Glickman, M. (1996). *Fountain house: Portraits of lives reclaimed from mental illness.* Center City, MN: Hazelden.

Gillette, N. P. (1965). Guest Editorial—Occupational therapy education and the curriculum study project. *American Journal of Occupational Therapy, 19,* 351–353.

Grove, E. (1969). Occupational therapy and the nurse. *Nursing Times, 65,* 141–143.

Halford, M. A. (1957). I had polio. *American Journal of Occupational Therapy, 11,* 129–130, 166.

Helming, F. (1964). What the nurse should know about OT. *Journal of Nursing Education, 3,* 7–8, 25–26.

Hightower, M. D. (1966). Independence through activities of daily living. *Delaware Medical Journal, 38,* 238–242.

Huddleston, O. L. (1956). Use of occupational therapy in physical rehabilitation. *Archives of Physical Medicine and Rehabilitation, 37,* 31–36.

Isaac, A. M. (1963). Re-education. *Journal of the Kansas Medical Association, 64,* 58–62.

Jones, M. (1953). *The therapeutic community.* New York: Basic.

Kaplan, W. (1989). *"The art that is life": The arts and crafts movement in America, 1985–1920.* Boston: Museum of Fine Arts.

Mazer, J., & Goodrich, W. (1958). The prescription: An anachronistic procedure in psychiatric occupational therapy. *American Journal of Occupational Therapy, 12,* 165–170.

McLean, F. M. (1949). Occupational therapy in the management of poliomyelitis. *American Journal of Occupational Therapy, 3,* 20–27.

Mental Retardation Facilities and Community Mental Health Centers Construction Act (1963), Pub. L. 88–164.

Meyer, A. (1922). Philosophy of occupation therapy. *Archives of Occupational Therapy, 1,* 1–10.

Murphy, L. S. (1951a). Editorial—Disemphasizing crafts. *American Journal of Occupational Therapy, 5,* 39.

Murphy, L. S. (1951b). Editorial—Occupation or therapy. *American Journal of Occupational Therapy, 5,* 117–118.

Pattison, H. A. (1922). The trend of occupational therapy for the tuberculosis. *Archives of Occupational Therapy, 1,* 19–24.

Peters, C. O. (2005). *Power and professionalism in occupational therapy.* Doctoral dissertation, New York University, New York.

Poole, M. A., & Kassalow, S. (1968). Manpower survey report: Wisconsin Occupational Therapy Association. *American Journal of Occupational Therapy, 22,* 304–308.

Reed, K. L. (2006). Occupational therapy values and beliefs: The formative years, 1904–1929. *OT Practice, 11*(7), 21–25.

Reed, K. L., & Peters, C. (2006). Occupational therapy values and beliefs: Part II. The great depression and war years: 1930–1949. *OT Practice, 11*(18), 17–22.

Reilly, M. (1962). Eleanor Clarke Slagle Lecture—Occupational therapy can be one of the great ideas of 20th century medicine. *American Journal of Occupational Therapy, 16,* 1–9.

Rood, M. S. (1956). Session on neurology: Neurophysiological mechanisms utilized in the treatment of neuromuscular dysfunction. *American Journal of Occupational Therapy, 10,* 220–225.

Shields, C. S., Oelhafen, W. R., & Sheeham, H. R. (1952). The role of occupational therapy in the physical medicine management of physical disabilities. *Southern Medical Journal, 45,* 395–400.

Starr, D. (1982). *The social transformation of American medicine.* New York: Basic.

Stattel, F. M. (1966). The occupational therapist in rehabilitation: Projections toward the future. *American Journal of Occupational Therapy, 20,* 144–150.

West, W. L. (1951). From the executive director. *American Journal of Occupational Therapy, 5,* 60–63.

Zamir, L. J. (1966). Editorial—Whither occupational therapy. *American Journal of Occupational Therapy, 20,* vii, 195.

Kathlyn L. Reed, PhD, OTR, FAOTA, MLIS
Associate Professor, Texas Woman's University–Houston Center
Chairperson, Ethics Commission (2006–2010)

Christine Peters, PhD, OTR/L
Associate Professor, Pacific University
Member, AOTA's Mental Health Evidence-Based Literature Review Resource Advisory Group (2007–2008)

CHAPTER 13

Is It Possible to Be Ethical?

In the wake of recent corporate scandals, the topic of ethics is gaining new attention. But is it possible to act ethically while meeting the needs and expectations of everyone involved in a dilemma? This chapter presents a step-by-step process for ethical decision making that aims at consensus among all those involved in an ethical dilemma.

One common complaint about ethics is that most ethical dilemmas seem too complicated to be solved. Although it is true that ethical dilemmas can often become quite complex, especially in today's technological, global community, resolving ethical dilemmas need not be viewed as an impossible task. To claim at the outset that ethics simply cannot be accommodated is to set oneself up for failure. Even the most difficult of ethical dilemmas can be sorted through and resolved with enough time, patience, and careful reflection.

This article offers a model for ethical decision making that strives to help its users reach consensus. Although many in the public forum are fond of the claim that we can all just "agree to disagree," such an approach simply cannot work when one has entered into a therapeutic relationship, thereby making a professional promise to assist someone in the pursuit of health and optimal occupational performance. Therapy is a collaborative effort, and consensus is an implicit part of collaboration.

STRIVING FOR CONSENSUS

To clarify the need for consensus in the therapeutic relationship, we must understand what it means. Let me begin with what consensus is not. Consensus is not 100%, total agreement. Anyone could rightly question whether, in a pluralistic society, total agreement can ever be achieved. Further, consensus cannot be completely equated with compromise. Most will recognize that compromise involves giving up something you believe or hold as a value. However, one of the foundational points of ethics is that each person must maintain personal integrity, meaning that to remain ethical there are some things that each of us should not be asked to give up. Each of us must guard the sanctity of our own conscience. Ethics never obligates one to sacrifice his or her own integrity.

What, then, does consensus entail? I suggest that authentic consensus is achieved when all parties involved in a debate, dispute, or dilemma can accept and live with the decision being offered. By the phrase "live with," I mean that the decision under consideration does not violate one's integrity and conscience. Such a decision may not be one's top choice—to that degree, there is some give and take in arriving at consensus. But all involved must be able to accept the decision and follow through with the recommended course of action. Given this, the task of reaching a consensus must involve dialogue with all those involved.

Dialogue, of course, takes time, and so this phase is often where problems arise. Many are under the impression that ethical decisions must be made quickly and on the spur of the moment. This attitude may partly reflect the influence of capitalism on contemporary American society. The business community tells us we need to be ready to respond to the global market at any time, that opportunities only come along once and can be lost in a minute, and that in the world of business the slow always lose. And so we live in a world of overnight shipping, 24-hour stores, e-commerce, and fast food. Naturally, many assume that ethical decision making must follow the same model—be quick and responsive to the marketplace of dilemmas.

But is this presumption true? No. We all remember the story of the tortoise and the hare. Speed has its uses, but it can also breed recklessness. Remember such marketing fiascoes as New Coke and Pepsi Clear? In a hospital emergency room, decisions often need to be made quickly (although rarely as fast as a popular television drama portrays them). But for most health care and therapy, there is indeed time to carefully study and reflect before making a decision—if one but takes the time, or requests it of others. Indeed, it is even better from a business standpoint to take some time before acting instead of spending twice as much time after the fact trying to clean up whatever mess has been made. And some decisions, like the *Challenger* shuttle disaster, can never really be "cleaned up."

The first step in sound ethical decision making is to take the time to reflect on one's actions from the perspective of ethics. I often hear from people who have found themselves seemingly trapped in very complex ethical dilemmas when they never even realized that what they had been doing had ethical implications—it was just business, just billing, just legal, just personal, etc., etc., etc. Furthermore, the truly complicated ethical dilemmas that we so often hear about on newsmagazine shows rarely arise from a single action—more often, they are the result of a series of smaller, but still unethical, actions. Carefully reflecting on one's day-to-day actions can go a long way toward avoiding these larger dilemmas.

A MODEL FOR ETHICAL DECISION MAKING

Even the most careful people can find themselves facing an ethical dilemma—either one of their own doing or one into which they have been dragged. So how can one resolve a complex ethical dilemma? With so many different theories of ethics to choose from, how can one really figure out the best way to act? Is ethics just a crapshoot—roll the dice and take your chances? Again, my response is no! What is needed is a way to sort through the complexity of a moral dilemma. To this end, I offer the following model for ethical decision making.

This model has developed through a collaborative effort with other professionals, and I have presented it in ethics courses and workshops. I do not offer it as the only way to solve ethical dilemmas, but merely as one possible guide for sorting through the complexity of some of the challenges we find ourselves facing from day to day. As such, this model is a response to the claim that ethics is often too complex to really address. Using a model can help one break the dilemma into manageable pieces, thereby reducing the complexity of the situation. It is also worth noting that using a model for thinking through a problem will not necessarily make ethics "simple." Indeed, most often the difficult part of ethics is following through on the decision one has reached— knowing what is right and doing what is right are two different things. The goal of this model is to present an orderly way of approaching an ethical dilemma so that one can have a firmer foundation from which to make an ethical decision as well as increased confidence in following through with that action.

AM I FACING AN ETHICAL DILEMMA?

The process of ethical decision making begins, quite naturally, with the realization that one may be facing an ethical dilemma. I start the model with this question, however, because at times what may appear to be an ethical problem may actually be more of a legal matter, a personnel issue, or some other kind of dilemma (although at times laws and policies are broken and concurrently ethical principles are violated). So the first question is, Does the situation involve a violation of the American Occupational Therapy Association (AOTA) *Occupational Therapy Code of Ethics and Ethics Standards (2010)* (referred to as the "Code and Ethics Standards"; AOTA, 2010)? Does the problem impinge on your personal integrity and conscience? If so, then you may be facing an ethical dilemma, and you should begin to clarify the situation.

What Are the Relevant Facts, Values, and Beliefs?

As you begin to examine the situation causing the dilemma, you should carefully examine all the pertinent facts—which also means sorting through those factors that are irrelevant. In many cases, ethical problems arise, in part, because one or both parties do not know all the facts. In such cases, getting the facts straight at the outset may lead to a quick resolution.

It is also important to try to identify the values at stake in the dilemma—both your own and those of everyone else directly involved. Values are those things we hold dear, and when values clash, ethical dilemmas arise. A misunderstanding, or outright ignoring, of others' values will only worsen the situation, putting resolution and consensus further out of reach.

Finally, what are the beliefs guiding everyone involved? Beliefs and values are both subjective, and so they will vary from person to person. But recognizing different beliefs can lead to understanding—even when disagreement over the beliefs remains. Being clear about the facts, values, and beliefs involved in an ethical dilemma will help pave the way for dialogue among all those involved.

Who Are the Key People Involved?

Next, identify the people involved in the dilemma. It can also be helpful to prioritize each person's role. For example, in all dilemmas surrounding the therapeutic relationship, the client being served should always remain at the forefront of the dialogue. As part of identifying the key people involved, it is also helpful to consider what might be called the "ripple effect" in ethics—those people not directly involved at that precise moment, but who nonetheless will be affected (e.g., future clients, other students or faculty, other members of a clinic or hospital, other professionals, the school district). Be thorough, so as not to leave anyone out of consideration. True dialogue cannot take place if everyone does not have a seat at the table.

State the Dilemma Clearly

As you begin to sort through the details of the situation under consideration, you must be able to bring the problem into focus. A helpful format for structuring the dilemma is to form a question identifying the possible ethical conclusions: "Is it (or *was* it) *permissible, impermissible,* or *obligatory* to _____?" (Beabout & Wenneman, 1994). Stating the dilemma in this manner leaves the issue under consideration open ended and allows for honest dialogue and debate. Being able to state the dilemma also provides direction for the dialogue. If you are in a situation that involves multiple problems, it is best to focus on the most pressing issue in need of resolution first. The other problems can be addressed at a later time. Care should be taken not to lump too many problems together, because doing so just adds to the confusion of sorting through complex problems. It is better to sort through each problem on its own so as not to miss anything important. This kind of careful reflection can also help avoid future problems of a similar nature.

ANALYZE

What Are the Possible Courses of Action?

After it is clear that you are indeed facing an ethical dilemma and you have identified the key factors and people involved with the problem, you can begin to search for a resolution. The first step in moving toward a consensus is to identify possible courses of action. For example, in every situation, you could always just do nothing. Even if you were in a situation in which you absolutely knew you were going to do something, it is helpful to recognize that doing nothing is always an option.

Laying out the possible actions facilitates being thorough in your reflections, and considering all the possibilities can help keep you from missing something important. People having serious dilemmas often point out that they did not realize all of their options before ending up in their present situation. We hear people say, "What was I thinking?" But the problem may have been that they were not thinking—at least not thoroughly enough to avoid trouble. Taking time for reflection will add to the dialogue involved with resolving the situation at hand.

What Conflicts Could Arise From Each Action?

After the possible courses of action are identified, they must be analyzed. The task here is to consider the impact of each action as reasonably as possible. It is also important to consider the possible course of action from the vantage point of each of the key people involved with the dilemma. Granted, we cannot always predict how people will react, but the point here is not to play fortune-teller; rather, the idea is to consider the consequences of your actions—both for yourself and for everyone else involved.

Through the process of identifying the conflicts involved with certain actions, you will begin to see why certain actions are not viable—because they are impractical, because there is something preventing them from occurring, or even because they can now be seen as unethical. With such an analysis you will be able to explain and, if necessary, defend your actions. The ultimate goal of this analysis, then, is to identify a single course of action, or a connected series of actions, that will resolve the dilemma. It is this proposed course of action that will then be evaluated for its adherence to ethical standards.

EVALUATE

The final part of the ethical decision-making process is evaluation of the proposed course of action. For this part of the process, I am going to work backward, so to speak, beginning with an examination of one's self-interests, to a consideration of one's social roles, then finally to a consideration of the Code and Ethics Standards and general ethical principles. This part of the model reflects the model proffered by Gregory Beabout and Daryl Wennemann (1994) in *Applied Professional Ethics,* which builds on developmental psychologist Lawrence Kohlberg's ideas about moral development but also considers a critique of Kohlberg's work that incorporates notions of Carol Gilligan's "ethics of caring." The reason for this approach is that we must be careful not to justify our decisions through a simple process of rationalization. Beginning with the Code and Ethics Standards and principles may give the appearance of not being fair in our deliberations and not recognizing that at times we have a personal interest in a decision or in fulfilling a social role that is pressuring us to act. To avoid any such problems, it helps to begin with self-interest and build toward general ethical principles. That way, it will be clearer that your principles are supporting the decision at the highest levels of moral reasoning, as opposed to your own interests.

Self-Interests (Level I)

The simple fact is that each of us has personal interests at stake in the actions we perform.

This alone is not necessarily a problem. We all want to give and receive good things, while at the same time we want to avoid having bad things happen to us. When a therapist creates a technically sound intervention that is also successful, it is quite natural to feel good about this accomplishment. Most people who enter the profession of occupational therapy do so because they want to help people. The problem arises when a person focuses only on his or her own interests, especially to the detriment and neglect of others. For example, spending $200 on a weekend golfing trip is not in itself unethical. But it would be if a parent did so at the expense of necessary food and clothing for his or her children. The first case is clearly an example of self-interest; the second evolves into selfishness. Therefore, it is important to recognize one's personal interests in a situation so as to recognize which interests are appropriate and which are not.

Some people believe that we should all act at the level of self-interest. This ethical theory is known as egoism and has been defended by people such as novelist Ayn Rand. The idea behind the theory is to maximize one's personal happiness. But the problem is that our interests always conflict. I might want to speed to get home faster, but I don't want to get a ticket. If I am an egoist, and I decide to be safe and not speed, then when I get home without a ticket I think, "I could have sped and been home 20 minutes ago—there weren't any cops out tonight!" But if I speed and get a ticket, then I chastise myself, saying, "I knew this would happen—I should have been more careful!" In short, every action that holds some promise of benefit also brings with it some risk or hardship. The dieter wants to eat the doughnut but not gain weight. The two interests are incompatible. And so, when one begins to thoroughly reflect on all the options that go into making a decision, it becomes clear that acting solely out of personal interest will not bring satisfactory results. Nor will this approach help us attain a consensus; rather, it only divides us.

Identify your interests, admit that they are there, then move on to a higher level of moral reasoning.

Social Roles (Level II)

After you move past the narrow focus of self-interest, you begin to realize that you belong to various communities. These communities are broad and include family, work, religious group, political affiliation, and friends. You will also begin to realize that the members of these groups have certain expectations of each other. These expectations establish our social roles. With our social roles come obligations. At this level, then, one moves out of the purely individualistic thinking of self-interest and begins to recognize that other people also matter. Regarding the needs and interests of others moves us to consider how our actions affect others in the groups to which we belong so as to further the interests and needs of the group over our own. It is helpful to identify your social roles in a dilemma and to clarify the expectations that may be influencing your thinking.

Clearly, social roles provide a better and more satisfactory perspective for ethics than pure self-interest. Yet this level does have its limitations because our social roles often conflict. A promotion at work that requires travel may bring added income for your family, helping to fulfill the social role of provider. But the travel required will also reduce time spent with the family, which detracts from the social roles of spouse and parent. Because each of us has so many different social roles, trying to use these roles as a basis for making a decision is often difficult—clear solutions can be hard to find.

A second problem with this level is that it is not all-inclusive. Whereas our social roles call us to consider the other members of our groups, they do not necessarily move us toward the needs and interests of those who fall outside our social groups. If I am a Democrat, do I have to care about a Republican? If I am

Baptist, should I care about those who are Jewish? Is my only priority to care for my family, or do I have any obligations toward people in other countries? At this level there is nothing that pushes us to look past our own social groups to a more global perspective. In the end, we can see that each of us has multiple social roles, and those roles tend to cause tension in our lives. Resolving these conflicts requires a higher level of moral reasoning, one that can help us prioritize our roles and bring them into harmony. This higher perspective can also draw us to a more inclusive view of humanity that challenges us to recognize the needs and rights of all.

Code and Ethics Standards (Level II)

The highest level of moral reasoning is the level of universal moral principles, such as those embodied in the Code and Ethics Standards. These are principles that apply to all occupational therapy personnel, regardless of race, gender, and creed. The spirit of the Code and Ethics Standards is not limited only to members of AOTA, but extends an obligation of respect and care toward all.

As you continue to reflect on the proposed course of action, having identified personal interests and social roles, evaluating the action using the Code and Ethics Standards will bring you toward resolution. Do the Code and Ethics Standards explicitly require that the action under consideration be performed? Do the Code and Ethics Standards explicitly forbid the proposed course of action? If the Code and Ethics Standards are not explicit, what is the spirit of the Code and Ethics Standards regarding the situation? Use the Code and Ethics Standards and the ethical principles within them to support your decision or to show why the decision is unethical and should not be carried out. In doing so, you will recognize how personal interests and social roles are brought into harmony through the higher, unifying perspective of the Code and Ethics Standards.

Ethical Principles (Level III)

You can often further support a good decision with more general ethical norms, such as justice, beneficence, autonomy, and so forth, which form the philosophical basis for the Code and Ethics Standards. Appealing to general ethical principles is especially helpful when dealing with people who are not members of the profession and who have no specific obligations toward the Code and Ethics Standards. By pointing out the general societal norms that further support the decision at hand, you can show that action was not based solely on the role of occupational therapy (which would be Level II thinking), but rather was truly based on ethical principles. Additionally, an appeal to general ethical principles helps foster dialogue and will help further the spirit of the Code and Ethics Standards in the public forum.

PROCEED: YES OR NO

In the end, the final question to ask is, Does your proposed course of action lead to consensus? If yes, then proceed, knowing that the decision can be supported and defended. If no, then return to the analysis portion of the model and review your evaluations. Perhaps there were more options that you did not consider, or another course of action could be proposed for evaluation.

CONCLUSION

We should not be alarmed when we find that we have no consensus and that we must continue our ethical deliberations and dialogue. The process of ethical decision making can indeed be involved, especially as a situation becomes more serious. I offer the model worksheet in Figure 13.1 because in difficult cases it can help to sit down and organize one's thoughts on paper. The worksheet may even prove useful in a group setting to foster dialogue and to help reach consensus.

If time does not allow for further consideration, then you must do the best you can and be open to reflection and critique in the future.

Am I facing an ethical dilemma here?

➤ 1) What are the relevant facts, values, _____
   and beliefs?   _____
                                         _____

➤ 2) Who are the key people involved?   _____
                                         _____
                                         _____

➤ 3) State the dilemma clearly.   _____
                                         _____
                                         _____

Analysis ◄·······························

➤ 1) What are the possible courses   _____
   of action one could take?   _____
                                         _____

➤ 2) What are the conflicts that   _____
   arise from each action?   _____
                                         _____

Proposed Course of Action

Evaluate:

➤ 1) Ethical principles: _____
   Level III   _____
                                         _____

➤ 2) Code and Ethics Standards: _____
   Level II   _____
                                         _____

➤ 3) Social roles: _____
   Level II   _____
                                         _____

➤ 4) Self-interests: _____
   Level I   _____
                                         _____

**Does your proposed course
of action lead to consensus?**   **If yes—then proceed . . .**

                                      ·· ·If no . . .

FIGURE 13.1. Model for Ethical Decision Making.

Remember, becoming a virtuous person takes time and experience. It is a lifelong endeavor. That does not mean we can be cavalier with our decisions now and straighten up later. But it does mean that we most likely will not get everything right the first time around. Through our life experiences, we all grow and develop. The same is true of our ethics. The decisions we make affect our future selves. Good decisions pave the way for more good decisions, and bad decisions must be dealt with if we are to improve ourselves and our world.

REFERENCES

American Occupational Therapy Association. (2010). Occupational therapy code of ethics and ethics standards (2010). *American Journal of Occupational Therapy, 64*(6 Suppl.), S17–S26. doi:10.5014/ajot.2010.64S17

Beabout, G. R., & Wennemann, D. J. (1994). *Applied professional ethics.* New York: University Press of America.

ACKNOWLEDGMENTS

Many thanks go to Robin Bowen, EdD, OTR, FAOTA, and Shelly Chabon, PhD, CCC-SLP. Drs. Bowen and Chabon are members of Rockhurst University and have collaborated with me on the development of this model of ethical decision making. Both have also presented this model with me at professional conferences. I especially thank them for their gracious permission to publish this model for use by members of AOTA.

John F. Morris, PhD
Public Member, Commission on Standards and Ethics (2001–2004)

CHAPTER 14

Unethical and Illegal: What Is the Difference?

Members of the American Occupational Therapy Association (AOTA) often ask if something is unethical, illegal, or both. This is not a simple question with a single answer, and the answer depends on several factors. *Ethics* is a branch of applied philosophy and is the study of rules of conduct and the general nature of morals as applied to individual choice. *Law* is a body or system of rules used by an authority to impose control over a system or people. The major issue is whether the unethical action has been adopted by a legislature as being unlawful. Basically, unless the law mandates that the conduct is illegal, violations of ethical principles and standards will not result in criminal sanctions or fines. Therefore, it is best if occupational therapy practitioners check with their state's regulatory board to inquire about the legality or illegality of an act.

Associations frequently develop codes of ethics, policies, or other guidelines that specify standards of practice and conduct that is commonly recognized and accepted to be illegal, immoral, or unacceptable in a particular profession. These codes often set forth certain rules of conduct that describe aspirational goals to be achieved by all members. The *Occupational Therapy Code of Ethics and Ethics Standards (2010)* (referred to as the "Code and Ethics Standards"; AOTA, 2010b) is such a code. It is hoped that members aspire to do good and act in an ethically responsible manner. Members are expected to adhere to standards set forth in the Code and Ethics Standards to protect the recipients of services. Although the Code and Ethics Standards constitute a type of self-regulation within the Association and profession, the *Enforcement Procedures for the Occupational Therapy Code of Ethics and Ethics Standards* provide a regulatory component (AOTA, 2010a). Violations of the Code and Ethics Standards can result in certain sanctions imposed by the Association on its members, including reprimand, censure, probation, suspension, and revocation of membership in the association.

Not every violation of the Code and Ethics Standards also is a violation of the law. An act is considered illegal if it is contrary to a law. Therefore, only if the violation prescribed by the Code and Ethics Standards also is a violation of the law will the violator be subject to criminal sanctions and penalties.

An example of an unethical and illegal practice is the following: An occupational therapy practitioner who engages in a sexual relationship with a minor or with a client who has mental impairments would be breaching Principles 2C and 2D (nonmaleficence) of the Code and Ethics Standards. Principle 2C states, "Occupational therapy personnel shall avoid relationships that exploit the recipient of services, students, research participants, or employees physically, emotionally, psychologically . . . or in any other manner that conflicts or interferes with professional judgment and objectivity." Principle 2D further states that "occupational therapy personnel shall avoid engaging in any sexual relationship or activity, whether consensual or nonconsensual, with any recipient of service . . . while a relationship exists as an occupational therapy practitioner [or] educator. . . ." It is widely acknowledged that engaging in sexual relations with a minor also is committing a criminal act.

An example of unethical behavior as defined by the Code and Ethics Standards, but not necessarily illegal behavior, could be a violation of Principle 5F (Procedural Justice), which states, "Occupational therapy personnel shall take responsibility for maintaining high standards and continuing competence in practice, education, and research by participating in professional development and educational activities. . . ." An occupational therapy practitioner could fail to function within the parameters of his or her competence and not seek continuing education (CE) even though the techniques that he or she was taught in school have drastically changed. New technology and emerging practice areas demand that all practitioners keep abreast of current evidence-based research and trends; however, failure to participate in CE may not be considered a criminal violation. It should be noted, however, that if the state regulatory board requires CE to maintain one's license to practice, then failure to meet CE requirements may subject the occupational therapy practitioner to license suspension or other sanctions.

Ethics and law are indeed strange bedfellows. Ethics deals with making ethical decisions and morally good choices (not necessarily right or wrong), and law usually deals with justice, right, and wrong (not necessarily morally good choices). Occupational therapists, occupational therapy assistants, and students must gather the facts and, when an ethically appropriate course of action is unclear, seek guidance from multiple sources. These sources may include the state regulatory board, the peer occupational therapy community, the state association, ethics committees, human resources personnel and workplace policies and procedures, AOTA, the National Board for Certification in Occupational Therapy, and legal counsel. All can provide information and different perspectives to assist in ethical decision making.

REFERENCES

American Occupational Therapy Association. (2010a). Enforcement procedures for the *Occupational Therapy Code of Ethics and Ethics Standards*. *American Journal of Occupational Therapy, 64*(6 Suppl.), S4–S16. doi:10.5014/ajot.2010.64S4

American Occupational Therapy Association. (2010b). Occupational therapy code of ethics and ethics standards (2010). *American Journal of Occupational Therapy, 64*(6 Suppl.), S17–S26. doi:10.5014/ajot.2010.64S17

Penny Kyler-Hutchison, MA, OT/L, FAOTA
Manager, AOTA Ethics Program

Amy Mah
Paralegal, AOTA Office of General Counsel

Deborah Yarett Slater, MS, OT/L, FAOTA
AOTA Staff Liaison to the Ethics Commission

CHAPTER 15

Legal and Ethical Practice: A Professional Responsibility

If your employer asks you to provide daily maintenance for a patient's hearing aid after he or she has been instructed and is independent in its care, or to include lower-extremity lymphedema management in your treatment program until the vacant physical therapy position is filled, is it legal? Is it ethical? Is it within the occupational therapy scope of practice? Staffing patterns, emerging practice settings, alternative treatment modalities, programmatic models of care, and blurring of single-discipline supervisory models have left occupational therapists and occupational therapy assistants seeking clarification in defining their roles and their legal and ethical responsibilities. When there is divergence between legal and ethical obligations, it can be difficult to ascertain where the final authority resides.

Recently, many of the questions that come to the American Occupational Therapy Association (AOTA) share a general theme: "My supervisor is asking/demanding that I do _____ [fill in the blank with a treatment intervention]. They think it's insubordination if I refuse, but I think I'm being asked to do something unethical. Or is it just unreasonable? Who is right?"

In many cases, supervisors or administrators have different expectations and understandings of "what occupational therapy is" than do occupational therapists or occupational therapy assistants themselves. Further, even if an intervention is within the legal scope of practice of occupational therapy, should it be done by that practitioner with that client? Questions about personal competency and doing the right thing to benefit the client must also be considered. How can practitioners understand their legal scope of practice and their responsibility to uphold the profession's ethical principles while communicating the appropriate role of occupational therapy to their consumers, colleagues, administrators, and payers?

COMMON CONCERNS

The following are samples of the types of questions relating to ethics, legal issues, and scope of practice that are often received at AOTA:

- In my facility, a physical therapist was treating a patient for balance deficits and hit the outpatient reimbursement cap. Can I pick up the patient for occupational therapy and continue to work on balance but with occupational therapy goals?
- What can I do with respect to video fluoroscopy, functional capacity evaluations, and other particular programs or interventions?
- The physical therapist in my facility is leaving. Can I treat lower-extremity lymphedema (I'm trained and credentialed in this area) until they hire a new physical therapist?
- My state practice act does not specifically state that occupational therapists work with back pain clients or provide back treatment. As a result, one of our major payers won't pay for back treatment. How can I prove that this is appropriate occupational therapy intervention?

- Is trachea suctioning within the occupational therapy scope of practice? I have a client who needs it. What about monitoring oxygen saturations?
- Do occupational therapists have to be certified to provide dysphagia services?
- I work in a rural area where staffing is difficult. I'm the only occupational therapist, working with several physical therapists. To provide continuity for my clients when I'm sick or on vacation, if I can't find an occupational therapist replacement and the physician has referred for occupational therapy/physical therapy, can I write in my evaluation that the patient will be treated by a physical therapist if indicated by the occupational therapist?
- Are lymphedema and wound care within the occupational therapy scope of practice? If so, do I need certification? What type, and where do I get it?
- What are the legal and ethical implications of working in a driving program, and what competency and level of training are required for staff?

Other questions often arise around adding services (e.g., becoming a durable medical equipment provider, providing complementary or alternative medicine like massage or acupuncture) to an existing private practice or setting up a separate business in these areas. Is there a conflict of interest when a practitioner has access to a ready-made pool of potential patients or clients who are already in a therapeutic relationship with him or her? For example, in these cases the practices may complement each other, but how can the business owner ensure that clients' rights of autonomy and informed consent are safeguarded (AOTA, 2010a, Principle 3)? As a general principle in evaluating this situation, consider that full and open disclosure of any competing businesses from which the therapist may realize financial gain is important to preserve patient rights, as are policies and procedures to avoid conflicts of interest.

Role delineation between disciplines can be another practice challenge in settings where certain referral patterns exist because of organizational history and where occupational therapy education and clinical training are not well understood. Role blurring can be a result of staffing shortages, pressure to maintain productivity within clinical departments, department leadership, and lack of confidence on the part of occupational therapy personnel in understanding and articulating the occupational therapy domain and scope of practice.

As the complexities and venues of practice grow and new specialty areas emerge, the search for guidelines for appropriate legal and ethical practice will intensify. These questions generally do not have a direct, simple answer. Rather, a reasoning process or decision matrix for addressing these dilemmas is more appropriate and can be applied to a variety of settings and practice challenges. A number of resources are available to answer these questions.

DETERMINING SCOPE OF PRACTICE

The first step in the reasoning process is to understand what is meant by *scope of practice*. The foundation of a profession's domain has legal, professional, ethical, and educational components. Specifically, a profession's domain or scope of practice derives from three basic elements: (1) a body of knowledge historically included in the educational preparation of the discipline, (2) a clearly established history of application in practice as reflected in the professional literature, and (3) the legal framework created by state practice acts. It is important to understand the relationship of these elements to each other because they support occupational therapy practice and are the basis for delineated scope of practice language in state law.

Education

The Accreditation Council for Occupational Therapy Education (ACOTE, 2007a, 2007b, 2007c) standards define entry-level skills and competencies that students should acquire during the educational and fieldwork process, thereby establishing the baseline occupational therapy body of knowledge. However, many practice areas, particularly as specialization and knowledge grow, require additional training (which may include hands-on practicums) to ensure competency. Competency must be documented and upgraded regularly to maintain a consistent skill level and to provide state-of-the-art care. It is also necessary to meet the requirements of regulatory agencies that want proof of current competency, particularly in high-risk procedures.

Principle 5F of the *Occupational Therapy Code of Ethics and Ethics Standards (2010)* (referred to as the "Code and Ethics Standards"; AOTA, 2010a) speaks specifically to this ethical obligation: "Occupational therapy personnel shall take responsibility for maintaining high standards and continuing competence in practice, education, and research." In addition, an ethical mandate to "do good" or do the right thing ("Principle 1. Occupational therapy personnel shall demonstrate a concern for the well-being and safety of the recipients of their services") and, above all, do no harm ("Principle 2. Occupational therapy personnel shall intentionally refrain from actions that cause harm") reinforces the need for basic and continuing education to maintain and enhance knowledge and skills. Principle 1G of the Code and Ethics Standards provides additional support for competency in less established areas: "Occupational therapy personnel shall take responsible steps . . . and use careful judgment to ensure their own competence and weigh potential for client harm when generally recognized standards do not exist in emerging technology or areas of practice."

Application in Practice

The second component of defining a scope of professional practice is an identifiable history of application. Although certain aspects of occupational therapy practice are well documented in the literature, others that reflect newer or less traditional approaches to practice or atypical settings are not. Relevant literature or research studies showing the efficacy of certain interventions, combined with practitioner competency, may satisfy the test for inclusion in the occupational therapy scope of practice, especially where statutory language is very broad and nonspecific. This history may be especially important when a particular approach would not be defined as "usual and customary" practice by the average clinician.

However, a more basic consideration, particularly when an administrator or supervisor is requesting that an occupational therapy practitioner provide more medically related or maintenance-type interventions, is the appropriateness of such a request. The recipient of such services should require the skills unique to an occupational therapist or occupational therapy assistant, and the treatment plan should focus on objective, measurable goals to be met within a reasonable timeline. This guideline reflects Medicare criteria for appropriate intervention and payment but is also useful as an internal gauge of whether occupational therapy services should be provided and within what parameters.

Legal Framework

State licensure laws legally define a profession's scope of practice or domain. Although occupational therapy is regulated in all states, the District of Columbia, Puerto Rico, and Guam, several of these entities have less stringent forms of regulation, such as certification, registration, or trademark. The primary goal of all forms of regulation is to protect consumers. However, only licensure defines and legally protects the occupational therapy scope of practice so that those who are not licensed cannot call themselves occupational therapists or occupational therapy assistants and cannot provide services delineated within the occupational therapy scope of practice. In 2010, licensure for occupational therapists existed in 48 states and for occupational therapy assistants in 46 states. Registration (Hawaii and Colorado) may contain a definition of occupational therapy but does not define a scope of practice, so others may, under some circumstances, use occupational therapy interventions if they do not call these services "occupational therapy."

It is every occupational therapist's and occupational therapy assistant's professional responsibility to have a copy of his or her state licensure law (or other regulatory document) and to be familiar with its contents, as well as to access updates as they occur. This is also an ethical responsibility, as per Principle 5 of the Code and Ethics Standards ("Occupational therapy personnel shall comply with institutional rules, local, state, federal, and international laws and AOTA documents applicable to the profession of occupational therapy" (procedural justice). About 16 states have adopted some version of the AOTA Code and Ethics Standards (although not always the most current version). Other states have language pertaining to ethics or ethical practice within their statutes. State licensure laws define what can legally be done by practitioners licensed in that state, so in that regard licensure laws are the final authority. However, laws can be subject to interpretation, especially because it is virtually impossible (and undesirable) to enumerate in detail every possible appropriate occupational therapy evaluation or intervention.

Members of a state licensure board may assist in clarifying what they consider to be within the occupational therapy scope of practice as defined in the licensure law. A good test is to determine whether most occupational therapy practitioners would, if called to testify in a court case, verify that the area in question is "usual and customary practice" (although this test becomes more difficult as innovative practice areas emerge that are not yet in the mainstream).

In addition to statutory language, educational criteria for accredited occupational therapy programs, support from the literature and Association and other documents, and evidence of competency may assist practitioners in supporting their actions as being within an appropriate occupational therapy scope of practice. In the case of less mainstream practice areas, these criteria, as well as alignment with occupational therapy philosophy (as outlined in the next section), will be particularly relevant.

Practitioners also need to understand payer policies and other laws and regulations that govern their practice. This information includes Medicare rules about supervision, documentation, and coding and billing, as well as other legal information that relates to their client population or practice setting. Because these guidelines change frequently, it is important to visit the Centers for Medicare and Medicaid Services Web site (http://www.cms.gov/) frequently, as well as to use announcements and updates on the AOTA Web site (www.aota.org) from the Federal Affairs, State Policy, and Reimbursement groups. Additional resources, particularly on potential or pending legislation and other activities that affect practice and education, can be found in AOTA's monthly electronic *Scope of Practice Issues Update*. The following AOTA documents provide important guidance in supporting current and evolving practice parameters:

- *Occupational Therapy Practice Framework: Domain and Process* (AOTA, 2008)
- *Occupational Therapy Code of Ethics and Ethics Standards (2010)* (AOTA, 2010a)
- ACOTE accreditation standards (ACOTE, 2007a, 2007b, 2007c)
- *Standards for Continuing Competence* (AOTA, 2010c)
- *Scope of Practice* (AOTA, 2010b)
- Position papers on the specific topic available on the AOTA Web site (http://www.aota.org/Practitioners/Official/Position.aspx).

Reasoning Through Legal and Ethical Practice Challenges

The purpose of the preceding discussion is to provide resources and foundational knowledge to understand and articulate the legal and ethical occupational therapy scope of practice. However, because many of the questions posed earlier in this article do not necessarily have a straightforward, definitive answer, a framework for decision making may be useful to assist in the reasoning process regarding whether an action is part of the occupational therapy scope of practice in which definitive opinions cannot be obtained. The following are some questions for self-reflection:

- Was this body of knowledge part of my educational curriculum?
- Am I competent to provide this intervention based on past education or current or continuing education?
- Is my knowledge in this area current and adequate to provide competent services?
- Is this intervention or practice usual and customary among occupational therapy practitioners, and would many of them agree? If not, is it defensible and consistent with the occupational therapy scope of practice using criteria previously outlined?
- Have I sought clarification from the state licensure board in interpreting less well defined areas of the occupational therapy scope of practice?
- Have I sought resources like AOTA position papers or official documents relating to this area of practice (or done a literature search to provide evidence for my practice interventions)?
- Is this occupational therapy? How does this relate to the philosophy of occupational therapy? Am I using occupation to promote engagement in meaningful activities and participation in life roles?

The last question may be the most critical. Despite the fact that an intervention is legal and ethical, it still may not be in line with the philosophical tenets of the occupational therapy profession. As articulated in the *Framework,*

> the defining contribution of occupational therapy is the application of core values, knowledge, and skills to assist clients (people, organizations, and populations) to engage in everyday activities or occupations that they want and need to do in a manner that supports health and participation. (AOTA, 2008, p. 626)

As the profession's roles and contributions to society continue to evolve, the concepts outlined in the *Framework* can prove invaluable in facilitating the reasoning process to respond to scope of practice challenges.

Conclusion

The evolution of new patient populations, intervention strategies, and practice settings inevitably poses challenges to ensuring that practice is in line with legal, ethical, and philosophical guidelines and regulations. The occupational therapy profession has much to offer if occupational therapy practitioners, regardless of their roles and practice settings, have the knowledge and understanding of the underpinnings that define our profession and are able to clearly articulate it to consumers, colleagues, and outside publics.

References

Accreditation Council for Occupational Therapy Education. (2007a). Accreditation standards for a doctoral-degree-level educational program for the occupational therapist. *American Journal of Occupational Therapy, 61,* 641–651.

Accreditation Council for Occupational Therapy Education. (2007b). Accreditation standards for a master's-degree-level educational program for the occupational therapist. *American Journal of Occupational Therapy, 61,* 652–661.

Accreditation Council for Occupational Therapy Education. (2007c). Accreditation standards for an educational program for the occupational therapy assistant. *American Journal of Occupational Therapy, 61,* 662–671.

American Occupational Therapy Association. (2008). Occupational therapy practice framework: Domain and process (2nd ed.). *American Journal of Occupational Therapy, 62,* 625–683. doi:10.5014/ajot.62.6.625

American Occupational Therapy Association. (2010a). Occupational therapy code of ethics and ethics standards (2010). *American Journal of Occupational Therapy, 64*(6 Suppl.), S17–S26. doi:10.5014/ajot.2010.64S17

American Occupational Therapy Association. (2010b). Scope of practice. *American Journal of Occupational Therapy, 64*(6 Suppl.), S70–S77. doi:10.5014/ajot.2010.64S70

American Occupational Therapy Association. (2010c). Standards for continuing competence. *American Journal of Occupational Therapy, 64*(6 Suppl.), S103–S105. doi:10.5014/ajot.12010.64S103

FOR MORE INFORMATION

- AOTA *Scope of Practice Issues Update, State Policy Update,* and *Federal Issues* newsletters are available at www.aota.org/Pubs/Enews.aspx.
- The Centers for Medicare and Medicaid Services has a wealth of information at www.cms.gov.

Deborah Yarett Slater, MS, OTR/L, FAOTA
AOTA Staff Liaison to the Ethics Commission

CHAPTER 16

Ethics in Practice: Whose Responsibility?

The resurgence in the job market for both occupational therapists and occupational therapy assistants is good news to educators, students, and practitioners alike. In some cases, sign-on bonuses and other incentives seem to be making a comeback. This would appear to be a positive sign for the profession, but is it coming at a price?

For a number of years, reimbursement in all clinical settings has generally been capitated, often at a level that barely covers costs and expenses. It is usually linked to a diagnostic category that estimates the resources required to care for the client. These resources include equipment, nursing, therapy, medical supplies, room and board, and so forth. Salaries, although increasing only in small increments, represent a significant expense against limited and fixed reimbursement. The cost of advances in technology has also added to rising expenditures. As a result of these various factors, it has become increasingly difficult for facilities to break even or to make even a modest profit. But publicly held companies, even in health care, need to show profits to their shareholders.

In an effort to earn income, given all the regulatory and other constraints, some facilities and contract staffing companies have mandated productivity requirements, documentation guidelines, and general rules about clinical management of clients that appear to be based primarily on administrative decisions to meet designated financial goals. These requirements often do not rely on the clinical judgment of therapists or take into account the individual needs or capabilities of the client. As health care focuses on business practices and profits, there has been "an erosion of the appropriate professional moral climate from service to self-interest in all of its forms . . . and the opposite of moral courage: indifference and apathy" (Davis, 2005, p. 215).

Although this trend seems to be more prevalent in skilled nursing facilities (SNFs) under the prospective payment system, and especially in contract staffing companies that provide employees for these facilities, it is also reported in other settings. Recently, an increasing number of questions have arisen from American Occupational Therapy Association (AOTA) members about their employers' administrative practices and directives. The questions center on ethical and legal concerns related to client safety, personal liability and licensure, and potential Medicare fraud. These situations may include

- Admitting clients who are independent, then requiring therapists to "be creative" in developing goals and treatment plans
- Admitting clients for rehabilitation who are very acute or unstable, placing them in very high resource utilization group (RUG) categories to maximize reimbursement, then mandating that therapists provide the hours

of therapy these categories require. This may happen in spite of the client's inability to tolerate extensive therapy, and according to some reports, therapists are asked to record rest periods as minutes of treatment

- Having nonclinical administrators or clinical directors in other disciplines dictate the frequency or length of treatment without input from the evaluating or treating occupational therapist
- Asking a new therapist to "fill in" missing documentation (on clients they have not treated or who may already have been discharged), which should have been done by an occupational therapist or occupational therapy assistant at the time of treatment, so the facility can bill for those sessions after the fact
- Not permitting clinicians to discharge clients when their goals have been met unless the discharge is "approved" by an administrator (extending length of stay and reimbursement)
- Requiring excessive group treatment and calling it "concurrent treatment" when it is not appropriate to meet the client's goals
- Therapists and clients alike feeling like "failures" for their inability to achieve the prescribed minutes of therapy and having to provide explanations for the shortfall.

These situations can lead to loss of autonomy in clinical decision making, a potential feeling of disrespect from colleagues, and in many cases, ethical and legal unrest. The dilemmas and stress increase when practitioners are told that these practices are acceptable, perhaps the industry standard, and that "others" can meet these demands. An additional source of concern is members who report that less experienced practitioners don't seem to recognize that there is a problem with these directives. Practitioners may believe that when they are following a supervisor's or administrator's directive, any behavior is acceptable, and they and their licenses are protected.

In fact, each occupational therapist and occupational therapy assistant has a personal and professional responsibility to know and understand regulations that govern his or her practice. Principle 5 of the *Occupational Therapy Code of Ethics and Ethics Standards (2010)* (referred to as the "Code and Ethics Standards"; AOTA, 2010a) states that "Occupational therapy personnel shall comply with institutional rules, local, state, federal, and international laws and AOTA documents applicable to the profession of occupational therapy." This principle includes state practice acts where applicable, Medicare and other payer regulations, and so forth. Understanding regulations is as much a part of one's job and professional role as clinical knowledge. Lack of knowledge is not an acceptable excuse and will not stand up to ethical or legal scrutiny. Practitioners must provide treatment, document, and bill according to Medicare requirements for coverage of occupational therapy services (e.g., skilled services that are reasonable and necessary to meet realistic, objective goals in a specified time frame). In addition, there are clear rules about group treatment that apply to Medicare Part A in SNFs: The group may not exceed four patients and may not exceed 25% of each client's total treatment time.

The Code and Ethics Standards can provide assistance in responding to these situations. Principle 6B of the Code and Ethics Standards states that any form of communication (which includes written documentation) should not contain "false, fraudulent, deceptive, misleading, or unfair statements or claims." Principle 1H of the Code and Ethics Standards also provides relevant guidance: "Occupational therapy personnel shall terminate occupational therapy services in collaboration with the service recipient or responsible party when the needs and goals of the recipient have been met or when services no longer produce a measurable change or outcome." These official documents, as well as relevant payer regulations, can provide support for practitioners confronting potentially unethical situations or managers who create them.

At a more fundamental level, professionals have the public's trust and operate with relative freedom and autonomy because they have a code of ethics and are generally considered altruistic. Situations like those reported directly challenge two core ethical concepts: beneficence and nonmaleficence. Principle 1 of the Code and Ethics Standards states, "Occupational therapy personnel shall demonstrate a concern for the well-being and safety of the recipients of their services." Principle 2 states, "Occupational therapy personnel shall intentionally refrain from actions that cause harm." Therefore, clinicians have a responsibility to provide treatment that will, in their judgment, benefit the client and not do any harm and then to accurately document and bill for the services delivered.

Dealing with organizational pressures to use financial goals as the basis for action can be stressful and may result in negative consequences. These consequences can be severe and have both legal (e.g., fines, prison time) and ethical (e.g., reprimand, censure) implications. However, moral courage requires not only identifying ethical dilemmas and knowing what is good and right, but also doing what is good and right (Davis, 2005). Rather than self-serving behaviors or excuses to justify one's actions, the moral imperative to action stems from true altruism or caring about others (Davis, 2005). Whistleblower laws can provide some protection from retribution, but job loss or demotion may, in some cases, be realistic deterrents. Although practitioners can face difficult choices, being prepared with creative problem-solving skills and objective strategies may assist in responding to potentially unethical, and sometimes illegal, directives.

A first step may be to educate employers and colleagues. They should understand that it is in their best interest, as well as a legal requirement, to be compliant with regulations and that doing so will protect them against liability. Many resources are available from AOTA, including official documents such as the *Occupational Therapy Code of Ethics and Ethics Standards (2010)* (AOTA, 2010a); *Scope of Practice* (AOTA, 2010b); *Standards of Practice for Occupational Therapy* (AOTA, 2010c); and *Guidelines for Supervision, Roles, and Responsibilities During the Delivery of Occupational Therapy Services* (AOTA, 2009). This *Reference Guide to the Occupational Therapy Code of Ethics and Ethics Standards* contains Advisory Opinions and other articles relating to ethical challenges in practice situations. Staff in the Ethics Office at AOTA are also available to discuss ethical dilemmas and provide assistance in resolving them (e-mail ethics@aota.org). In addition, knowledge and availability of relevant Medicare and other payer regulations, as well as current written updates, are critical components of every practitioner's professional library. These are available on the AOTA Web site in the "Reimbursement" section and on the Centers for Medicare and Medicaid Services (CMS) Web site (www.cms.hhs.gov/default.asp?). CMS also maintains a hot line in the Office of the Inspector General and provides information on how to report alleged fraud at http://www.oig.hhs.gov/fraud/hotline/.

Practitioners are expected to be familiar with, make others aware of, and apply the Code and Ethics Standards in their everyday practice. Given the business-driven focus in the health care industry, practitioners are likely to encounter ethical and legal dilemmas in their workplace. It is ultimately a personal and professional responsibility not only to recognize unethical situations but also to take action to expose and correct them to the extent possible.

References

American Occupational Therapy Association. (2009). Guidelines for supervision, roles, and responsibilities during the delivery of occupational therapy services. *American Journal of Occupational Therapy, 63,* 797–803. doi:10.5014/ajot.63.6.797

American Occupational Therapy Association. (2010a). Occupational therapy code of ethics and ethics standards (2010). *American Journal of Occupational Therapy, 64*(6 Suppl.), S17–S26. doi:10.5014/ajot.2010.64S17

American Occupational Therapy Association. (2010b). Scope of practice. *American Journal of Occupational Therapy, 64*(6 Suppl.), S70–S77. doi:10.5014/ajot.2010.64S70

American Occupational Therapy Association. (2010c). Standards of practice for occupational therapy. *American Journal of Occupational Therapy, 64*(6 Suppl.), S106–S111. doi:10.5014/ajot.2010.64S106

Davis, C. (2005). Educating adult health professionals for moral action: In search of moral courage. In R. B. Purtilo, G. M. Jensen, & C. B. Royeen (Eds.), *Educating for moral action: A sourcebook in health and rehabilitation ethics* (pp. 215–224). Philadelphia: F. A. Davis.

ADDITIONAL RESOURCES

- **AOTA Ethics Office:** ethics@aota.org; 301-652-6611, ext. 2930
- **Centers for Medicare and Medicaid Services:** http://www.cms.hhs.gov/default.asp?
- **"Reimbursement" section of the AOTA Web site:** http://www.aota.org/Practitioners/Reimb.aspx
- **Purtilo, R. B., Jensen, G. M., & Royeen, C. B. (2005).** *Educating for moral action: A sourcebook in health and rehabilitation ethics.* Philadelphia: F. A. Davis.

Deborah Yarett Slater, MS, OT/L, FAOTA
AOTA Staff Liaison to the Ethics Commission

Copyright © 2005, by the American Occupational Therapy Association. This chapter was originally published in *OT Practice,* October 17, 2005, pp. 13–15. It has been revised to reflect updated AOTA official documents, recent legislation, Web sites, AOTA style, and additional resources.

CHAPTER 17

The Ethics of Productivity

Occupational therapy practitioners have a legal and ethical responsibility to their clients, regardless of facility policies. Productivity measures can be an effective management tracking tool, ensuring that departments are run efficiently and enabling accurate budgeting. But in the hands of overly aggressive administrators or supervisors, they sometimes are used as a tool to push the reimbursement envelope and supersede professional judgment about how clients receive occupational therapy services. In spite of organizational directives about frequency, duration, and one-on-one versus group intervention, every occupational therapist and occupational therapy assistant has a professional responsibility to ensure that he or she is in compliance with legal statutes and ethical principles when providing care.

Productivity targets are frequently achieved through the use of alternatives to one-on-one intervention. These alternatives can include what Medicare defines as *concurrent therapy* or *dovetailing*, allowing the practitioner to work with more than one client in the same treatment area. According to the *Resident Assessment Instrument (RAI) User's Manual* (an instrument developed by the Centers for Medicare and Medicaid Services [CMS], 2010, for the minimum data set in nursing homes), for Medicare Part A, therapists may treat no more than two patients concurrently, and the total time spent with the two patients must be split according to the actual time spent with each patient. However, the treatment of two or more patients under Medicare Part B is documented as group treatment. Concurrent therapy is not permitted under Medicare Part B.

In the skilled nursing facility prospective payment system Final Rule, CMS stated that concurrent therapy is a legitimate mode of delivering therapy, it should be an adjunct to individual (1:1) delivery, and it should represent an exception rather than the standard of care. The examples provided in the RAI clarify CMS's expectation that the client is receiving a substantial amount of true one-on-one therapy in addition to the therapy provided concurrently. In addition, CMS has stated that the decision of whether concurrent therapy is to be used should be made at the treating therapist's discretion and should not be based on company policy or productivity concerns ("Prospective payment system and consolidated billing," 2009).

Group therapy is another method of providing care to multiple clients at the same time. Skilled nursing facility Part A rules require that group therapy be limited to 25% of the patient's weekly therapy and that there be only four or fewer clients per group per supervising therapist or therapy assistant ("Prospective payment system and consolidated billing," 1999). Medicare rules emphasize that although concurrent therapy is allowable, the decision to use it must be based on the therapist's judgment when clinically appropriate and documented as part of the client's plan of treatment. Practitioners should check these resources periodically for updates as policies and regulations do change.

The *Standards of Practice for Occupational Therapy* (American Occupational Therapy Association [AOTA], 2010b) outline the appropriate components of the service delivery process. With support from the *Occupational Therapy Code of Ethics and Ethics Standards (2010)* (referred to as the "Code and Ethics Standards"; AOTA, 2010a) and relevant legal statutes, they also define best practice. These documents can assist practitioners in making appropriate decisions about how to render care. After evaluation, occupational therapists develop plans of care that specify frequency, duration, and types of intervention that best match the collaborative goals set by therapists with their clients. The plan of care may incorporate not only one-on-one direct service but, where appropriate, may also reflect the use of group or concurrent therapy as elements of the intervention plan. However, individualized, one-on-one intervention should be part of every client's plan of care for the following reasons:

- The collaboration between the client and the therapist to identify meaningful goals and the strategies to attain them is, by nature, an individualized, developmental process.
- The treatment plan should be reassessed and revised at different points in the course of rehabilitation on the basis of the client's response to intervention.
- Group or concurrent therapy does not allow for the therapist who is overseeing multiple patients to adapt the activity to provide the "just-right" challenge based on individual performance or response.

"Reductionist" therapy interventions, such as basic exercises, are easily adapted to group or concurrent therapy but often are not occupation based. Practitioners should consider the following questions when deciding whether to use group or concurrent therapy:

- Am I choosing to provide treatment concurrently or in a group because that form of treatment is the most effective method of providing the necessary intervention and is, therefore, in the client's best interests?

or

- Am I selecting group or concurrent therapy because these interventions are easiest and result in the ability to "treat" many more clients than a labor-intensive, one-on-one service delivery model?

Organizations may mandate that all clients be treated in groups or that several be treated concurrently. This mandate is clearly designed to maximize billable hours and extend staff as much as possible. Staff at these organizations report that administrators also claim that this practice is perfectly legal. It is true that there is nothing inherently unethical or illegal in using these service delivery models as part of an overall occupational therapy plan of care. However, an ethical issue can arise when these models make up the bulk of the occupational therapy intervention or when the client's needs are not appropriate for this model.

It is the role of the occupational therapist, using clinical judgment, to determine an appropriate mix of group, concurrent, and individual interventions as supported by the goals and outcomes that he or she has identified with the client. It is also the role and ethical responsibility of the therapist to personally know, understand, and interpret payer and other rules and regulations that govern the delivery of services. Copies of the relevant statutes, program transmittals, and so forth should be available in clinical departments for reference and support if challenged. It is not acceptable for practitioners to permit external, sometimes nonclinical, staff or administrators to supersede their own clinical judgment. That said, it is also a professional responsibility to incorporate a mix of service delivery models that will most efficiently meet the therapy goals so limited staffing resources can be allocated appropriately and fairly. Again, the key is that the decisions must be clinically based.

Occupational therapy practitioners sometimes have a unique challenge in that their focus on occupational performance may present an even greater challenge to productivity. For example, repetitive exercises done independently by a client are inherently less time consuming than doing a kitchen activity that includes all steps involved in preparing a meal, something that a client is likely to require to return home and live independently. The nature of the profession is to provide occupation-based evaluation and collaborative goal setting to ensure that therapeutic interventions translate to actual performance in real-life, meaningful activities for that client in their natural environment. The purpose of these types of intervention is to ultimately facilitate greater engagement and participation within that client's daily life and roles as well as in the community.

CASE EXAMPLE

An occupational therapist is hired to work 8 hours of as-needed coverage in a local skilled nursing facility over the weekend. Upon arrival, he finds coverage notes indicating that he is to complete 20 Medicare Part A treatments and 3 occupational therapy evaluations. Overwhelmed, he contacts the facility rehabilitation director to ask for clarification. The director advises him to "dovetail," or provide concurrent therapy for, 5 clients at a time, seeing each cluster of clients for a 1-hour period. This approach will allow the therapist to complete all 20 treatments in 4 hours and will leave the other half of his workday free to complete the evaluations.

In examining the goals and clinical issues of some of the clients on his caseload, the occupational therapist suggests that one-on-one therapy visits may be more appropriate for some of the treatments. The director replies that this is the facility "protocol," and if the occupational therapist cannot fulfill the demands of the policy, then perhaps he should find another place to work. The therapist is torn between doing what he believes to be the clinically appropriate

course of action and satisfying the expectations of the work site. *(Case example submitted by Pam Toto, PhD, OTR/L, BCG, FAOTA)*

DISCUSSION

So how do intervention models that use group therapy or concurrent therapy fit with the client-centered approach occupational therapy practitioners promote? Are occupational therapy personnel working to increase employer reimbursement or to benefit their clients? Can both of these mandates be satisfied? Are they using intervention models that maximize the number of clients who can be "treated" at once so staff numbers can be kept unrealistically low and reimbursement can be kept relatively high? These questions present true ethical dilemmas because an organization must be financially viable, yet clients trust occupational therapy practitioners to provide only the services they believe will be effective for clients' particular clinical situations and for only as long as clients benefit from these services. AOTA frequently receives inquiries from members who are challenged to meet productivity requirements that seem arbitrary (or are based on the number needed to hit reimbursement targets) while providing what they consider to be ethical treatment in line with the philosophy of occupational therapy.

How should occupational therapy practitioners make clinical decisions, and what constitutes "best practice"? In addition to the *Standards of Practice for Occupational Therapy* (AOTA, 2010b), the Code and Ethics Standards provide guidance that ensures that the best interests of the client are served. They also serve as support for practitioners' right to autonomy in making clinical decisions based on their knowledge, competence, and status as a professional. Several principles of the Code and Ethics Standards are particularly relevant. Principle 1 states, "Occupational therapy personnel shall demonstrate a concern for the well-being and safety of the recipients of their services," and Principle 4E is related: "Occupational therapy personnel shall make efforts to advocate for recipients of occupational therapy services to obtain needed services through available means." Occupational therapy practitioners have an ethical obligation to promote good for their clients and provide what they believe is in clients' best interests to address their performance and other needs.

An equally central principle of ethical treatment is to prevent harm (Nonmaleficence). Principle 2F requires that occupational therapy personnel "avoid any undue influences . . . that may compromise the provision of occupational therapy services. . . ." Likewise, Principle 2I requires that they "avoid compromising client rights or well-being based on arbitrary administrative directives by exercising professional judgment and critical analysis." This principle applies to physician orders that may conflict with what an occupational therapist or occupational therapy assistant believes will benefit the client or are counter to current best practice and evidence. It also applies to administrative mandates that violate clinical judgment about what will benefit clients.

Principles 5 (Procedural Justice) and 6 (Veracity) of the Code and Ethics Standards also speak to ethical imperatives that are relevant to practice. Principle 5 requires occupational therapy personnel to be knowledgeable about and compliant with laws, rules, policies, and so forth, whether local, state, federal, or institutional, that are applicable to delivering occupational therapy services, including payer regulations. This Principle obligates occupational therapists and occupational therapy assistants to ensure that their employers are also aware of the ethical requirements of the profession. Further, Principle 6B prohibits the use of "false, fraudulent, deceptive, misleading, or unfair statements or claims." Therefore, practitioners cannot document group or concurrent therapy services as if one-on-one, individual services were actually provided, and they should not allow their employers to do so, either.

Principle 1B of the Code and Ethics Standards, "Occupational therapy personnel shall provide appropriate evaluation and a plan of intervention for all recipients of occupational therapy services specific to their needs," also addresses facility administrators who may direct practitioners to put all clients into groups or provide treatment when no physician referral or evaluation has been done first, as is required. Of course, services should be terminated "when needs and goals of the recipient have been met or when services no longer produce a measurable change or outcome" (Principle 1H).

In short, all aspects of the service delivery process, from the initial evaluation including the plan of care to discharge, must be provided with the client's goals and benefit in mind, supported by the practitioner's clinical judgment and objective documentation. This process is necessary to meet coding and billing regulations for legitimate payment for services. Principle 5N calls on occupational therapy personnel to work with their employers to develop policies and procedures to ensure that they are legal, in compliance with regulations, and consistent with the Code and Ethics Standards.

When conflict or potential ethical violations occur within an organization, occupational therapy personnel should first attempt to resolve them internally (Principle 7D). If that is not successful or appropriate, Principle 7C obliges occupational personnel to "take adequate measures to discourage, prevent, expose, and correct any breaches of the Code and Ethics Standards, and report any breaches of the former to the appropriate authorities." This Principle implies an obligation to ensure not only that one's facility is in compliance with legal and ethical mandates, but that one's clinical colleagues are as well.

A challenging reimbursement environment has the potential to give rise to unrealistic productivity requirements that are illegal or unethical. Occupational therapy practitioners should remember that they have an obligation to exercise their professional judgment in making clinical decisions and to be in compliance with the

Standards of Practice for Occupational Therapy (AOTA, 2010b), the Code and Ethics Standards, and applicable laws, regardless of organizational, supervisory, or peer pressure.

REFERENCES

American Occupational Therapy Association. (2010a). Occupational therapy code of ethics and ethics standards (2010). *American Journal of Occupational Therapy, 64*(6 Suppl.), S17–S26. doi:10.5014/ajot.2010.64S17

American Occupational Therapy Association. (2010b). Standards of practice for occupational therapy. *American Journal of Occupational Therapy, 64*(6 Suppl.), S106–S111. doi:10.5014/ajot.2010.64S106

Centers for Medicare and Medicaid Services. (2010, September). *Revised long term care Resident Assessment Instrument (RAI) user's manual for the minimum data set (MDS)* (Version 3.0). Retrieved December 9, 2010, from http://www.cms.gov/NursingHomeQualityInits/45_NHQIMDS30Training Materials.asp

Prospective payment system and consolidated billing for skilled nursing facilities: Final rule. (1999, July 30). *Federal Register, 64,* 41643–41683.

Prospective payment system and consolidated billing for skilled nursing facilities for FY 2010: Final rule. (2009, August 11). *Federal Register, 74,* 40288–40395.

ADDITIONAL RESOURCES

- **Medicare rules about concurrent therapy (dovetailing) and group therapy:** See the Reimbursement Section of the AOTA Web site at http://www.aota.org/Practitioners/Reimb/Pay/Medicare.aspx
- **Reporting violations of Medicare rules:** Find information on reporting facilities that intentionally disregard Medicare rules at http://www.medicare.gov/FraudAbuse/HowToReport.asp
- **American Occupational Therapy Association. (2011).** *Reference manual of the American Occupational Therapy Association, Inc.: Official documents* (16th ed.). Bethesda, MD: Author.
- **Jacobs, K., & McCormack, G. L. (Eds.). (2011).** *The occupational therapy manager* (5th ed.). Bethesda, MD: AOTA Press.

Deborah Yarett Slater, MS, OT/L, FAOTA
AOTA Staff Liaison to the Ethics Commission

To Err Is Human! Common Practice Errors and Preventive Strategies in Occupational Therapy

To err is human. As with other health care professionals, occupational therapy practitioners sometimes make errors and even cause harm to clients as well as to themselves (American Occupational Therapy Association [AOTA], 2001; National Board for Certification in Occupational Therapy, 2000; Scheirton, Mu, & Lohman, 2003). Although errors are inevitable, the costs of human tragedy for clients, practitioners, and others highlight the urgent need for error reduction and prevention. A first step in error reduction and prevention is to describe and understand common errors that occupational therapy practitioners make in practice. This understanding will allow practitioners to select appropriate prevention strategies.

Since 2000, the authors of this article have conducted a series of research projects on occupational therapy practice errors, supported by the Health Future Foundation and the National Patient Safety Foundation. Specifically, we examined the types, root causes, and impact of practice errors and preventive strategies in physical rehabilitation and geriatrics practice settings (Scheirton et al., 2003). In this article, we synthesize our findings and discuss their implications.

COMMON OCCUPATIONAL THERAPY PRACTICE ERRORS

Practice errors can be categorized in different ways (see Table 18.1). One is to consider the severity, from minor to severe. Examples of minor errors include ripping fingernails, causing a client unnecessary fatigue, scratching a client's skin, or fabricating unfit splints. More severe errors consist of a client falling during a transfer and being injured and rupturing tendons or fracturing bones and a clinician pulling out a catheter during a transfer, treating the wrong client or the wrong site, burning the client when applying a hot pack, causing urine backflow, and even contributing to a client's death.

Errors also can be categorized as technical or moral. *Technical errors*, which concern certain methods, skills, or approaches within the scope of practice, often cause physical harm to clients. Technical errors include things like causing damage by using improper passive range of motion techniques, exceeding client limitations after a hip replacement, experiencing an equipment malfunction, and so forth. *Moral errors* concern behaviors that (a) undercut the basic fabric of the professional–client relationship or (b) are inconsistent with the *Occupational Therapy Code of Ethics and Ethics Standards (2010)* (AOTA, 2010a) and *Standards of Practice for Occupational Therapy* (AOTA, 2010b). Examples of moral errors consist of failing to refer clients to the most appropriate provider or for the most appropriate services, providing unneeded service to obtain payment or reimbursement, being unable to provide needed services due to impairments or lack of knowledge and skills, and creating unrealistic expectations about a client's prognosis.

TABLE 18.1. Classification of Occupational Therapy Practice Errors

CLASSIFICATION	CATEGORIES	EXAMPLES
Severity	Minor	The therapist was transferring a client and had a poor grip on the gait belt when the client began to fall. The therapist readjusted his hold and ripped off his own thumbnail while simultaneously hitting the client.
	Severe	The therapist left a client unattended on a commode chair. The client tried to get up and fell off, hitting his head, which eventually led to his death.
Domain	Technical	A client requested a home evaluation after a hip replacement surgery. The therapist transported the client to her home. While the therapist was getting a walker for the client, the client independently got out of the car and popped the affected hip.
	Moral	The therapist conducted an evaluation, and the intervention was provided by an occupational therapy assistant who did not follow the treatment plan written by the therapist. The occupational therapy assistant required the client to use adaptive equipment that was inappropriate to the level of functioning. The client began to think negatively and felt disabled as a result of the adaptive equipment, which he did not need to use.
Occupational therapy process	Referral	The therapist failed to read the physician's orders.
	Evaluation	While establishing the client's occupational profile, which includes taking the medical history, the therapist failed to clarify the client's weight-bearing status.
	Intervention planning	The therapist failed to consider the layout of the client's bathroom when ordering a transfer bench, and it did not fit.
	Intervention	While the therapist was working on cooking activities with the client standing, the client lost her balance and fell.
	Discontinuation of service	The therapist discontinued a splint for a client recovering from a fracture without a physician's order.
Act	Omission	The therapist failed to perform a driving evaluation for a client who stated his intentions to resume driving.
	Commission	The therapist underestimated the strength required to independently transfer a client, resulting in a client fall.
Scope	Individual	The therapist allowed the client to do tasks independently without direct supervision, when it was unsafe.
	Systemic	During a room exchange, the therapist failed to transfer all of the client's name-marked items, leading to future confusion.

REFERENCE GUIDE TO THE OCCUPATIONAL THERAPY CODE OF ETHICS AND ETHICS STANDARDS

Errors can be further classified on the basis of the occupational therapy process as delineated in the *Occupational Therapy Practice Framework: Domain and Process* (e.g., evaluation, intervention, outcomes; AOTA, 2008). We found that the vast majority of practitioners' errors occur during the intervention phase (Scheirton et al., 2003).

Errors can also occur as a result of an act of omission or an act of commission. *Omission* is the failure to do something one can and ought to do or the failure to do the right thing. For example, failing to communicate the deteriorating mental status or disorientation of a client to other health care professionals, which results in the client falling, is an error of omission. An error of *commission* is a direct action that is wrong or incorrect, such as performing the wrong procedure on a client.

Furthermore, errors can be classified as individual *(active)* or systemic *(latent)*. *Individual errors* are those for which a particular person is clearly responsible. *Systemic errors* are removed from the direct control of the person and frequently remain unnoticed or dormant until the resultant error occurs.

Root Causes

When an error occurs, most practitioners are extremely concerned and want to identify the underlying causes to understand how it could have happened and to prevent it from occurring again. However, the root causes of errors are multidimensional. They may involve human factors, equipment factors, controllable or uncontrollable environmental factors, and poorly structured organizations. The Joint Commission on the Accreditation of Healthcare Organizations (JCAHO, 2003) reported that many errors in health care are due to inadequate orientation, training, and education; communication failure; insufficient staffing; or distraction. The major reported causes of error in occupational therapy are similar: misjudgment of the situation, inadequate preparation, lack of experience, inadequate training and knowledge,

miscommunication among professionals, lack of attention, heavy workload, and others (Lohman, Mu, & Scheirton, 2003).

Many of these causes of errors can be viewed as the result of problematic systems or process failures, to which there can be contributing factors. For example, inadequate preparation may involve a lack of necessary training, the quality of the training program, and the level of competence or proficiency testing following the training (JCAHO, 2002). Miscommunication may occur when there is a hierarchical culture that inadvertently creates barriers to sharing information. In fact, some reported practice errors in occupational therapy are caused by the practitioner's reluctance to raise concerns or question the physician or other health care professionals involved with the client's care (Scheirton et al., 2003). This example raises further concerns since preventing, alleviating, or eliminating harm is an ethical concern as well. Many errors in occupational therapy are due to inadequate supervision of staff or unrealistic workloads. Heavy workload is a human resource and a supervisor issue and not just an individual occupational therapy practitioner problem.

Furthermore, when occupational therapy practitioners cause errors, it is assumed that if they pay more attention or are more careful in the future, these errors will not occur again. Again, this approach points only to the individual as the source of error. In a complex system such as health care delivery, however, errors are inevitable regardless of how skilled, well intentioned, or careful the individual practitioner may be. The potential for disastrous outcomes to occur in complex systems is well documented (Reason, 1990). Rarely is there just one isolated cause of error; rather, a series of events occur that ultimately result in the error.

Reason (1990) used a Swiss cheese model to illustrate how the random chance of multiple errors can create organizational accidents or system errors. In this model, latent conditions lie dormant in a system and become evident when they combine with other factors, thus wreaking havoc and posing a threat to the system. In hindsight, we often refer to these as "accidents waiting to happen." Alternatively, unsafe acts that are committed by practitioners who are in direct contact with the client or system are referred to as active errors and "are felt almost immediately" (Reason, 1990, p. 173). These active errors "nibble away at the cheese," making more holes in a system's defense. To illustrate, it would normally be impossible to place a stick straight through a block of Swiss cheese via the holes, because they do not line up. But when latent conditions combine with active errors, the system (or cheese) is "eaten away," creating more holes. The eventual alignment of holes is a perfect trajectory of opportunity for error and harm (JCAHO, 2002). Most adverse events that result in harm to clients involve this combination of active and latent conditions (Reason, 1990).

ERROR PREVENTION AND IMPLICATIONS

Fortunately, there are effective strategies to prevent or reduce errors. The most significant is to take a proactive, rather than a reactive, approach. Examples of proactive preventive approaches include, but are not limited to, establishing policies and procedures related to client safety, modifying existing safety protocols, cultivating a nonpunitive work culture, and critically considering the client mix to determine the most appropriate error prevention approaches. These strategies involve an administrative focus on safety and error prevention. For example, a facility manager may establish specific safety protocols for splint application. But for these protocols to work, the manager must also create a nonpunitive work environment where practitioners feel comfortable reporting and learning from errors. Policies and procedures must also be developed to address problems, and compliance must be mandated. A nonpunitive atmosphere promotes open and honest sharing and discussion to encourage

practitioners to learn from errors. In fact, research suggests that practitioners value the learning opportunity when errors occur, and as a result they make constructive changes to their future practice (Lohman et al., 2003; Scheirton et al., 2003). Critically examining the client mix is another proactive approach. An example would be to establish a skin care program to help prevent skin breakdown after determining from an elder's medical history the potential for that problem.

A number of specific and discrete strategies can also be used by administrators and practitioners to prevent and reduce errors. For instance, administrators can strengthen the orientation process for new occupational therapists, occupational therapy assistants, and students. During the orientation, participants can be informed of situations in which errors have occurred or are prone to occur, the procedures that need to be followed when errors do occur, and the processes that need to be undertaken to ensure that staff members learn from the situation.

Providing frequent in-service training can improve practitioners' clinical competence. In-service training is a proactive approach to preventing and decreasing practice errors that occur due to lack of knowledge or lack of experience. It may also be instituted to generate ideas, strategies, and standards to reduce errors if a quality assurance review suggests particular trends. This training should also address areas identified as causative factors on the basis of facility data. For example, our research findings identified a lack of therapist assertiveness with physicians as a causative factor for client errors. Providing an in-service program focused on assertiveness training was one approach for reducing these errors. Another is creating a culture that supports assertiveness under certain conditions. In situations where therapists' poor judgment is a factor, in-service training could review case studies and potential interventions to hone clinical decision-making skills.

Professional educational programs should enhance their curriculum content pertaining to error reduction and client safety. Professional training should also teach future occupational therapy practitioners to be assertive in encouraging communication and collaboration among other health care professionals through an interdisciplinary care management process (JCAHO, 2005). Offering an interprofessional course that focuses on client safety and error prevention is one way to promote effective communication and team building with other health care professionals. It is also important for educational programs to require critical analysis and active learning components to prepare students for the ambiguity of the practice environment. Students learn through activity by doing, including continual exploration and interaction with others. An example of active learning is to role-play the handling of certain error scenarios.

TABLE 18.2. Error Examples, Possible Causes, and Preventive Strategies

ERROR EXAMPLES	POSSIBLE CAUSES	PREVENTIVE STRATEGIES (Select those most appropriate to the setting)
Falls	Distraction, lack of attention, misjudgment, insufficient staffing, inadequate training	■ Cultivate a nonpunitive work culture to encourage reporting and learning from errors
Skin breakdown as a result of a splint being on too long	Insufficient staffing, poor communication, inexperience, insufficient monitoring	■ Create policies and procedures and require staff to follow them
Not reviewing and verifying chart information	Poor communication, heavy workload, unavailability of chart	■ Conduct a critical review of client mix
Treating the wrong client	Poor verification and communication, lack of attention	■ Hold department orientation and training for all new staff
Hot pack on too long, resulting in burn	Lack of attention, heavy workload, inadequate knowledge	■ Provide frequent in-services ■ Establish department/institution programs for areas of concern (e.g., falls prevention plan)
Ruptured tendon	Lack of attention, misjudgment, inexperience, inadequate knowledge	■ Provide staff in-services on how to generally work with different treatment approaches (e.g., with a splint program)
Not involving the client in the care plan	Misjudgment, inexperience	
Applying a serial cast on a person with poor sensation, resulting in pressure sores	Lack of attention, misjudgment, inexperience, inadequate knowledge	■ Maintain appropriate staff levels ■ Verify clients before beginning intervention
Making assumptions about an elder, such as cognitive impairment	Misjudgment, poor communication, inexperience	■ Secure assistance when needed
False documentation	Inexperience, lack of assertiveness, inadequate knowledge, or unethical behavior	■ Provide assertiveness training

Another major error preventive mechanism, recommended by the National Institute of Medicine, is to establish a comprehensive client safety program in individual health care settings (Aspden, Corrigan, Wolcott, & Erickson, 2004). For example, a nursing home could establish a splint safety program in which precautions and wearing schedules are clearly communicated to all staff. In any facility, the operations manager can make sure that the equipment is in good repair.

Error prevention and reduction should target the particular causes of the errors (see Table 18.2). For example, if a client fall was caused by poor judgment by the occupational therapist, a suggested preventive strategy is to teach therapists when it is appropriate to secure additional help with transfers and to create a trigger list of criteria that might warrant help (e.g., client weighs more than 200 pounds). If the error involves treating the wrong client, a suggested prevention strategy is to have all clients wear, and practitioners verify, identification bracelets.

CONCLUSION

Although researchers have been studying practice errors by physicians, nurses, and pharmacists for some time, there is still much to be learned about occupational therapy errors. There is a need to continue to establish baseline data on errors and to implement changes and evaluate improvement. There is also a need to create a learning culture in which errors are not "swept under the carpet" so that authentic learning can take place. Client safety and error-reduction education and training should be made available to all occupational therapy practitioners. Knowledge is power, and learning from errors gives the practitioner and other health care professionals the tools necessary to improve client safety.

REFERENCES

American Occupational Therapy Association. (2001). *Ethics officer report: Comparison of occupational therapy insurance claims and ethics complaints.* Bethesda, MD: Author.

American Occupational Therapy Association. (2008). Occupational therapy practice framework: Domain and process (2nd ed.). *American Journal of Occupational Therapy, 62,* 625–683. doi:10.5014/ajot.62.6.625

American Occupational Therapy Association. (2010a). Occupational therapy code of ethics and ethics standards (2010). *American Journal of Occupational Therapy, 64*(6 Suppl.), S17–S26. doi:10.5014/ajot.2010.64S17

American Occupational Therapy Association. (2010b). Standards of practice for occupational therapy. *American Journal of Occupational Therapy, 64*(6 Suppl.), S106–S111. doi:10.5014/ajot.2010.64S106

Aspden, P., Corrigan, J. M., Wolcott, J., & Erickson, S. M. (Eds.). (2004). *Patient safety: Achieving a new standard for care.* Washington, DC: National Academies Press.

Joint Commission on the Accreditation of Healthcare Organizations. (2002). *Failure mode and effects analysis in health care: Proactive risk reduction.* Oakbrook Terrace, IL: Author.

Joint Commission on the Accreditation of Healthcare Organizations. (2003). *Root cause analysis in health care: Tools and techniques* (2nd ed.). Oakbrook Terrace, IL: Author.

Joint Commission on Accreditation of Healthcare Organizations. (2005). *Essentials for health care: Patient safety* (3rd ed.). Oakbrook Terrace, IL: Author.

Lohman, H., Mu, K., & Scheirton, L. (2003). Occupational therapists' perspectives on practice errors in geriatric practice settings. *Occupational Therapy in Geriatrics, 21*(4), 21–39.

National Board for Certification in Occupational Therapy. (2000). *Investigations program manager report, NBCOT cases (complaints) broken down by state in the past 5 years (1995–1999).* Gaithersburg, MD: Author.

Reason, J. (1990). *Human error.* New York: Cambridge University Press.

Scheirton, L., Mu, K., & Lohman, H. (2003). Occupational therapists' responses to practice errors in physical rehabilitation settings. *American Journal of Occupational Therapy, 57,* 307–314.

Keli Mu, PhD, OTR/L
Assistant Professor, Creighton University
Medical Center

Helene Lohman, OTD, OTR/L
Associate Professor, Creighton University
Medical Center

Linda Scheirton, PhD
Associate Dean, Academic Affairs
Associate Professor, Creighton University
Medical Center

This chapter was originally published in the 2006 edition of the *Reference Guide to the Occupational Therapy Code of Ethics*. It has been revised to reflect updated AOTA official documents, Web sites, AOTA style, and additional resources.

CHAPTER 19

Combating Moral Distress

The complex nature of today's health care environment often constrains occupational therapy practitioners from taking a course of action believed to be ethically indicated (Brandt, 2007). These constraints may result in moral distress. Andrew Jameton (1984) was the first to examine concepts of moral distress as they applied to nursing practice and ethical decision making. As defined by Jameton, *moral distress* relates to the painful feelings and psychological disequilibrium that result from a moral conflict in which one knows the correct action to take, but constraints prevent implementation of the action.

Although institutional constraints were initially identified as the key contributor to moral distress among nurses, ongoing research has shown that a number of variables, both internal and external, have led to an increase in this phenomenon—which is not unique to any one health care discipline (Gutierrez, 2005; Hamric, Davis, & Day Childress, 2006; Redman & Fry, 2000; Sundin-Huard & Fahy, 1999). In addition, with the evolution of the health care environment, identifiable sources of moral distress have expanded beyond the institution itself to include clinical situations and external and internal factors (Hamric et al., 2006). Recognized clinical situations that can affect moral distress relate to unnecessary intervention, prolonging the dying process, and inadequate informed consent of clients. External factors identified in the nursing literature include systemic issues such as the pressure to do more with less, reimbursement constraints, low staff-to-patient ratios, and lack of time. Internal factors, as identified by Hamric et al. (2006), include feelings of powerlessness, lack of knowledge or understanding, and moral sensitivity.

Moral sensitivity may help providers identify ethical dimensions of care because this characteristic stems from an innate ability to empathize with others; however, increased moral sensitivity may also heighten a provider's feeling of injustice. These factors, whether clinical, internal, or external, lead to a perceived inability among health care providers to be patient advocates and to act in a way that not only reflects clinical judgment but is also ethically indicated.

MORAL DISTRESS AND OCCUPATIONAL THERAPY

Although the sources of moral distress for occupational therapy practitioners may differ slightly from those identified for nurses, there are more similarities than differences. Attention must be paid to these sources and their related negative outcomes in order to ensure ethical delivery of care within the profession and the protection of occupational therapy practitioners. Because situations leading to moral distress can be personally and professionally challenging, practitioners should seek assistance to clarify and explore options to address them. A variety of sources, including the

American Occupational Therapy Association (AOTA) and institutional ethics committees, are available to assist with these complex issues.

One of the key functions of AOTA's Ethics Commission (EC) is education related to identifying and making decisions about ethical dilemmas. The EC provides ethics resources through a variety of methods, including feedback on specific questions (through ethics@aota.org or phone conversations), the *Reference Guide to the Occupational Therapy Code of Ethics and Ethics Standards,* and a continuing education course on *Everyday Ethics: Core Knowledge for Occupational Therapy Practitioners and Educators* (AOTA, n.d.). In increasing numbers, practitioners call or e-mail their questions, seeking advice on whether their concerns are, in fact, ethical dilemmas and on strategies for analyzing and addressing them.

In recent years, organizational ethics has emerged as one of the most prevalent concerns for occupational therapy practitioners as judged by the number of questions received by AOTA. The moral distress felt by practitioners when their ethical principles are challenged appears to be so significant that the EC presented its "Everyday Ethics" workshop at AOTA's 2008 Annual Conference & Expo on just that topic. The EC wanted to explore moral distress more broadly among the Association's members and to look at whether similar concerns and outcomes exist for members of other professions. In preparation for their Conference presentation, the EC developed a survey to identify major causes of moral distress and how these causes may influence a practitioner's clinical practice and psychosocial well-being. Questions were formulated by analyzing ethics-based inquiries to the EC staff liaison, as well as by reviewing sources of moral distress identified in the nursing literature. The survey was distributed to AOTA members via the Special Interest Section listservs and other Association publications for 1 month in spring 2008, before the Conference.

Although this was not a random sample, there were more than 100 responses, far more than expected, and consistent themes clearly emerged from those who chose to respond. In fact, the survey results confirmed that the issues that prompt practitioners to contact the EC represent those that most frequently arise in the workplace. For example, in response to the survey question "As an occupational therapist or an occupational therapy assistant, have you experienced distress related to any of the following issues?" the strongest responses (more than half the respondents, combining "commonly" and "occasionally") were to such items as

- Reimbursement constraints (70%)
- Conflict with organizational policies (70%)
- Excessive pressure to meet productivity standards (61%)
- Lack of administrative support (59%)
- Questionable or unrealistic clinical decisions by others (57%)
- Patients who decline treatment (57%)
- Decision making regarding patient discharge (55%)
- Excessive pressure to increase billable hours (54%)
- Compromised care due to pressure to decrease costs (53%).

Not surprisingly, the survey results indicated that sources of moral distress among occupational therapy practitioners were most closely related to external factors. External factors are often market-based, such as the pressure to do more with less, a lack of resources, and increased productivity standards. Occupational therapy is often provided in settings that depend on delivery of services as a source of revenue. Therefore, practitioners may experience moral distress from the same sources that have been linked to distress in physicians. According to Walter Davis, MD, physicians may become "morally distressed when institutional or third-party payer pressures to contain or reduce costs seem to compromise patient care" (quoted in Hamric et al., 2006, p. 21).

Other professionals, such as nurses, may feel financial pressure indirectly; however, occupational therapy practitioners, like physicians, may be more apt to experience this pressure directly as they personally deal with payment for their services. Other external sources of moral distress related to organizational policies and differing professional opinions affect occupational therapy practitioners because practitioners are often required to deliver care in a team environment, within a system, and in many cases through physician referral.

These externally based factors mirror the queries received by the AOTA EC staff liaison. An overarching theme is the use of reimbursement considerations to override clinical judgment about the quantity and type of therapy intervention the client actually needs in order to address occupational performance deficits and goals. From an ethical perspective, it is easy to see how reimbursement considerations can place practitioners in untenable situations when their primary concern—providing only what the client needs (Principle 1, Beneficence, of the *Occupational Therapy Code of Ethics and Ethics Standards [2010]*, referred to as the "Code and Ethics Standards"; AOTA, 2010)—is overshadowed by more lucrative intervention models. Reimbursement considerations can translate to inappropriate or too-frequent group intervention when one-on-one therapy may be indicated. They can impede appropriate discharge from services when goals have been met or clients can no longer make therapeutic progress. They can also lead to potentially fraudulent documentation and billing as practitioners try to reconcile clinical status with service delivery models that support administrative directives. Maximizing reimbursement wherever feasible in a tight health care environment is essential for the organization to survive. However, doing so can also put practitioners in a position where they not only feel ethical angst, but also may actually be noncompliant with external regulatory standards. Practitioners must become familiar with applicable local, state, and federal laws so

they do not jeopardize their license and ability to practice, as reflected in Principle 5, Procedural Justice, of the Code and Ethics Standards.

The effect of these organizational issues on occupational therapy practitioners can be significant. Members who contact AOTA with such dilemmas are clearly troubled, and some eventually resign from a job that provoked a daily struggle to maintain ethical and legal practice. In response to the survey question "When you have experienced distress, has it resulted in any of the following outcomes?" 38% (combined responses of "commonly" and "occasionally") stated that they had resigned from their position. Among the responders, 62% were at least exploring other employment opportunities, and 33% had contemplated leaving the field. These statistics speak to the long-term, potentially negative implications of moral distress. In 56% of the responses, practitioners also identified fragmented client care as a result of organizational issues. Painful feelings, such as guilt, anger, and depression, were expressed by 53% of the respondents, and 60% identified perpetuation of power imbalances as additional negative outcomes.

The results of the occupational therapy survey mirror the negative consequences associated with moral distress in nursing practice, ranging from fragmented care, to inappropriate use of resources, to a shrinking professional pool (Gutierrez, 2005; Hamric et al., 2006; Peter & Liaschenko, 2004; Redman & Fry, 2000; Sundin-Huard & Fahy, 1999). Moral distress has even been identified as potentially the "most pervasive and pressing problem in academic health care," seriously threatening the practitioner's moral integrity (Hamric et al., 2006). And although it has been "argued that moral distress has a pervasive quality intrinsically connected to health care practice" (Austin, Lemermeyer, Goldberg, Bergum, & Johnson, 2005, p. 39), it is important to recognize that as a result of this connection there is a vast and substantial literature exploring strategies for reducing moral distress and the negative consequences associated with this phenomenon (Austin et al., 2005; Erlen, 2001; Gutierrez, 2005; Hamric et al., 2006).

Strategies for Addressing Moral Distress

Although moral distress may be an inevitable byproduct of health care work, there are strategies that all occupational therapy practitioners can use to limit the negative consequences and feelings of powerlessness. These strategies, which are addressed below, include recognizing moral distress, implementing educational strategies, facilitating interdisciplinary research, improving communication, creating healthy organizational work environments, and promoting ethical leadership.

Recognize Moral Distress

First and foremost, it is necessary to recognize and identify moral distress when it occurs. Recognizing that moral distress is prevalent within occupational therapy practice makes it easier to identify. Those who demonstrate increased moral sensitivity and a reliance on relationships may be particularly prone to experiencing moral distress (Austin et al., 2005). Moral distress can be especially problematic for occupational therapy practitioners who use relationship building as a cornerstone of practice by establishing rapport with their clients. Moral distress can manifest itself as "physical, emotional, psychological, and cognitive symptoms; these symptoms can originate from different situations and occur through different processes" (Austin et al., 2005, p. 36), making them sometimes difficult to recognize.

It is important to understand that context will influence whether common sources of moral distress result in associated negative outcomes. For example, an occupational therapist may encounter moral distress when reimbursement constraints prevent a client from receiving needed services. However, the same occupational therapist may not feel moral distress if he or she knows that the client has another way to obtain treatment; the distress is variable depending on the context and the outcome of the conflict. Therefore, identifying sources of moral distress in the delivery of occupational therapy services is important, but it is only one aspect of this phenomenon in practice.

Implement Educational Strategies

Because personal and professional values are often developed before one's initiation into clinical practice, Gutierrez (2005) encouraged dialogue among medical and nursing students in academic settings to encourage collaboration and communication before entering the workforce. This concept should be applied to all health professions, including occupational therapy. Academic programs need to reflect the diverse environments in which occupational therapy practitioners actually work. When students are educated in integrated settings, they are more able to adequately engage in professional dialogue outside of an academic environment. Similarly, it is easy to criticize physicians and other health care professionals for lack of referrals or for not understanding occupational therapy practice, but when these professionals have not been educated on the role of occupational therapy, it is difficult to place blame. Strategies for communication need to originate in educational settings, where health care professionals are socialized (Austin et al., 2005). By encouraging collaboration and ethical dialogue across disciplines in academic settings, a precedent is set for ongoing integration of services in the health care environment.

Facilitate Interdisciplinary Research

Collaboration among disciplines can be extended to address the need for interdisciplinary research with regard to ethical conflict. Moral distress research has revealed that "all members of the health care team can benefit from a more in-depth understanding of moral distress" (Austin et al., 2005, p. 44); however, moral distress among occupational therapy practitioners has not been sufficiently explored in the interdisciplinary research. As long as the interdisciplinary team not only experiences moral distress but also acts as a potential source of it, research must be integrated in order to truly affect outcomes related to this phenomenon.

Improve Communication

Communication continues to be the underlying factor in decreasing negative consequences associated with moral distress: "Improving communication between the patient, family, and health care team would aid collaboration between practitioners and provide support for [providers] to voice and implement moral judgment" (Gutierrez, 2005, p. 238). Encouraging open dialogue facilitates a safe context for voicing moral discord between providers and also between providers and administrators (Gutierrez, 2005). In addition, if families and clients are involved in this open dialogue, different value sets can be explored. The health care provider's values may still differ from those of the family, but understanding why a family or client is making a certain choice, and having the opportunity to voice concerns or differences of opinion in a respectful way, can substantially decrease the antagonism and frustration associated with moral distress. Divergent opinions may still exist, but the harmful feelings associated with moral distress are less likely to occur.

Create a Healthy Work Environment

Healthy organizational work environments are imperative for making ethical decisions and reducing negative outcomes associated with moral distress. Although communication is arguably the most important strategy for addressing issues of moral distress, increased communication will occur only when organizational decision making provides support for it: "Efforts at high administrative levels to analyze and improve existing decision making and communication systems may assist in increasing communication and collaboration"

(Gutierrez, 2005, p. 239). Unfortunately, transparency in communication is not always embraced within health care organizations. Some administrators have yet to shed a "'blame and shame' approach to dealing with serious issues; transparency can't happen without culture change," and "transformation in health care won't happen without transparency" (GE Healthcare, 2005, p. 6). Open and respectful dialogue cannot occur when the parties are not aware of the ground rules for providing care and are unable to accurately present all options to clients and families.

Providers must be able to openly explain policy-related limitations to clients and offer other options for care. For example, occupational therapy practitioners understand that they cannot discontinue treatment on the basis of the client's inability to pay without exploring other options. However, organizational constraints may affect the way in which services are provided, such as availability of free care, payment scheduling, charity care (reduced rates, etc.), bill write-off, and alternative care options. When possible, therapists should offer to continue providing services on an out-of-pocket basis, or, if there is potential for alternate funding sources, they should work with the client to explore these. Therapists should also be familiar with organizational processes that will affect the cost of treatment and refer clients to the institution's financial services department to determine whether charity care or discounted rates are available. Practitioners should also explore whether there are other community services that can meet the needs of that client, including pro bono clinics in the area.

Work environments are also influenced by the providers themselves, who can personally ensure ethical delivery of care, thereby promoting an ethical work environment. If health care providers demand healthy work environments and consistently choose organizations that support best practice, organizations will facilitate an institutional culture that works to alleviate the negative outcomes associated with moral distress and other ethical conflicts.

Promote Ethical Leadership

Closely tied to healthy work environments is ethical leadership. Leaders must understand the benefits of a healthy work environment and promote a culture that not only espouses the importance of ethical, quality-driven health care, but also implements policies that support high standards, even in difficult situations. Ethical occupational therapy leaders and managers have to advocate for appropriate staffing. To be successful in this effort, they must make a case for additional clinicians based on clinical outcomes and the needs of the clients. It is also the manager's responsibility to understand organizational culture and how occupational therapy services will be most supported within that culture and mission.

For example, administrators in an acute care facility may want to limit the number of occupational therapy staff to keep the salary budget down. However, if an occupational therapy manager can demonstrate that by increasing occupational therapy intervention patient length of stay can be reduced, and that these reduced days more than offset the salaries of the additional staff, there is a greater likelihood that staffing requests will be supported. Simply by increasing occupational therapy staffing, one can potentially have a positive impact on clinical outcomes, client satisfaction, physician satisfaction, and the organization's profit margin, all of which will work toward decreasing moral distress. Leaders in occupational therapy must also recognize their role within the context of where services are provided. Learning to effectively speak the language to advocate for healthy work environments and improved client outcomes is a critical management responsibility.

Conclusion

Practitioners who are in ethically challenging work environments face difficult decisions. Even when a practitioner has tried to decrease sources of moral distress and implemented strategies as outlined in the literature, difficult choices regarding employment and organizational fit may continue to persist. Ultimately, the practitioner may be faced with very personal decisions based on values, circumstances, ability to promote change within the system, and so forth. Practitioners should seek assistance in analyzing and exploring options to address ethical dilemmas that cause moral distress and ultimately affect our primary responsibility, which is to provide individualized, beneficial care to our clients.

References

American Occupational Therapy Association. (2010). Occupational therapy code of ethics and ethics standards (2010). *American Journal of Occupational Therapy, 64*(6 Suppl.), S17–S26. doi:10.5014/ajot.2010.64S17

American Occupational Therapy Association. (n.d.). *Everyday ethics: Core knowledge for occupational therapy practitioners and educators* [CE on CD]. Bethesda, MD: Author.

Austin, W., Lemermeyer, G., Goldberg, L., Bergum, V., & Johnson, M. (2005). Moral distress in healthcare practice: The situation of nurses. *HEC Forum, 17*(1), 33–48.

Brandt, L. C. (2007). AOTA Ethics Commission advisory opinion: Organizational ethics. *OT Practice, 12*(21), 15–19.

Erlen, J. A. (2001). Moral distress: A pervasive problem. *Orthopaedic Nursing, 20*(2), 76–80.

GE Healthcare. (2005). *Establishing a framework for organizational transformation in healthcare: Performance solutions.* Waukesha, WI: General Electric Company.

Gutierrez, K. M. (2005). Critical care nurses' perceptions of and response to moral distress. *Dimensions of Critical Care Nursing, 24*(5), 229–241.

Hamric, A. B., Davis, W. S., & Day Childress, M. (2006, Winter). Moral distress in health care professionals: What is it and what can we do about it? *The Pharos, 69,* 16–23.

Jameton, A. (1984). *Nursing practice: The ethical issues.* Englewood Cliffs, NJ: Prentice Hall.

Peter, E., & Liaschenko, J. (2004). Perils of proximity: A spatiotemporal analysis of moral distress and moral ambiguity. *Nursing Inquiry, 11*(4), 218–225.

Redman, B. K., & Fry, S. T. (2000). Nurses' ethical conflicts: What is really known about them? *Nursing Ethics, 7*, 361–366.

Sundin-Huard, D., & Fahy, K. (1999). Moral distress, advocacy and burnout: Theorising the relationships. *International Journal of Nursing Practice, 5*, 8–13.

ADDITIONAL RESOURCES

American Occupational Therapy Association. (n.d.). *Everyday ethics: Core knowledge for occupational therapy practitioners and educators* [CE on CD]. Bethesda, MD: Author.

Purtilo, R. B., Jensen, G. M., & Royeen, C. B. (2005). *Educating for moral action: A sourcebook in health and rehabilitation ethics.* Philadelphia: F. A. Davis.

Deborah Yarett Slater, MS, OT/L, FAOTA
Staff Liaison to the AOTA Ethics Commission

Lea Cheyney Brandt, OTD, MA, OTR/L
Program Director, University of Missouri School of Health Professions
Member at Large, Ethics Commission (2005–2008, 2008–2011)

CHAPTER 20

Ethics and Research: An Annotated Bibliography

RESPONSIBLE CONDUCT IN RESEARCH

Office of Research Integrity. (2007). *Guidelines for responsible conduct of research.* **Retrieved January 4, 2011, from http://www.pitt.edu/~provost/ethresearch.html#_Toc153961821**

These guidelines will help beginning and experienced investigators in the social and behavioral sciences follow ethical standards and avoid research misconduct. *Research misconduct* includes fabrication, falsification, or plagiarism, including misrepresentation of credentials, in proposing or performing research or reviewing or reporting results. Topics covered include order of authorship, storage and retention of data, and conflict of interest.

National Academy of Sciences, National Academy of Engineering, and Institute of Medicine. (2009). *On being a scientist: A guide to responsible conduct in research* **(3rd ed.). Washington, DC: National Academies Press.**

On Being a Scientist supplements the informal lessons in ethics provided by research mentors and thus is particularly useful to graduate students and junior investigators. Applicable to all forms of research, the book describes the ethical foundations of scientific practices and includes hypothetical scenarios and discussion providing guidance in ethical reasoning. Topics include sharing of research results, intellectual property, authorship and the allocation of credit, and the researcher's role in influencing society's health.

AUTHORSHIP

Authorship order reflects the effort and roles of the researchers. Many associations and journals list specific criteria for authorship. It is generally expected that each author has participated in the study process and writing of the paper. In fact, many journals require a signed statement from authors attesting that they have substantially contributed to the manuscript and/or approve it. Ideally, authorship should be agreed upon by all at the outset, preferably in writing. If everyone has worked equally, then a common approach is to list the authors alphabetically with the advisor being listed at the end.

HUMAN PARTICIPANTS

Practical Ethics Center, University of Montana. (2003). *Online research ethics course.* **Retrieved January 4, 2011, from http://ori.dhhs.gov/education/products/montana_round1/human.html**

This section of the ethics course reviews the history of using human subjects and the evolution of standards. Discussion addresses the importance of obtaining informed consent, avoiding coercion, obtaining approval from institutional review boards, protecting confidentiality, and considering special groups as participants (e.g., women, racial minority groups).

Bioethics Resources on the Web. (2007). *Human subjects research and IRBs.* **Retrieved January 4, 2011, from http://bioethics.od.nih.gov/IRB.html**

This Web site has many links to and examples of resources on using human subjects for research. It also covers the issues to consider when obtaining informed consent from children or from participants who have intellectual limitations.

WRITING

Office of Research Integrity, U.S. Department of Health and Human Services. (2009). *Avoiding plagiarism, self-plagiarism, and other questionable writing practices: A guide to ethical writing.* **Retrieved January 4, 2011, from http://ori.dhhs.gov/education/products/plagiarism/**

This self-paced module covers important topics such as appropriate paraphrasing, copyright law, appropriate citing of sources, and selective reporting of literature, methodology, or results. Other modules related to research misconduct are also available.

INTELLECTUAL PROPERTY RIGHTS

University of Ottawa. (2009). *Research ethics.* **Retrieved January 4, 2011, from http://www.grad.uottawa.ca/default.aspx?tabid=1388**

This Web site briefly describes intellectual property rights and implications for revenue sharing and publishing.

ETHICS TRAINING

National Institutes of Health. (2009). *Introduction to the responsible conduct of research.* **Retrieved January 4, 2011, from http://researchethics.od.nih.gov/CourseIndex.aspx**

This training module allows those who are not on the National Institutes of Health staff to browse through slides and topics covering scientific integrity, data management, publication and authorship, and conflict of interest. It also covers social issues related to research such as the mentor–trainee relationship and collaborative science.

Susan H. Lin, ScD, OTR/L
AOTA Director of Research

CHAPTER 21

Before You Sign on the Dotted Line

Thinking about contracting with a managed care company or vendor? Read this first—learn what you should know before you enter into any contract. Although the contents of this *Reference Guide* are focused on providing ethical guidance to address diverse situations that may occur in the student, educator, practitioner, and researcher roles, a number of alleged ethics complaints also stem from contract disputes. Contracts are legal documents, and these types of complaints reflect the intersection of ethical and legal issues. Therefore, information in this chapter is provided to assist the reader in understanding these separate but related issues.

How many times have you signed a contract or negotiated an agreement without really understanding, or perhaps even carefully reading, the contract's terms? If you are like many people, you may enter into contractual relationships without fully appreciating all the possible ramifications of quickly signing on the dotted line—ramifications that can be expensive and potentially damaging to both your career and your finances.

Whether you are about to sign a contract with a vendor, a managed care company, or anyone else, the first thing to remember is that the written contract you are asked to sign is most often drafted by the company's lawyers with that company's interest in mind, not yours. If you automatically sign without understanding the contract and obtaining the proper advice, you may be agreeing to terms that you will later regret.

One obvious way to avoid an unfavorable contract is to hire your own attorney to review the contract and, if necessary, negotiate its terms with the company. Of course, this will entail some expense on your part, but signing a bad contract could end up costing you much more in the long run.

Another thing to remember about contracts is that the laws governing the interpretation and implementation of contracts vary from state to state. It is important, therefore, that the lawyer reviewing your contract be familiar with the applicable state law.

Read what you are signing. This sounds elementary, but even if you are a sole practitioner signing a contract that has been drafted by a large company, you need to know and understand the terms to which you will be bound by the contract. In fact, by signing the agreement, the law generally assumes that you have read it and agreed with its terms.

There are certain terms that appear in various contracts but still may be unfamiliar to many occupational therapy practitioners. The laws of the various states may differ on the interpretation of these terms, however, so readers are cautioned to seek advice from an attorney in their state regarding how these terms would likely be applied to their particular contracts. A sampling of these contract terms are provided below.

Indemnification or Hold-Harmless Clause

Signing an indemnification or hold-harmless clause may make you responsible for paying another party's portion of damages and/or attorney's fees awarded in a subsequent legal action by another party. Imagine, for example, that a managed care company and a hospital are both sued for their decision in credentialing certain physician providers. If the contract between the two calls for the hospital to indemnify the managed care company, the hospital may be required to foot the entire bill, even though the managed care company shares some of the responsibility. Clearly, the financial consequences of signing a contract with an indemnification or hold-harmless clause can be significant. And your own insurer may refuse to cover those expenses. Many insurance companies expressly exclude coverage for claims that are contractually assumed, such as those arising through indemnification or hold-harmless agreements. An attorney reviewing these clauses as part of a contract will be better able to assess their scope and validity and advise you as to whether it is in your interest to agree to them. An attorney will also be able to explain the risk involved if you do.

Dispute Resolution

Many contracts spell out how a dispute between contracting parties will be resolved—not only where the dispute would be heard but also the law that would apply. These clauses are not as innocuous as they initially seem.

A choice of law clause establishes that the law of a certain state will apply to the interpretation and implementation of the contract. Does that really matter? It could. Suppose you are contracting with a company based in New Hampshire, but you live in Montana. If the contract calls for New Hampshire law to be applied, you could find yourself having to find a lawyer who knows New Hampshire state law if a contract dispute arises.

A choice of forum or forum selection clause sets out where a dispute will be heard. Using the above example, if the contract also contains a New Hampshire choice of forum clause, the Montana therapist could end up having to travel to New Hampshire to litigate a dispute.

A contract might also contain an arbitration clause that requires disputes to be brought to arbitration rather than to court. This type of clause could bar an occupational therapy practitioner from going to court, and if the practitioner files a court action, it could be dismissed in favor of arbitration. The decision of the arbitrators also may be binding on the parties, leaving little room for subsequent appeals to the court.

Termination and Renewal

In certain contracts, such as managed care contracts, the life span of the contract may be set forth in writing. If so, the terms should be tailored to the needs of the contracting parties— that is where the advice and assistance of an attorney can be invaluable when drafting the contract. You don't want to be in the position of losing money on the contract without any recourse.

Some contracts call for automatic renewal if notice of cancellation is not given, requiring some close monitoring of the dates by the practitioner. Also, the contract may specify the ways the contract can be terminated by the parties with or without cause. These provisions should be reviewed by an attorney to ensure that they are fair to the practitioner and conform to local state law.

Compensation

Managed care contracts can contain a variety of different payment structures—fee for service, discounted fee for service, capitation, per diem, and per case structures. Each of these carries varying degrees of risk to the practitioner. They should be carefully reviewed before the contract is signed to ensure that the payment terms make financial sense to the practitioner. Some managed care company contracts allow the company to change the payment rate from time to time. Again, an attorney reviewing the contract may be able to negotiate terms that define or control the circumstances under which the company may make changes to protect your interests.

Occupational therapy practitioners who treat clients covered by Medicare and Medicaid have another issue for concern—complying with the federal fraud and abuse provisions, which include the Federal Anti-Kickback Law, the False Claims Act, and the Federal Physician Self-Referral Laws (Stark); the latter was expressly made applicable to occupational therapy practitioners as of January 1995. Under the federal fraud and abuse provisions, occupational therapy practitioners may be both civilly and criminally liable for, among other things, making false claims or statements for any benefits or accepting or offering kickbacks or rebates in return for obtaining a referral, service, or item to be paid by Medicare, Medicaid, or any other federal health care program. Referrals to practices in which the health care practitioner has an interest are also prohibited. The penalties for violating these laws include civil monetary fines, criminal penalties, and exclusion from participation in Medicare and Medicaid.

There are some so-called safe harbors built into the fraud and abuse provisions. The interpretation and application of the safe harbors, however, are complicated. The consequence of an incorrect analysis could be significant liability. Therefore, contracts in which Medicare and Medicaid funds may be expended, including managed care contracts and contracts with vendors, should be carefully reviewed by an attorney for adherence to those laws.

INTEGRATION CLAUSES

Integration clauses generally state that the written terms of the contract reflect the full and final agreement between the parties. If you discussed certain terms before the contract was signed and they don't show up in the written contract, those terms may not be considered part of the agreement. A court may not even allow you to present evidence of those discussions should a dispute arise.

Make sure that the contract includes all of the terms of the agreement. If the contract lists certain exhibits or describes separate documents, be sure to have read and consented to the terms in those documents. Many contracts also contain clauses that limit or bar subsequent modifications to the contract, making it important to ensure that the contract fully reflects your agreement.

These are just a few of the many contract terms that can surprise the unwary occupational therapy practitioner. Contracts can contain other terms of equal importance that require the same level of scrutiny. Seek appropriate advice, and know what you are agreeing to before you sign any contract.

Rita Burghardt, OTR, JD
Attorney, Piper & Marbury, LLP, New York

Leslie Stein Lloyd, Esq.
AOTA Regulatory Counsel

Copyright © 1996, by the American Occupational Therapy Association. This chapter was originally published in *OT Week*, June 20, 1996, pp. 12–13. It has been revised to reflect updated AOTA official documents, Web sites, AOTA style, and additional resources. Rita Burghardt thanks Lisa Taylor, Esq., for her assistance with this article.

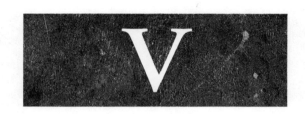

ADVISORY OPINIONS

CHAPTER 22

Balancing Patient Rights and Practitioner Values

INTRODUCTION

Clinical reasoning in occupational therapy involves art, science, and ethics, according to Joan Rogers (1983). The relationship between rights and duties is one of the ethical issues that may arise in clinical practice. The art and science of care delivered by occupational therapy personnel relate directly to the correlation between rights and duties. The rights of a person who presents for intervention should be met with a trained practitioner's duty to provide care that benefits that individual.

The following question is raised: Do circumstances exist whereby occupational therapy personnel can ethically refrain from providing services? Although there is an overarching professional duty to provide benefit to clients, there may be unsafe situations in which the practitioner may ethically refrain from providing service. In addition, the practitioner may feel unsafe due to a significant difference of personal values that impedes therapeutic interaction. Some argue that there are situations in which the practitioner's moral duty or personal values will outweigh the patient's right to receive services. However, in a diverse society, ideas of right and wrong vary as much as the individuals themselves.

It is increasingly difficult to identify what constitutes an ethical right of conscience in health care and the limits of decisions based on conscience (Stein, 2006). Although some may agree with the provider's right to refrain from care in scenarios in which the practitioner has a personal moral conflict with a patient, moral consensus as to the provider's rights versus responsibilities has not been reached. Therefore, the practitioner must be prudent and diligent in differentiating between a conflict of values and a truly unsafe environment in order to obtain a balance with the rights of the patient.

Many occupational therapy practitioners have experienced working with difficult patients who are uncooperative, appear to lack motivation, or are in some way repugnant. This may be manifested by harsh and inappropriate language spoken during the therapy session or complete unresponsiveness. A homebound patient unable to perform daily hygiene activities or who does not have anyone responsible for overseeing such basic needs as nutrition and cleansing may become offensive to the practitioner. In these situations it is important to separate personal feelings of aversion from the treatment protocol and to deliver the prescribed care.

Occupational therapy practitioners must acknowledge the dignity of patients regardless of their unpleasant nature or condition. Within the boundaries of the provider–patient relationship, the continuation of care is essential in upholding the ethical guidelines of patient autonomy and beneficence. In other words, patients have choices about personal behaviors and are entitled to receive the benefit of services and care. However, if environmental conditions exist that truly jeopardize the practitioner's safety, he or she has the right to refrain from providing services in that context.

CASE SCENARIOS

Scenario 1: Conflict of Values

Keisha, an occupational therapist working in home care, meets her new patient, Rafaella, who recently had a hip replacement as a result of long-standing rheumatoid arthritis. Rafaella is currently estranged from her husband, who has been abusive in the past. On the second visit, the therapist notices a large bruise on her neck, which Rafaella has attempted to cover up with a scarf. The therapist inquires as to how she got bruised, and Rafaella responds that she fell out of bed, but she seems withdrawn and does not make eye contact while speaking. The therapist is concerned about the situation and suspects abuse.

As Keisha continues to treat Rafaella, they establish a therapeutic relationship, and Rafaella discloses that her husband continues to stop by when he is intoxicated and can become physically abusive. Keisha encourages Rafaella to file a police report and get a restraining order. Rafaella adamantly refuses this advice, stating that she still loves her husband and would not want to get him into trouble. The occupational therapist questions her ability to continue treating Rafaella because she does not feel that she can support Rafaella's choice to remain in an abusive relationship.

Scenario 2: Unsafe Environment

One day, while Keisha is treating Rafaella, her estranged husband arrives with alcohol on his breath, is verbally abusive, and staggers around the house. Keisha notices a gun in his waistband. The husband confronts Keisha and orders her to leave, yelling that he will shoot if she returns. Keisha feels that she cannot continue to treat Rafaella in her home because she fears for her own safety. Keisha also fears for Rafaella, but she feels she has done all she can to encourage Rafaella to seek assistance from the police.

DISCUSSION

Although both of these scenarios portray a situation in which the provider, Keisha, questions her duty to continue treating Rafaella, her professional ethics may require her to act differently based on the circumstances at hand. The moral dilemma facing Keisha stems from conflicts between the client's and the professional's autonomy and from Keisha's obligation of beneficence. Respect for an individual's autonomy, or the right to make his or her own decisions (self-determination), has historically pervaded the field of ethics. Respect for the client's autonomy requires the practitioner to acknowledge the individual as a moral agent and to recognize the client's "right to hold views, to make choices, and to take actions based on personal values and beliefs" (Beauchamp & Childress, 2009, p. 103). The overriding question is, How far does this right extend? Does respect for client autonomy require the practitioner to place himself or herself in a situation in which he or she is in danger? Although patient autonomy plays a significant role in the ethical delineation of services, according to Fleming (2005), "a successful and ethically grounded [provider]–patient relationship presumes respect for autonomy, bolstered by good communication and shared decision-making that requires careful balancing of the values and beliefs of both participants" (p. 263). Neither scenario supports abandonment of the patient; instead, both scenarios call for communication and decision making, as described by Fleming.

Following this line of thinking, in Scenario 1 Keisha needs to work with Rafaella to facilitate a safe environment. However, if Rafaella does not ultimately agree to Keisha's involvement in changing her environment, according to Principle 3 of the *Occupational Therapy Code of Ethics and Ethics Standards (2010)* (referred to as the "Code and Ethics Standards"; AOTA, 2010), occupational therapy personnel are required to "respect the right of the individual to self-determination." Moral objections to a person's life or lifestyle would not warrant discontinuation of services. Therefore, Keisha must respect Rafaella's autonomy and does not have an ethical right to refrain from providing services based on her moral objections regarding Rafaella's decision. However, if there is a law that requires a health care practitioner to report abuse (e.g., of children or elderly clients), then the occupational therapy practitioner must do so regardless of the autonomy principle.

Scenario 2 also calls for shared decision making between the client and the provider. However, Keisha can ethically remove herself from the immediate situation, which violates her own rights as a provider. Keisha is not ethically required to subject herself to danger in order to serve her clients. However, Keisha does have an extended responsibility to acknowledge their provider–patient relationship and thus work with Rafaella to find a safe place in which to continue therapy services. This extended responsibility of the provider is supported through Principle 1, Beneficence, of the Code and Ethics Standards, which requires occupational therapy personnel to "demonstrate a concern for the well-being and safety of the recipients of their services." In addition, Principle 4E requires the practitioner to "make efforts to advocate for recipients of occupational therapy services to obtain needed services through available means." Again, through shared decision making and communication, Keisha should partner with Rafaella to ensure access to services in the safest environment available.

SUMMARY AND CONCLUSION

The actions of a practitioner must benefit the health of the patient in addition to acknowledging the autonomy of the patient as established by his or her right to be informed, privacy, and confidentiality. The recipient of occupational therapy services has duties, and the provider has rights that affect the therapeutic relationship. For example, the recipient has the duty to arrive on time for therapy,

follow through with intervention plans, and pay for services rendered. Occupational therapy personnel have the right to work in safe environments and in clinical settings that support the ethical nature of their role with clients.

Given these parameters, when questions arise regarding rights versus responsibilities of the provider, one must thoughtfully determine which justifiable course of action to take. Practitioners must be grounded not only by a moral conscience to do what is right, but also by the courage to proceed and ensure the best interests of the patient. This may require occupational therapy personnel to apply a framework of ethical decision making. Such action highlights the specific details of the case, assessment of the patient's condition, and determination of realistic alternatives for intervention, if needed. Therapeutic interventions should be interrupted only after all potential avenues to continue care have been exhausted. Acknowledging these moral obligations within the provider–patient relationship clearly delineates the role of occupational therapy personnel.

REFERENCES

American Occupational Therapy Association. (2010). Occupational therapy code of ethics and ethics standards (2010). *American Journal of Occupational Therapy, 64*(6 Suppl.), S17–S26. doi:10.5014/ajot.2010.64S17

Beauchamp, T. L., & Childress, J. F. (2009). *Principles of biomedical ethics* (6th ed.). New York: Oxford University Press.

Fleming, D. A. (2005). Futility: Revisiting a concept of shared moral judgment. *HEC Forum, 17*(4), 260–275.

Rogers, J. C. (1983). Clinical reasoning: The ethics, science, and art (Eleanor Clarke Slagle Lecture). *American Journal of Occupational Therapy, 37,* 601–616.

Stein, R. (2006, July 16). A medical crisis of conscience: Faith drives some to refuse patients medication or care. *Washington Post,* p. A01.

Lea Cheyney Brandt, OTD, OTR/L
Member at Large, Ethics Commission
(2005–2008, 2008–2011)

Donna F. Homenko, PhD, RDH
Public Member, Ethics Commission
(2005–2009)

This chapter was originally published in the 2008 edition of the *Reference Guide to the Occupational Therapy Ethics Standards*. It has been revised to reflect updated AOTA official documents, Web sites, AOTA style, and additional resources.

CHAPTER 23

Cultural Competency and Ethical Practice

VIGNETTE 1

Joan, a pediatric therapist, is asked to make a home visit to a Vietnamese child who was recently burned. On examination of the child, she notes red, round, coin-sized marks over the child's back. She never asks the mother about the marks. After leaving the home, Joan wonders if the mother is using a traditional healing treatment. She asks herself, "How can I give this child ethical and quality care while allowing the mother to continue with this harmful practice?"

INTRODUCTION

People face problems, dilemmas, and issues with ethical significance that necessitate action or nonaction every day. Doing the right thing in practice is always a challenge. In an increasingly pluralistic society, health care providers are finding themselves confronting choices that may depend more on moral and ethical values than on medical knowledge. Joan's dilemma is not a question of what intervention method she should use, but whether she can provide quality ethical care. Culturally competent practitioners realize that behaviors are shaped and defined differently by every culture. Rather than being distressed by another culture's health practice, a culturally competent practitioner welcomes collaboration and cooperation in making sound ethical decisions.

This advisory opinion outlines and discusses the provisions within the most recent version of

Occupational Therapy Code of Ethics and Ethics Standards (2010) (referred to as the "Code and Ethics Standards"; American Occupational Therapy Association [AOTA], 2010) that address culturally competent services. Vignettes are presented to demonstrate the range of ethical concerns that cultural encounters can generate. This advisory opinion was developed to provide guidance to the AOTA membership so that they can provide ethically and culturally appropriate services to all populations while recognizing their own cultural or linguistic background or life experience and that of their clients, colleagues, or students.

CULTURAL COMPETENCE

Cultural competence is a journey, rather than an end. It refers to the process of actively developing and practicing appropriate, relevant, and sensitive strategies and skills in interacting with culturally different persons (AOTA, 1995). It is a set of congruent behaviors, attitudes, and policies that come together in a system or agency or among professionals and enable that system or agency or those professionals to work effectively in cross-cultural situations (Cross, Bazron, Dennis, & Isaacs, 1989). Cultural competence entails

> understanding the importance of social and cultural influences on patients' health beliefs and behaviors; considering how these factors interact at multiple levels of the health care delivery system; and fi-

nally, devising interventions that take these issues into account to assure quality health care delivery to diverse patient populations. (Betancourt, Green, Carrillo, & Ananeh-Firempong, 2003, p. 297)

Clinically, cultural competence means having the self-awareness, knowledge, skills, and framework to make sound, ethical, and culturally appropriate decisions. It is the integration and transformation of knowledge about individuals and groups of people into specific standards, policies, practices, and attitudes used in appropriate cultural settings to increase the quality of services, thereby producing better outcomes (Davis & Donald, 1997). In Vignette 2 below, the therapist does not take into account the socioeconomic level, living environment, or culture of Mrs. Jones before training her to use a variety of adaptive equipment. A culturally competent practitioner is not afraid to ask the client culturally pertinent questions up front.

Competence in practice means learning new patterns of behaviors and effectively applying them in appropriate settings. Examples include the following (Wells & Black, 2000):

- Involving the extended family in the intervention process
- Addressing elderly persons more formally (by their last name and title) than younger clients
- Acknowledging and working with traditional and/or faith healers
- Being cautious about touching
- Engaging in small talk at the beginning of a session, which is considered good manners and keeps one from appearing rushed
- Conducting the session in the preferred language of the client or arranging for a professional interpreter
- Adding culturally related questions during the evaluation process.

Cultural competence is key to effective therapeutic interactions and outcomes. It implies a heightened consciousness of how clients experience their uniqueness and deal with their differences and similarities within a larger social context. It enhances the occupational therapy provider's knowledge of the relationship between sociocultural factors and health beliefs and behaviors. It equips providers with the tools and skills to manage these factors appropriately, with quality occupational therapy delivery as the gold standard. Cultural competence is an evolving and developing process that depends on self-exploration, knowledge, and skills.

VIGNETTE 2

Mrs. Jones is in her mid-60s and of Hispanic ethnicity. She is dependent for her existence on food stamps and Supplemental Security Income benefits. Somewhat hard of hearing, she has a slight tremor in her voice and arthritis in her hands. The three-bedroom house in which she lives is in poor condition and is unkempt. For meals she relies on her neighbors and junk food.

Mrs. Jones is admitted to the rehabilitation unit after experiencing a mild stroke that leaves her impaired on the right side. Her treatment sessions consist of transfer training, learning one-handed cooking, and dressing with adaptive equipment. A variety of equipment and devices are recommended and ordered for her. At the discharge planning session, the occupational therapist states in her report, "Mrs. Jones has refused all the equipment even though she is able to use it safely and properly."

ETHICAL CONFLICTS

Several Western bioethical principles and concepts may be in opposition to certain values and beliefs of other cultures, presenting ethical conflicts and dilemmas. Culture affects many therapist–client interactions, but the participants may not perceive the interactions as culturally or ethically related. Western bioethics places the self at the center of all decision making (autonomy). However, many cultures place the family, community, or society above the rights of the individual. The disclosing (truth-telling) of a diagnosis of serious illness or disability to the client is not universally accepted. Many believe that the family, not the client, should make important health care decisions. Some people believe that health is maintained and restored through positive language. When disclosing risks of a treatment or approach, health care providers speak in a negative way (informed consent). Questions of race, ethnicity, and cultural beliefs are part of the equation when resources are finite or scarce (justice). Some cultures believe that it is the duty of the family to care for its sick member (self-independence). When the therapist promotes independence in self-care or activities of daily living, the role of the family may be negated (Wells, 2005).

Ethical dilemmas can be further complicated by the unequal distribution of power in the relationship between the client and therapist. Clients and families faced with medical decisions are often subject to being over- or underinfluenced by the health care system and providers (power and dominance). The therapist–client relationship is one in which the therapist has the ultimate responsibility for developing conclusions and proposing treatment. These issues can lead to dilemmas in which the practitioner must either accede to the family's wishes or withdraw care. Respect for autonomy grants clients, who have been properly informed in a manner appropriate to the client's beliefs and understanding, the right to refuse a proposed treatment (Wells & Black, 2000).

THE ISSUE

In view of the changing demographics in the United States, occupational therapists and occupational therapy assistants will have the opportunity to work with growing numbers of increasingly diverse clients. They will encounter individuals with different values and belief systems about health, well-being, illness, disabilities, and activities of daily living. They will develop evaluation and intervention plans for consumers

who may not speak their language; who differ from them in socioeconomic and educational level, ethnicity and race, and religion; and who have diverse beliefs about and reactions to illness. Clients and families, as well as practitioners, bring many different cultures to the therapeutic setting. The interaction of clients and practitioners embodies a form of multiculturalism in which several cultures—including the health care profession, institution, family, community, and traditional culture—are all merged (Genao, Bussey-Jones, Brady, Branch, & Corbie-Smith, 2003). Therefore, every therapeutic interaction is a cross-cultural interaction. It is this overlap and interaction of cultures and dialects that can create ethical conflicts and dilemmas in providing occupational therapy services.

Without cultural competence, one can easily imagine the possible adverse consequences that can result when distrust, miscommunication, and misunderstanding interfere with the therapeutic relationship. The outcome can range from frustration, confusion, or shame to anger in the client, family, and practitioner. Cultural incompetence can result in compromised quality of care, noncompliance by the client, inability to recognize differences, fear of the new or unknown, denial, and inability to look in-depth at the individual needs of the client and his or her family (Wells & Black, 2000). Alternatively, cultural competence can produce a positive outcome for the client and a feeling of professional satisfaction in the practitioner from knowing that he or she helped a client at a time of need.

Individual cultural beliefs affect how occupational therapy practitioners approach, speak to, and measure outcomes with clients. Within a personal context, occupational therapy practitioners tend to make assumptions and judgments about individuals based on their particular culture, ethnicity, race, religion, sexual orientation, language, disability, or life experiences, and such assumptions and judgments can lead to improper intervention. In the clinical environment, responsibility for making sound ethical decisions rests with the individual practitioner. Ethical situations can arise when the behavior of the practitioner is in conflict with the behavior of the client or family. When two values present themselves and a participant chooses one rather than another, that participant is saying, on the basis of his or her own cultural context and beliefs, that one value is more valuable than another (Iwama, 2003). Problems arise when the participants have a different interpretation of illness and treatment and use language or decision-making frameworks differently. As individuals and professionals, occupational therapists and occupational therapy assistants take a particular action based on their own sense of right and wrong, values, knowledge, and skills.

APPLICATION OF THE CODE

Professional codes of ethics provide a moral framework for and define the ideal standard of practice. They and associated documents provide guidelines and standards for resolving ethical conflicts, dilemmas, and issues. The relevant ethical principles of the Code and Ethics Standards that are valid for culturally competent occupational therapists, occupational therapy assistants, and students are as follows:

Principle 1. Occupational therapy personnel shall demonstrate a concern for the well-being and safety of the recipients of their services. (Beneficence)

Principle 4. Occupational therapy personnel shall provide services in a fair and equitable manner. (Social Justice)

Occupational therapy personnel shall

F. Provide services that reflect an understanding of how occupational therapy service delivery can be affected by factors such as economic status, age, ethnicity, race, geography, disability, marital status, sexual orientation, gender, gender identity, religion, culture, and political affiliation.

Principle 4F speaks directly to the prohibition of discrimination in the delivery of professional services. This principle holds the welfare of occupational therapy clients as paramount. Occupational therapists and occupational therapy assistants must consider all relevant contexts that influence the performance, skill, and patterns that determine the behaviors of their clients. According to the *Occupational Therapy Practice Framework: Domain and Process* (AOTA, 2008), "the expectations, beliefs, and customs of various cultures can affect a client's identity and activity choices and need to be considered when determining how and when services may be delivered" (p. 651). The entire process of service delivery begins with a collaborative relationship with the client and family; therefore, incompetence in cross-cultural interaction, knowledge, and skill can lead to unethical decision making.

Principle 1E. Occupational therapy personnel shall provide occupational therapy services that are within each practitioner's level of competence and scope of practice. . . .

Principle 3I. Occupational therapy personnel shall take appropriate steps to facilitate meaningful communication and comprehension in cases in which the recipient of service, student, or research participant has limited ability to communicate (e.g., aphasia or differences in language, literacy, culture).

Principle 5F. Occupational therapy personnel shall take responsibility for maintaining high standards and continuing competence in practice, education, and research . . . to improve and update knowledge and skills.

Principles 1E, 3I, and 5F remind practitioners of the importance and duty of lifelong learning to develop the knowledge and skills required to provide culturally appropriate service. They also speak to requiring occupational therapy practitioners to strive to deliver culturally competent services to an increasingly broad range of clients. They hold practitioners accountable for continuing their professional development and seeking knowledge throughout their careers, which is required to provide culturally competent care. In addition, Principles 5G and 5H prohibit delegation of tasks that are beyond the competence of the designee and require that the certified individual provide adequate supervision, especially important when linguistic differences exist and bilingual assistants, aides, and interpreters are used.

> Principle 7. Occupational therapy personnel shall treat colleagues and other professionals with respect, fairness, discretion, and integrity. (Fidelity)

Principle 7 provides guidance on interactions with individuals, colleagues, and students from diverse backgrounds. It calls on practitioners to "respect the traditions, practices, competencies, and responsibilities of their own and other professions" (Principle 7A). Culturally diverse students and practitioners bring a special skill and knowledge to the profession. They are entitled to professional equity and should not be exploited or debased because of their differences. They should not be held to different expectations, roles, or behaviors. Discrimination in any professional interaction and against any individual with whom an occupational therapy practitioner interacts ultimately debases the profession and harms all those within the practice.

DISCUSSION

The Code and Ethics Standards recognize that culture may influence how individuals cope with problems and interact with each other. The way in which occupational therapy services are planned and implemented needs to be culturally sensitive to be culturally effective. Cultural competence builds on the profession's ethical concepts of beneficence, nonmaleficence, autonomy, confidentiality, social and procedural justice, veracity, and fidelity, adding inclusion, tolerance, and respect for diversity in all its forms.

The direct service provider, educator, supervisor, researcher, and professional leader must be mindful of the impact of cultural diversity in interactions with clients, families, students, and colleagues. Some materials and approaches may be inappropriate and even offensive to some individuals. Clients and families may choose complementary and alternative medicine or traditional or faith healing practices as opposed to mainstream therapeutic approaches. Colleagues and students approach issues and events from their own cultural perspective.

Cultural competence requires occupational therapy practitioners to enter into the therapeutic relationship with an awareness of their own culture and cultural biases, knowledge about other cultures, and skills in cross-cultural communication and intervention (Wells & Black, 2000). Practitioners need a nonjudgmental attitude toward unfamiliar beliefs and health practices. They should be prepared to be open and flexible in the selection, administration, and interpretation of intervention approaches. They must be willing to negotiate and compromise when conflicts arise. And when cultural or linguistic differences may negatively influence outcomes, practitioners must be ready to refer to or collaborate with others who have the needed knowledge, skill, and experience. Cultural competence requires occupational therapy practitioners to detect and prevent exclusion or exploitation of diverse clients and to monitor cultural competence in their agencies, policies and procedures, and delivery systems.

VIGNETTE 3

You are attending a lecture about a disabling condition and its effect on specific populations. A multitude of groups and populations are presented and discussed. The only time that gay men and lesbians are mentioned is in connection with the total number of deaths resulting from the condition. When asked by an attendee about the effects of this condition on the gay and lesbian population, the speaker ignores the individual and goes on to another question.

Caution must be taken not to attribute stereotypical characteristics to individuals. Rather, an attempt should be made to gain a better understanding of the culture of clients, colleagues, and students. Practitioners should devise a plan to continually acquire the training and education necessary to be culturally competent. The Code and Ethics Standards clearly show that occupational therapists and occupational therapy assistants have an ethical responsibility to be culturally competent practitioners.

CONCLUSION

To effectively reach diverse populations, the field of occupational therapy must have culturally competent professionals. Cultural competence is a basic reminder to all practitioners of their responsibility in protecting the rights of clients and their families and in acting as their advocates. Recognizing the link among trust, cultural competence, and the therapeutic relationship is critical to providing ethical care. Being culturally competent can help occupational therapy practitioners develop intervention approaches, health delivery systems, and health policies that fully recognize and include the effects of culture on the ethics of health decisions. It can aid practitioners in integrating fair and equitable services for all people and ensuring the holistic, contextual, and need-centered nature of such services. It can assist practitioners in achieving their goals of providing sound ethical decision making, practice, and care to all persons.

Ethical considerations dictate that cultural competence should be considered in activities such as hiring practices, teaching, evaluation, and supervision of staff and students. There is an equally important need for all occupational therapists and occupational therapy assistants to continually improve their level of cultural competence and to establish a mechanism for the evaluation of competence-based practice. Guided by the Code and Ethics Standards, occupational therapists and occupational therapy assistants should take a leadership role not only in disseminating knowledge about diverse client groups but also in actively advocating for fair, equitable, and culturally appropriate treatment of all clients served. This role should extend within and outside the profession. In the principles of the Code and Ethics Standards, therapists have a framework to guide their decisions when cultural conflicts arise.

REFERENCES

American Occupational Therapy Association, Multicultural Task Force. (1995). *Definition and terms*. Bethesda, MD: Author.

American Occupational Therapy Association. (2008). Occupational therapy practice framework: Domain and process (2nd ed.). *American Journal of Occupational Therapy, 62*, 625–683. doi:10.5014/ajot.62.6.625

American Occupational Therapy Association. (2010). Occupational therapy code of ethics and ethics standards (2010). *American Journal of Occupational Therapy, 64*(6 Suppl.), S17–S26. doi:10.5014/ajot.2010.64S17

Betancourt, J. R., Green, A. R., Carrillo, J. E., & Ananeh-Firempong, O. (2003). Defining cultural competence: A practical framework for addressing racial/ethnic disparities in health and health care. *Public Health Report, 118,* 293–302.

Cross, T. L., Bazron, B. J., Dennis, K. W., & Isaacs, M. R. (1989). *Towards a culturally competent system of care: Vol. 1.* Washington, DC: CASSP Technical Assistant Center, Georgetown University Child Development Center.

Davis, P., & Donald, B. (1997). *Multicultural counseling competencies: Assessment, evaluation, education and training, and supervision.* Thousand Oaks, CA: Sage.

Genao, I., Bussey-Jones, J., Brady, D., Branch, W. T., & Corbie-Smith, G. (2003). Building the case for cultural competence. *American Journal of the Medical Sciences, 326*(3), 136–140.

Iwama, M. (2003). Toward culturally relevant epistemologies in occupational therapy. *American Journal of Occupational Therapy, 57*, 582–588.

Wells, S. A. (2005). An ethic of diversity. In R. B. Purtilo, G. M. Jensen, & C. B. Royeen (Eds.), *Educating for moral action: A sourcebook in health and rehabilitation ethics* (pp. 31–41). Philadelphia: F. A. Davis.

Wells, S. A., & Black, R. (2000). *Cultural competency for health professionals.* Bethesda, MD: American Occupational Therapy Association.

Shirley A. Wells, MPH, OTR, FAOTA
Chairperson, Commission on Standards and Ethics (2001–2004)

This chapter was originally published in the 2006 edition of the *Reference Guide to the Occupational Therapy Code of Ethics*. It has been revised to reflect updated AOTA official documents, Web sites, AOTA style, and additional resources.

CHAPTER 24

Ethical Considerations When Occupational Therapists Engage in Business Transactions With Clients

INTRODUCTION

Selling products to recipients of occupational therapy services requires an awareness of the various regulatory and ethical issues that guide how occupational therapists and occupational therapy assistants may engage in this business. Selling equipment and supplies to clients has become a common business activity for many occupational therapy practitioners.

However, careful consideration must be made to uphold an objective, professional, and therapeutic relationship with clients who require both goods and services. This relationship may become confusing and unclear when practitioners hold outside interests beyond the therapeutic interaction. Having a financial interest in a business venture such as product sales related to occupational therapy while providing occupational therapy services to the client may be perceived as a *conflict of interest*, which exists when there is a "conflict between the private interests and the official or professional responsibilities of a person in a position of trust" (*Merriam-Webster's Dictionary of Law*, 1996). When conflict of interest occurs in business matters such as these, a practitioner's professional integrity may be questioned if care has not been taken in how the equipment, supplies, or other items were sold to clients. Moreover, if financial benefits exceed acceptable reimbursement rates, this could be indicative of impaired or altered professional judgment by the practitioner.

THE ISSUES

A variety of products may be sold by occupational therapists directly to their clients, such as adaptive, durable medical, and exercise equipment, as well as books. Less common and sometimes questionable items, such as pain-relieving magnets and aromatherapy supplies, also may be sold to clients. Serious ethical questions can arise when selling products to clients while providing professional services. Thoughtful reflection on the responses to the following types of questions can be helpful in determining the appropriateness of this behavior:

- What types of products are being sold?
- If the item is related to a client's therapeutic goals, should the product be sold to the client by the therapist providing the services?
- Should the therapist hold ownership in the company from which the product is being sold?

The answers to these questions help clarify if financial interest in completing this transaction is influencing the therapeutic recommendation. These questions are not easily answered and are further complicated by the increased emphasis toward less-traditional occupational therapy practice settings. This emphasis has led to greater opportunities for occupational therapy practitioners to sell both goods and services to recipients of their services.

In situations in which an occupational therapy practitioner also assumes the role of product vendor, clients need to be assured that the practitioner has adhered to compliance regulations. For example, as a vendor, a practitioner may be required to provide the client with documentation of written warranty information; policies for complaints, questions, returns, and repairs; nondiscrimination policies; a consumer bill of rights; and the Health Insurance Portability and Accountability Act of 1996 compliance regulations. Practitioners need to be aware of all of the Federal Trade Commission and/or state consumer protection agency rules and regulations for product safety and liability.

Another area of concern is the potential for harm. What happens if a client is injured from the product a practitioner sold to him or her? Practitioners could be subjecting themselves to sanctions or exposure to professional liability issues from federal regulatory agencies such as the Center for Medicare and Medicaid Services (CMS; see www.cms.hhs.gov). The product may require specific standards of infection control such as those regulated by agencies such as the Joint Commission on the Accreditation of Healthcare Organizations (JCAHO, 2004–2005). Practitioners also may be required to meet prevailing industry standards as a product vendor, which may require additional state licensure. For example, durable medical equipment vendors must meet CMS standards if they want to bill CMS for the equipment. Items must be medically necessary and prescribed by a physician. The vendor must demonstrate adherence to a variety of rules and regulations including product safety, storage of equipment, patient bill of rights (i.e., right to refuse equipment), complaint process, and return policy.

The *Standards of Practice for Occupational Therapy* (AOTA, 2010b) support practicing according to Association and institutional policies and other relevant documents. When selling products, practitioners may be in a position to use their referral base as a source for potential customers. In such cases, it is critical to use this source objectively, considering the existing trust that clients have in those who provide their therapy. Occupational therapy practitioners have an ethical obligation to inform clients of (i.e., disclose) outside business relationships that may give the appearance of conflict of interest and to assure service recipients that therapeutic decisions are devoid of coercion. Whether financial interest in the business transaction is for direct or indirect monetary gain, practitioners' disclosures must be completely transparent.

The *Occupational Therapy Code of Ethics and Ethics Standards (2010)* (referred to as the "Code and Ethics Standards"; AOTA, 2010a) require that practitioners disclose financial conflicts of interests that may involve clients (e.g., Principles 2C, 2J, 6B, and 7E). Because of the broad spectrum of this topic, several principles from the Code and Ethics Standards that are applicable to the issue of selling goods and services to clients are listed in the box.

Primary among the core values are justice and altruism. *Justice* refers to relating in a fair and impartial manner with clients and others, as well as complying with applicable rules and laws. It is important for practitioners to reflect on their therapeutic practice and business interests to ensure that the two are clearly separate and that clients have full disclosure and information on both. Practitioners have a duty and obligation to provide occupational therapy services in an altruistic manner to clients. Altruism is one of seven core concepts that guide the values, actions, and attitudes of occupational therapy practitioners (AOTA, 2010a).

Occupational therapy interventions should be goal directed, avoiding any perceived potential to exploit recipients of service for financial gain. Participating in activities outside of this focus may damage the therapeutic relationship according to Principle 2C of the Code and Ethics Standards. According to JCAHO (2004–2005), *exploitation* is defined as "taking an unjust advantage of another individual for one's own advantage or benefit" (p. GL7). Health care providers have an obligation to protect clients from real or perceived abuse, neglect, or exploitation by anyone. Individuals who operate a private occupational therapy practice and sell therapeutic supplies and equipment to clients must ensure that the items are necessary for the clients' return to function; that the amount charged for products is fair and reasonable according to industry standards and practices; and that disclosures meet all of the legal, federal, and professional requirements.

CASE SCENARIO AND DISCUSSION

An occupational therapist who works in a private practice setting also is part owner of a durable medical equipment company. She recommends to a client the need to purchase certain items to enhance functional performance in home safety and provides the client with the name of her company as a resource for this equipment. She does not tell the client of her financial holdings in this company, nor does she provide a list of other vendors who also can supply the same equipment.

The client follows the occupational therapist's instructions and purchases the equipment. Later, when the client receives the invoice for the equipment, he notices that the therapist is listed as an owner of the company. The client calls and expresses anger about the occupational therapist failing to inform him of her financial holdings in the company.

Disclosure of the occupational therapist's role in this company may have prevented the client from feeling exploited. It is possible that the situation could have been avoided by offering a list of other potential vendors from which the client could make the purchase. Doing so could avoid the perception of impropriety and enable the client to make an informed decision, which is supported by Principles 2C, 3, and 5P of the Code and Ethics Standards.

PRINCIPLES FROM THE *OCCUPATIONAL THERAPY CODE OF ETHICS AND ETHICS STANDARDS* APPLICABLE TO SELLING GOODS AND SERVICES TO CLIENTS

Principle 2. Occupational therapy personnel shall intentionally refrain from actions that cause harm. (Nonmaleficence)

Occupational therapy personnel shall:

C. Avoid relationships that exploit the recipient of services, students, research participants, or employees physically, emotionally, psychologically, financially, socially, or in any other manner that conflicts or interferes with professional judgment and objectivity.

G. Avoid situations in which a practitioner, educator, researcher, or employer is unable to maintain clear professional boundaries or objectivity to ensure the safety and well-being of recipients of service, students, research participants, and employees.

Principle 3. Occupational therapy personnel shall respect the right of the individual to self-determination. (Autonomy, Confidentiality)

Principle 6. Occupational therapy personnel shall provide comprehensive, accurate, and objective information when representing the profession. (Veracity)

Occupational therapy personnel shall:

B. Refrain from using or participating in the use of any form of communication that contains false, fraudulent, deceptive, misleading, or unfair statements or claims.

G. Describe the type and duration of occupational therapy services accurately in professional contracts, including the duties and responsibilities of all involved parties.

According to Principle 2J, occupational therapy personnel shall "avoid exploiting any relationship established as an occupational therapist or occupational therapy assistant to further one's own physical, emotional, financial, political, or business interests at the expense of the best interests of recipients of services. . . ." According to Brock (1990), "Disclosure would at least be unlikely to have as corrosive an effect on that trust as would clients learning of the same undisclosed and apparently hidden conflict" (p. 35). What would happen if this client were referred to the therapist in the future? Would the objective therapeutic relationship be compromised? Would the client respect the therapist's role as his health care provider (Fidelity)? The trust so critical to a therapeutic relationship may be breached and ultimately reflect negatively on the profession of occupational therapy and those that provide services (Principle 6E). In addition, the core value of truth is demonstrated by honesty and accuracy in attitude, actions, and provision of information (AOTA, 2010a).

Engaging in business ventures in a competitive health care environment obligates occupational therapy practitioners to become educated in all of the rules and regulations that govern these endeavors. Practitioners must become educated in the ethics of prudent practice as well as appropriate business behaviors such as disclosure when dual roles of practitioner and entrepreneur are assumed. For example, objectivity can become clouded if a practitioner prescribes a wheelchair for a client and also sells this equipment to the client. Are the practitioner's intentions to provide the proper basic wheelchair, or is the practitioner motivated by profit to provide the most expensive wheelchair covered by the client's insurance?

Medicare regulations stipulate that practitioners should not engage in "self-dealing." According to Goldman (2004), "self-dealing occurs when a decision-maker is motivated in part for personal gain, and not entirely on what is good for the company [or client]." Financial rewards can be quite tempting but may be a breach of the honesty and trust that are a professional responsibility toward those whom occupational therapy practitioners serve.

Further, occupational therapists "have a fiduciary responsibility to safeguard the well-being of beneficiaries, and health professionals may not engage in self-dealing" (Baker, Caplan, Emanuel, & Latham, 1999, p. 182). When potential conflicts arise, fiduciaries are required to make a full disclosure of the conflict. According to Edge and Groves (1999),

> A fiduciary relationship is a special relationship of loyalty and responsibility that is formed between the client and practitioner. The client has the right to believe that the practitioner will maintain a higher level of accountability in regard to health care than that expected from most other relationships. (p. 296)

A critical point made by Sulmasy (1993) about physicians and the selling of goods and services is that

> the patient is an exceptionally vulnerable person in the hands of the physician. The patient entrusts his body, his dignity, his secrets, and frequently his life to the physician. The physical effects of being ill compound this vulnerability, affecting to varying degrees the patient's decision-making, communicative, and motor capacities in ways that always limit, even if minimally, the autonomous agency of the individual who is sick. (p. 32)

According to Principle 2 of the Code and Ethics Standards, "Occupational therapy personnel shall intentionally refrain from actions that cause harm"; thus, Sulmasy's point of view is appropriate to occupational therapy practitioners as well.

CONCLUSION

This advisory opinion is not intended to exclude occupational therapists from entrepreneurial ventures; instead, it is intended to educate them on the numerous issues related to product sales and potential ramifications if these ventures are conducted in a manner contrary to industry standards. Business, professional, and legal issues should be considered when conducting business for profit with clients.

Occupational therapy practitioners' behavior is representative of the therapeutic relationships they seek to achieve as well as a demonstration and reflection of the profession of occupational therapy. Practitioners have an obligation to cause no harm, real or perceived, to clients and to retain public trust. Participation in behaviors that may cast a shadow or negatively reflect on the professional standards that practitioners seek to uphold should be avoided. As Jecker (2004) observed, "Professionalism extols attributes such as being knowledgeable and skillful; altruistic; respectful; honest; compassionate; committed to excellence and on-going professional development; and showing a responsiveness to the needs of clients and society that supersedes self-interest" (pp. 47–48). It is therefore always important for occupational therapy practitioners to ask, To what end do these interactions contribute to the therapeutic goals? As Purtilo and Haddad (2002) noted, "Our professional training provides us with the skills and obligation to maintain objectivity and transparency in all interactions. We must adhere to our professional boundaries and remain committed to maintain appropriate limits . . . with clients or their families" (p. 213).

REFERENCES

American Occupational Therapy Association. (2010a). Occupational therapy code of ethics and ethics standards (2010). *American Journal of Occupational Therapy, 64*(6 Suppl.), S17–S26. doi:10.5014/ajot.2010.64S17

American Occupational Therapy Association. (2010b). Standards of practice for occupational therapy. *American Journal of Occupational Therapy, 64*(6 Suppl.), S106–S111. doi:10.5014/ajot.2010.64S106

Baker, R., Caplan, A., Emanuel, L., & Latham, S. (1999). *The American medical ethics revolution.* Baltimore: Johns Hopkins University Press.

Brock, D. (1990). Medicine and business: An unhealthy mix? *Business and Professional Ethics Journal, 9,* 21–37.

Edge, R., & Groves, J. R. (1999). *Ethics of health care: A guide for clinical practice* (2nd ed.). New York: Delmar.

Goldman, S. (2004, April 25). Three pillars of ethics lead to strong, sound business. *Silicon Valley/San Jose Business Journal.* Retrieved November 21, 2010, from http://www.bizjournals.com/sanjose/stories/2004/04/26/editorial3.html?page=1

Health Insurance Portability and Accountability Act of 1996, Pub. L. 104–191. Retrieved May 21, 2010, from http://aspe.hhs.gov/admnsimp/pl104191.htm

Jecker, N. (2004). The theory and practice of professionalism. *American Journal of Bioethics, 4*(2), 47–48.

Joint Commission on Accreditation of Healthcare Organizations. (2004–2005). Glossary: Exploitation. In *Comprehensive accreditation manual for home care* (p. GL7). Washington, DC: Author.

Merriam-Webster's Dictionary of Law. (1996). Conflict of interest. Retrieved August 24, 2005, from http://dictionary.reference.com/search?q=conflict%20of%20interest

Purtilo, R., & Haddad, A. (2002). *Health professional and client interaction.* Philadelphia: W. B. Saunders.

Sulmasy, D. (1993). What's so special about medicine? *Theoretical Medicine and Bioethics, 14,* 27–42.

Darryl Austin, MS, OT/L
Practice Representative, Ethics Commission (2001–2008)

This chapter was originally published in the 2008 edition of the *Reference Guide to the Occupational Therapy Ethics Standards.* It has been revised to reflect updated AOTA official documents, Web sites, AOTA style, and additional resources.

CHAPTER 25

Ethical Considerations in Private Practice

INTRODUCTION

For occupational therapy practitioners with an entrepreneurial spirit and the desire to work independently, a private practice can provide a venue in which one can truly reap the benefits of one's work and provide services consistent with one's interests. For other practitioners, the close collaboration with a physician inherent in providing services "incident to" their practice is equally appealing.

Occupational therapy practitioners who work in private practice, as either a business owner or employee, must consider a variety of issues to ensure that they maintain an ethical practice. Although practitioners should follow ethical principles regardless of clinical setting, in private practice clinicians are generally more directly involved with and affected by organizational aspects and ethical issues related to business practices. Therefore, practitioners, whether owners or employees, need to understand that business stability and predictability of referrals are important; however, these must be balanced against their possible influence on clinical care. Whether working in independent practice or in a physician's office, the burden is on practitioners to ensure that they are making clinical decisions that are in compliance with core ethical principles related to benefiting the consumer or patient.

THE ISSUES

Four key issues related to private practice have ethical implications for practitioners:

1. Referrals
2. Access to care, continuity of care, and collaboration
3. Practice ownership
4. Documentation and billing.

Referrals

One of the critical factors in maintaining a viable business is solid and consistent patient referrals, preferably from a variety of sources. Market forces, physician preference, and competition in the community can affect both the number and types of referrals. However, when physicians own a therapy practice, some ethical issues can compromise the occupational therapy practitioner. Physicians may selectively refer patients on the basis of their relative economic value. For instance, the physician may refer patients with "good" insurance to the physician's own therapy practice while referring patients who are likely to generate less or no reimbursement to others. Physicians may also refer exclusively to practitioners in their own practice; although this referral may be because the physician has confidence in the skills of the occupational therapy practitioner, if it happens regardless of whether the practice or clinician is best qualified to treat that particular patient, then ethical issues can arise. In addition, some physicians may repeatedly refer the same patients for therapy even when those patients do not have significant rehabilitation potential. These situations can create ethical dilemmas for practitioners.

Even with external pressure, practitioners can ensure that they use objective assessments and data to support their clinical decisions about whether a patient can benefit from occupational therapy services and when it is appropriate to discontinue those services. Principle 1H of the *Occupational Therapy Code of Ethics and Ethics Standards (2010)* (referred to as the "Code and Ethics Standards"; AOTA, 2010) states that "Occupational therapy personnel shall terminate occupational therapy services in collaboration with the service recipient or responsible party when needs and goals of the recipient have been met or when services no longer produce a measurable change or outcome." Principle 1 (Beneficence) of the Code and Ethics Standards also emphasizes the ethical mandate to provide benefit to recipients of services. There are effective and ethical strategies to discharge clients appropriately when they no longer need direct services because their goals are no longer objective and cannot reasonably be achieved in a realistic timeframe or they do not meet reimbursement coverage criteria. The occupational therapy practitioner should consider options such as providing instruction in a home program, training caregivers, or planning subsequent screening and reevaluation if the patient's status changes.

Occupational therapy practitioners in independent practices have the responsibility to ensure that they objectively evaluate and develop plans of care for all patients that include the frequency and duration of intervention. Practitioners have an obligation to be certain that economic gain or a desire to satisfy referral sources does not unduly influence the type and amount of therapy provided. Utilization of services must carefully reflect the clinical status of the patient, collaborative goals, and potential for realistic and meaningful outcomes. Practitioners also have an obligation to be guided by external payer requirements.

Access to Care, Continuity of Care, and Collaboration

Access to care is an important ethical concept related to social justice. Principle 4E of the Code and Ethics Standards reminds occupational therapy practitioners of the ethical mandate to "make efforts to advocate for recipients of occupational therapy services to obtain needed services through available means." There are many issues that can affect access to care, and not all are in the practitioner's control, such as limited access in rural areas or restricted panels of insurance providers. What is important are the safeguards clinicians put in place to reinforce that consumers have access to appropriate, qualified providers and have adequate information about what providers are available.

Practitioners should always ensure their competence to provide particular services and provide patients with information about their qualifications. Practitioners can also ensure that their practices or the practices of the physicians from whom they accept referrals have transparent financial relationships, allowing patients to make informed choices about obtaining therapy. In all situations, practitioners must consider whether the patient has access to the most clinically appropriate therapy services available.

Practice Ownership

A key issue with ethical implications that can affect decisions is who owns the practice and what influences drive occupational therapy practitioners' practice patterns in that setting (e.g., payers, referral sources). In some cases, physicians employ occupational therapy practitioners in their office. The physician can bill and be reimbursed for therapy services provided by the practitioner using the physician's provider number with Medicare as long as certain requirements are met. In particular, the patient's course of treatment from that physician must relate to occupational therapy services, and the physician must provide direct supervision (i.e., be present in the office suite). However, when the physician employs an occupational therapy practitioner who is working in his or her office space, the occupational therapy practitioner will need to be aware of and prepared to address potential issues of undue influence on the duration, type, and frequency of therapy being provided according to Principles 2F, 2G, 2I, and 2J of the Code and Ethics Standards.

Some of the issues identified in the section on Referrals above also apply to private ownership issues. Inappropriate referrals and pressure to overutilize therapy when the patient no longer has viable goals can challenge an independent practitioner who is beholden to comply with a referral source who is also the employer. At the same time, the convenience of a therapy practice in a physician's office or in the same building can benefit patients, especially older individuals, and potentially facilitate continuity of care. Collaboration and good communication between the physician and occupational therapy practitioner—both keys to good patient outcomes—can occur regardless of location. The same challenges may exist for independent practice owners if they do not want to alienate referral sources that support the financial health of their business. An important way to address this challenge in an ethical manner is transparency: Patients must be able to make an informed decision about their options for receiving therapy, which means knowing the qualifications of providers and being aware of any financial gain for either the occupational therapy practitioner or the referring physician that may influence referral recommendations.

Private practice owners must also keep in mind certain applicable state and federal laws related to private practice and potential referral sources. Many referral relationships between physicians and therapists are legal. The two major bodies of federal laws and regulations that identify which types of referral relationships are illegal are the federal physician self-referral ("Stark") and anti-kickback laws. The term "Stark Law" commonly refers to Section 1877 of the Social Security Act, which prohibits physicians from referring patients to health care entities with which they (or their immediate family) have a financial relationship for services that Medicare or Medicaid might pay. This law was enacted in 1989 and modified in 1993, at which time Congress expanded the list of services to which the law applies to include occupational and physical therapy. The Stark Law has no intent requirement. Therefore, if an arrangement is entered into that implicates the Stark Law, the arrangement also must meet an exception to be legal.

The federal anti-kickback statutes under Section 1128 of the Social Security Act make it a crime for anyone to knowingly and willingly solicit, receive, offer, or pay any remuneration, directly or indirectly (including bribes, rebates, kickbacks, cash, or in-kind payments), in return for referring an individual for services under any federal health program or in return for purchasing, leasing, or ordering any good, facility service, or item paid under a federal health care program. The statute specifically exempts certain types of payments and business practices, called "safe harbors," including compensation paid to bona fide employees.

Penalties for violating these laws can be severe. Practice owners should use legal assistance to ensure compliance with applicable regulations when setting up a business—particularly if a physician or other individual who may have a financial interest is involved.

Documentation and Billing

Every occupational therapy practitioner has a personal responsibility to be accurate and timely in compliance with documentation and billing standards and regulations, according to Principles 5, 6C, and 6D of the Code and Ethics Standards. However, the private practice owner has an additional responsibility to ensure that policies and procedures are in place for enforcing applicable regulations and standards with their employees because the owner is also responsible for the business elements of the organization. Policies and procedures may include regular medical record review or peer review, an in-service on appropriate documentation, timelines for completing documentation, and continuing education on current coding and billing requirements. Proper supervision is particularly critical to prevent situations in which an employee leaves the practice and documentation is incomplete or missing. Without documentation, treatment sessions cannot be billed and reimbursed, and other occupational therapy practitioners who have not treated those patients cannot "fill in" the missing portions of the record. These actions would be potential violations of Principles 5, 6B, and 6C of the Code and Ethics Standards. The record is a legal document, and the information it contains must be accurate. The private practice owner has responsibility for ensuring that employees follow this practice.

DISCUSSION

Private practice can be rewarding for occupational therapy practitioners who want the freedom to provide clinical services as they see fit and who have the requisite business expertise needed to run a viable business. For other practitioners, employment in a physician's office is a better match because they can have the benefits of independence in clinical practice without payment management and personnel issues. Regardless of the venue, occupational therapy practitioners must address ethical considerations to ensure compliance with professional standards.

Practitioners may also face challenges in identifying who holds the responsibility to inform consumers about potential ethical issues. These issues include conflicts of interest related to financial benefit to the referral source or practice owner, the provision for informed consent, and autonomy for consumers in choosing providers when they are referred for therapy. At the American Medical Association's (AMA's) Interim Meeting in November 2008, ethical guidelines on physician self-referral were adopted stating that physicians who refer patients for services at facilities in which they have a financial interest should disclose this interest to patients (O'Reilly, 2008). Further, physicians are advised to avoid any ownership or leasing arrangements that require patient referrals or prohibit recommending competitors. This new policy by the AMA may promote different practices by physicians.

Several principles from the Code and Ethics Standards are particularly relevant to the ethical concerns discussed:

- Principle 4E: "Occupational therapy personnel shall make efforts to advocate for recipients of occupational therapy services to obtain needed services through available means." It is the responsibility of occupational therapy practitioners, to the best of their ability, to provide guidance to patients about options for receiving the most appropriate and beneficial therapy from the most appropriate practitioner, regardless of the referral source. The owner of the practice—whether a physician or an occupational therapy practitioner—should not dictate how or where a patient receives therapy. Rather, the occupational therapy plan of care should be based on individual evaluation and clinical needs to maximize patient outcomes, according to Principle 1B.

- Principle 1I is also relevant and supports the concept of Principle 4E: "Occupational therapy personnel shall refer to other health care specialists solely on the basis of the needs of the client." Communication is crucial to identifying patients' desires and supporting autonomy in their decision making, whether in an occupational therapy practitioner's private practice or a physician's office.

- Principle 2F: "Occupational therapy personnel shall avoid any undue influences . . . that may compromise the provision of occupational therapy services, education, or research."
  - Principle 2J also supports the concept of Principle 2F: "Occupational therapy personnel shall avoid exploiting any relationship established as an occupational therapist or occupational therapy assistant to further one's own physical, emotional, financial, political, or business interests at the expense of the best interests of recipients of services, students, research participants, employees, or colleagues." This principle includes the need for practice owners to disclose to patients their ownership of the practice. Ethical principles that focus on benefits to the recipients of services must always guide the practitioner. In addition, practice owners need to ensure that they do not set up productivity targets and service delivery models geared to maximizing reimbursement without fully considering the impact on individualized and clinically relevant care. Designing programs or approaches to therapy provision with the intention only to increase profitability is not consistent with the client-centered philosophy of the profession of occupational therapy or with the profession's Code and Ethics Standards. Although economic issues are legitimate considerations, client-centered intervention must remain the central concept and should focus on individualized and meaningful goals to enhance function and participation.
- Principle 2I: "Occupational therapy personnel shall avoid compromising client rights or well-being based on arbitrary administrative directives by exercising professional judgment and critical analysis." This principle may be relevant for occupational therapy practitioners who receive repeated referrals from a particular referrer for patients who cannot

benefit from services (e.g., in a physician-owned practice) but have an insurance benefit that will continue to reimburse for therapy.

Several principles provide additional reinforcement for these concepts:

- Principle 7H: "Occupational therapy personnel shall be diligent stewards of human, financial, and material resources of their employers, and refrain from exploiting these resources for personal gain."
- Principle 2C: "Occupational therapy personnel shall avoid relationships that exploit the recipient of services, students, research participants, or employees physically, emotionally, psychologically, financially, socially, or in any other manner that conflicts or interferes with professional judgment and objectivity." Further, Principle 2G states that "occupational therapy personnel shall avoid situations in which a practitioner, educator, researcher, or employer is unable to maintain clear professional boundaries or objectivity to ensure the safety and well-being of recipients of service, students, research participants, and employees."
- Principle 5P mandates that personnel "maintain the ethical principles and standards of the profession when participating in a business arrangement as owner, stockholder, partner, or employee, and refrain from working for or doing business with organizations that engage in illegal or unethical business practices. . . ." Employees need to exercise due diligence in researching organizations for possible employment opportunities and must ensure that, after they are employed, the organization continues to follow ethical business practices. Employees need to protect their own license to practice and not get involved by association with illegal or unethical organizations. As business owners, occupational therapy practitioners have a similar responsibility to be aware of and follow applicable laws and ethical guidelines. Business owners should

never put their employees in an untenable position of involvement with fraud or questionable service delivery methods as a requirement for ongoing employment.

CONCLUSION

Regardless of the practice model, the best interests of the client must be kept at the forefront when providing clinical services. To ensure that they meet their ethical obligations, occupational therapy practitioners must maintain open communication and collaboration among all parties, transparency, and full disclosure to ensure autonomy in patient decision making and compliance with applicable laws and ethical principles to meet professional standards.

REFERENCES

American Occupational Therapy Association. (2010). Occupational therapy code of ethics and ethics standards (2010). *American Journal of Occupational Therapy, 64*(6 Suppl.), S17–S26. doi:10.5014/ajot.2010.64S17

O'Reilly, K. B. (2008). *AMA meeting: Doctors told to reveal financial stake in referrals.* Retrieved December 8, 2008, from http://www.ama-assn.org/amednews/2008/12/01/prsf1201.htm

Deborah Yarett Slater, MS, OT/L, FAOTA
Staff Liaison to the AOTA Ethics Commission

Ethical Considerations for the Professional Education of Students With Disabilities

INTRODUCTION

Assisting individuals with disabilities and valuing diversity are core tenets of the profession of occupational therapy. According to the American Occupational Therapy Association (AOTA, 2009b),

> The occupational therapy profession affirms the right of every individual to access and fully participate in society. . . . We maintain that society has an obligation to provide the reasonable accommodations necessary to allow individuals access to social, educational, recreational, and vocational opportunities. (pp. 819–820)

Most often the individual with a disability is a client, but sometimes the individual is a student in an occupational therapy educational program. Regardless of whether the student has a disability, educational programs must balance the needs of their students with their obligations to the future clients that program graduates will serve. Occupational therapy classroom and fieldwork educators must treat students fairly and act in accordance with the AOTA *Occupational Therapy Code of Ethics and Ethics Standards (2010)* (referred to as the "Code and Ethics Standards"; AOTA, 2010a) and federal and state laws.

This Advisory Opinion discusses ethical issues that may arise during the classroom and fieldwork portions of the educational process of occupational therapy students who have

disabilities. First, a brief background of key legislation is provided, including the Americans With Disabilities Act (ADA), Section 504 of the Rehabilitation Act of 1973, and the Family Educational Rights and Privacy Act (FERPA). Next, the Code and Ethics Standards are applied to two case studies that describe situations that may arise in the classroom and in fieldwork education. Last, the Advisory Opinion summarizes key issues. When the term *educational program* is used, it applies to both the academic and fieldwork portion of the educational program unless otherwise stated.

BACKGROUND

The ADA (1990) extended civil rights to individuals with disabilities. Similarly, the Rehabilitation Act of 1973, and specifically Section 504, defined exactly how services must be provided to people with disabilities who request assistance. These legislative mandates pertain to all aspects of American life, from housing and education to employment, recreation, and religion. In any situation where an otherwise qualified person might be prevented from achieving his or her potential due to a disability, ADA and the Rehabilitation Act demand assurances that opportunities be available for all.

The ADA and Section 504 of the Rehabilitation Act of 1973 are antidiscrimination acts, not entitlement acts. As such, they are outcome neutral, and the responsibility for initiating

147

accommodation rests with the student. The ADA and Section 504 require that individuals, such as those entering higher education, receive the opportunity to participate in educational and vocational endeavors for which they are otherwise qualified. An equal opportunity to participate does not mean that there will be equal outcomes. Just like their nondisabled peers, some students with disabilities will fail coursework and fieldwork. The ADA focuses on whether students with disabilities in higher education have equal access to an education. It is not intended to optimize academic success: "The intent of the law, again, was to level the playing field, not to tilt it" (Gordon & Keiser, 1998, p. 5).

Because the ADA's intention is to protect against discrimination based on a disability, a student can receive such protection only if he or she has substantial impairments that affect major life activities and he or she is found to be disabled relative to the general population (Gordon & Keiser, 1998). Some conditions warrant intervention but may not rise to the level of impairment as defined by the ADA. Furthermore,

> documentation of a specific disability does not translate directly into specific accommodations. Reasonable accommodations are individually determined and should be based on the functional impact of the condition and its likely interaction with the environment (course assignments, program requirements, physical design, etc.). As such, accommodation recommendations may vary from individual to individual with the "same" disability diagnosis and from environment to environment for the same individual. (Association on Higher Education and Disability, 2004b)

There are specific requirements for diagnosis and documentation in order to qualify for protection under the ADA as an individual with a disability. The diagnosis must be made and documented by a qualified professional, such as a physician, neuropsychologist, or educational psychologist, among others: "The general expectation is that people conducting evaluations have terminal degrees in their profession and are fully trained in differential diagnosis" (Gordon & Keiser, 1998, p. 13). The Association on Higher Education and Disability (2004a) provides additional information on best practices in documentation of a disability in higher education. The report based on the evaluator's findings must also be sufficient to allow for careful administrative review.

The coordination of the documentation and services for students with disabilities is usually managed through an administrative office at the college or university. This office is frequently called the Office of Disability Accommodations (ODA). The ODA determines if the student qualifies for accommodations and what accommodations are allowable by disability law and regulations.

The above process assumes that the student is aware of his or her disability and self-identifies. If a student chooses not to self-identify, he or she is within individual rights to pursue postsecondary education. However, such a student is not protected by the law. Simply stated, unless a student self-identifies as being eligible for protections under the ADA and Section 504, no associated privileges are afforded.

Because occupational therapy practitioners in their professional role assist people with impairments in their efforts to be successful, it is sometimes difficult for a faculty member to refrain from making special arrangements for a student who appears to have a disability but who has not self-identified or who has not completed the process to qualify for accommodations. However, educators must consider fundamental fairness to all students, including those who may struggle for a variety of other reasons but who do not qualify for special treatment.

It is not unusual for a disability to be discovered after a student enters professional school or even as late as Level II fieldwork. Sometimes students with learning or emotional disabilities have succeeded up to the point of professional school through extremely hard work and dedication. However, the demands of professional school and fieldwork can push such a student past his or her ability to compensate.

If the student is otherwise qualified, the educational program must determine if the student can perform the essential job function of being an occupational therapy student with or without reasonable accommodation. For a more complete discussion of essential job functions and reasonable accommodations in academic and practice settings, see Gupta, Gelpi, and Sain (2005). A variety of documents exist that contribute to understanding the essential job functions of an occupational therapist or occupational therapy assistant (AOTA, 2009a, 2010b, 2010c; U.S. Department of Labor, National O*NET Consortium, 2003, 2004).

In the field of health education, essential job functions are generally referred to as *technical standards*. Many occupational therapy programs include the technical standards as part of the admissions process (e.g., Medical College of Georgia, 2008; Samuel Merritt College, n.d.; Stony Brook University, 2004; University of Kansas, 2003; University of Tennessee, n.d.).

The last federal law relevant to this advisory opinion is the Family Educational Rights and Privacy Act, which protects the privacy of all students' educational records. Generally, "institutions must have written permission from the student in order to release any information from a student's educational record" (Van Dusen, 2004, p. 4). This protection of privacy applies to all students, regardless of disability.

Protection of confidential information is part of FERPA, the ADA, and Section 504. The Association on Higher Education and Disability (1996) stated that "disability related information should be treated as medical information and handled under the same strict rules of confidentiality as is other medical information" (p. 1). The student alone determines whether to share information, decides what information to share, and selects which faculty members may receive information: "The Department of Justice has indicated that a faculty member generally does not need to know what the disability is, only that it has been appropriately verified by the individual (or office) assigned this responsibility on behalf of the institution" (Association on Higher Education and Disability, 1996, p. 1).

APPLICATION TO PRACTICE: CASE STUDIES

Two case studies illustrate how to apply ethical reasoning to students with disabilities.

Case 1

Ashley is an occupational therapy student with a learning disability. Ashley is your advisee and in the first semester in the occupational therapy program. She makes an appointment with you and tells you about her learning disability and the difficulties she has had, shows you a psychological report describing her disability, and asks to be given extra time to complete exams and assignments. You advise her to go to the university's Office of Disability Accommodations. Ashley does not want to go to the ODA because she thinks that the university would label her as a student with a disability. You inform Ashley of the risks of not seeking accommodations and encourage her to reconsider. She leaves your office undecided.

You do not hear from Ashley again until after midterm exams, when she discovers she has a failing grade in two classes. She admits that she did not go to the ODA and states she thought she could make it on her own. Ashley says that one of her instructors gave her more time, and she can't understand why the other occupational therapy instructors did not. Ashley finally agrees to go to the ODA, but she also wants to be able to retake her midterm exams in the two courses she is failing. She wants more time for taking exams and turning in assignments. The ODA determines that Ashley does qualify as a student with learning disabilities and that her accommodations can include time and a half for exams, but she must turn in assignments on the dates they are due in the syllabi. She is also not allowed to retake the two midterm exams.

Your behavior as Ashley's advisor demonstrates understanding, caring, and responsiveness (core value: altruism) to Ashley's situation. By requiring Ashley to go to the ODA, you followed procedures (Code and Ethics Standards Principle 5, Procedural Justice), which requires that you are familiar with and comply with institutional rules and federal laws, in this case the ADA and Section 504. The instructor who gave Ashley more time on the exam before accommodations were in place demonstrated altruism but violated Principle 5 of the Code and Ethics Standards because university procedures stipulate that accommodations should not be given until the ODA determines that the student is entitled to them and specifies what the accommodations should be. Making accommodations without consulting the ODA may result in an unfair disadvantage for other students who may have extenuating circumstances affecting their performance by denying them an equal opportunity for extra time.

Principle 1 of the Code and Ethics Standards (Beneficence) applies to all faculty involved in this case. Specifically, Principle 1J reads, "Occupational therapy personnel shall provide occupational therapy education, continuing education, instruction, and training that are within the instructor's subject area of expertise and level of competence." Although academic and fieldwork educators may typically think of competence in terms of educating students without disabilities, knowledge of laws related to educating students with disabilities is also required.

Case 2

Tanisha is preparing for her first Level II fieldwork experience. She has a diagnosis of anxiety disorder for which she has received ac-commodations during the academic portion of her education. As the academic fieldwork coordinator, you encourage Tanisha to contact the ODA to determine what accommodations she would qualify for during clinical education. Tanisha states that she does not want to reveal to the fieldwork site that she has a disability because she plans to apply for jobs in this city after graduation. She says she feels more confident now and wants to prove to herself that she can perform without assistance. After you explain the risks and benefits of disclosure, Tanisha decides not to disclose or ask for accommodations from her clinical site.

You contact Tanisha after Week 2 to review her progress. Tanisha says things are OK. At Week 4, Jeremy, Tanisha's clinical educator, calls you to say that he is concerned about Tanisha's difficulty with time management and turning in documentation on time. He says that Tanisha's level of knowledge appears solid but that she sometimes "shuts down" in stressful situations. Jeremy asks if Tanisha has some learning or emotional issues that he should know about. He wants your advice on how to help Tanisha be more successful.

As the academic fieldwork coordinator, you must consider the ethical principle of Autonomy and Confidentiality (Principle 3). Principle 3G is especially applicable to this case:

> Occupational therapy personnel shall ensure that confidentiality and the right to privacy are respected and maintained regarding all information obtained about . . . students . . . . The only exceptions are when a practitioner or staff member believes than an individual is in serious foreseeable or imminent harm. Laws and regulations may require disclosure to appropriate authorities without consent.

In a similar fashion, Fidelity (Principle 7B) requires that "occupational therapy personnel shall preserve, respect, and safeguard private information about employees, colleagues, and students unless otherwise mandated by national, state, or local laws or permission to disclose is given by the individual." Veracity (Principle 6E) also applies to this case: "Occupational therapy personnel shall accept responsibility for any action that reduces the public's trust in occupational therapy." Principle 6E creates tension between your duty to your student and your duty to consumers of occupational therapy services. However, you realize that you have a greater obligation to avoid breaching confidentiality with Tanisha, as you do not have evidence at this point that Tanisha's behavior is putting clients at risk. If you had information to indicate that clients were at risk, you would have a greater obligation to protect the clients and to focus on Tanisha's lack of competence in the area of client safety.

You must also consider Procedural Justice (Principle 5), which requires you to be familiar and comply with institutional rules and federal laws, which in this case are the ADA, Section 504, and FERPA. Lastly, you consider Principle 1K, which states that "occupational therapy personnel shall provide students and employees with information about the Code and Ethics Standards, opportunities to discuss ethical conflicts, and procedures for reporting unresolved ethical conflicts." It is important that you model ethical conduct for Jeremy and Tanisha.

A more thorough discussion of ethical dilemmas involving confidentiality of students with disabilities during fieldwork education can be found in an article by Brown and Griffiths (2000). AOTA's Web site also provides useful information on this topic, including the following question and answer:

Does the academic program have to tell the fieldwork setting that the student has a disability? The academic program is not required to, nor should it, inform the fieldwork site of a student's disability without the student's permission. It is the student's decision whether or not to disclose a disability. The academic fieldwork coordinator will counsel students on the pros and cons of sharing this type of information prior to beginning fieldwork. If a student decides not to disclose this information, the academic fieldwork coordinator is legally not allowed to share that information with the fieldwork setting.

A fieldwork setting cannot refuse to place a student with a disability unless that student is unable to perform the essential job functions with or without reasonable accommodations. To refuse placement solely on the student's disability is discriminatory and illegal. (AOTA, 2000)

After considering the Code and Ethics Standards and other documents, you decide you cannot directly answer Jeremy's question about a disability, but you could brainstorm with Jeremy about strategies that might help Tanisha be more successful. You could encourage Jeremy to document Tanisha's difficulties and to give her frequent and specific feedback. If these suggestions don't correct the problems, a learning contract or site visit could be considered. You could contact Tanisha to assist her with making an informed decision by providing her with the potential risks of nondisclosure. However, as an autonomous person with freedom to exercise choice and self-direction, Tanisha must make the final decision. Autonomous persons can and do take risks. Tanisha may be risking failure of her first Level II fieldwork, but taking the risk is her choice. Wells and Hanebrink (2000) noted that

the decision to disclose or not to disclose as well as when and how to disclose is solely the right of the student. The fieldwork site can be held accountable only from the point in which they are informed or receive a request for accommodation. (p. 9)

Education programs should provide clinical sites with information about educating students with disabilities and the requirements of the ADA and Section 504 in regard to education and encourage sites to call the academic fieldwork coordinator when questions arise. The *AOTA Self-Assessment Tool for Fieldwork Educator Competency* (AOTA, n.d.) is a potential resource for educating fieldwork educators in general. Under Administration Competencies, Item 11 is pertinent to this discussion: "The fieldwork educator defines essential functions and roles of a fieldwork student, in compliance with legal and accreditation standards (e.g., ADA, Family Educational Rights and Privacy Act, fieldwork agreement, reimbursement mechanism, state regulations, etc.)" (p. 7).

DISCUSSION

Occupational therapy faculty and fieldwork educators must remain mindful of their obligations both to their occupational therapy students and to the clients those students will someday serve. Patient safety is always paramount. However, there will be students who can become competent occupational therapists despite their disabilities if given reasonable accommodations. Although the student has rights and responsibilities, so do the academic and clinical sites:

> The institution is always responsible for students who are participating in its programs whether on or off campus. The question is whether the institution has primary or secondary responsibility. The institution has the ultimate responsibility for the provision of reasonable accommodation. The intern site generally assumes the duty for providing accommodation on site; the institution, however, must monitor what happens in that environment to ensure that its students are not discriminated against and are provided necessary accommoda-

tions. . . . Students with disabilities have a right under ADA (Title II) to be seen first as capable people with marketable skills and only secondarily as people who happen to have disabilities. (Scott, Wells, & Hanebrink, 1997, pp. 44, 46)

According to the Northeast Technical Assistance Center (1999), faculty should not

> make assumptions about a student's ability to work in a particular field. Most often, concerns that students may not be able to "cut it" are based on fears and assumptions, not facts. Remember, too, that employers are also required to comply with the ADA.

REFERENCES

American Occupational Therapy Association. (2000). *Most frequently asked fieldwork questions.* Retrieved January 14, 2008, from http://www.aota.org/Educate/EdRes/Fieldwork/NewPrograms/38242.aspx

American Occupational Therapy Association. (2009a). Guidelines for supervision, roles, and responsibilities during the delivery of occupational therapy services. *American Journal of Occupational Therapy, 58,* 797–803. doi:10.5014/ajot.63.6.797

American Occupational Therapy Association. (2009b). Occupational therapy's commitment to nondiscrimination and inclusion. *American Journal of Occupational Therapy, 63,* 819–820. doi:10.5014/ajot.63.6.819

American Occupational Therapy Association. (2010a). Occupational therapy code of ethics and ethics standards (2010). *American Journal of Occupational Therapy, 64*(6 Suppl.), S17–S26. doi:10.5014/ajot.2010.64S17

American Occupational Therapy Association. (2010b). Scope of practice. *American Journal of Occupational Therapy, 64*(6 Suppl.), S70–S77. doi:10.5014/ajot.2010.64S70

American Occupational Therapy Association. (2010c). Standards of practice for occupational therapy. *American Journal of Occupational Therapy, 64*(6 Suppl.), S106–S111. doi:10.5014/ajot.2010.64S106

American Occupational Therapy Association. (n.d.). *The American Occupational Therapy Association self-assessment tool for fieldwork educator competency.* Retrieved November 24, 2007, from http://www.aota.org/Educate/EdRes/Fieldwork/Supervisor/Forms/38251.aspx

Americans With Disabilities Act of 1990, Pub. L. 101–336, 42 U.S.C. § 12101.

Association on Higher Education and Disability. (1996). *Confidentiality and disability issues in higher education* [Brochure]. Huntersville, NC: Author.

Association on Higher Education and Disability. (2004a). *Best practices resources.* Retrieved May 21, 2010, from http://www.ahead.org/resources/best-practices-resources

Association on Higher Education and Disability. (2004b). *Principles: Foundation principles for the review of documentation and the determination of accommodations.* Retrieved May 21, 2010, from http://www.ahead.org/resources/best-practices-resources/principles

Brown, K., & Griffiths, Y. (2000). Confidentiality dilemmas in clinical education. *Journal of Allied Health, 29,* 13–17.

Family Educational Rights and Privacy Act, 20 U.S.C. § 1232g, 34 CFR Part 99 (1974).

Gordon, M., & Keiser, S. (1998). *Accommodations in higher education under the Americans With Disabilities Act (ADA): A no-nonsense guide for clinicians, educators, administrators, and lawyers.* DeWitt, NY: GSI Publications.

Gupta, J., Gelpi, T., & Sain, S. (2005, August). Reasonable accommodations and essential job functions in academic and practice settings. *OT Practice,* pp. CE1–CE7.

Medical College of Georgia. (2008). *Technical standards for occupational therapy.* Retrieved November 21, 2010, from http://www.mcg.edu/sah/ot/standards.html

Northeast Technical Assistance Center. (1999). *Nondiscrimination in higher education.* Retrieved

January 21, 2007, from http://www.netac.rit.edu/publication/tipsheet/ADA.html

Rehabilitation Act of 1973, Pub. L. 93–112, 29 U.S.C. § 701 *et seq.*

Samuel Merritt College. (n.d.). *Occupational therapy technical standards.* Retrieved July 3, 2007, from http://www.samuelmerritt.edu/occupational_therapy/technical_standards

Scott, S. S., Wells, S., & Hanebrink, S. (1997). *Educating college students with disabilities: What academic and fieldwork educators need to know.* Bethesda, MD: AOTA Press.

Stony Brook University. (2004). *Technical standards for admission and continuation in the occupational therapy program.* Retrieved June 7, 2007, from http://www.hsc.stonybrook.edu/shtm/ot/tech-standards.cfm

University of Kansas. (2003). *Occupational therapy education department policy: Technical standards and essential functions for occupational therapy students.* Retrieved November 24, 2007, from http://alliedhealth.kumc.edu/programs/ot/documents/PDF/techstds_preadm.pdf

University of Tennessee. (n.d.). *Technical standards for students in occupational therapy.* Retrieved July 3, 2007, from http://www.uthsc.edu/allied/ot/tech_standards.php

U.S. Department of Labor, National O*NET Consortium. (2003). *Summary report for occupational therapists.* Retrieved January 14, 2008, from http://online.onetcenter.org/link/summary/29-1122.00

U.S. Department of Labor, National O*NET Consortium. (2004). *Summary report for occupational therapy assistants.* Retrieved January 14, 2008, from http://online.onetcenter.org/link/summary/31-2011.00

Van Dusen, W. R. (2004). *FERPA: Basic guidelines for faculty and staff: A simple step-by-step approach for compliance.* Retrieved January 21, 2007, from http:// www.nacada.ksu.edu/Resources/FERPA-Overview.htm

Wells, S. A., & Hanebrink, S. (2000). Lesson 11: Students with disabilities and fieldwork. In *Meeting the fieldwork challenge: AOTA self-*

paced clinical course. Bethesda, MD: American Occupational Therapy Association.

Linda Gabriel, PhD, OTR/L
Education Representative, Ethics Commission (2003–2009)

Betsy DeBrakeleer, COTA/L, ROH
OTA Representative, Ethics Commission (2005–2008)

Lorie J. McQuade, MEd, CRC
Public Member, Ethics Commission (2004–2007)

This chapter was originally published in the 2008 edition of the *Reference Guide to the Occupational Therapy Ethics Standards*. It has been revised to reflect updated AOTA official documents, Web sites, AOTA style, and additional resources.

CHAPTER 27

Ethical Considerations Relevant to Emerging Technology-Based Interventions

INTRODUCTION

The use of new intervention techniques and emerging areas of practice create the potential for various ethical concerns. Decisions about selecting the most appropriate, safe, and effective interventions should be made on the basis of judicious clinical reasoning, sound judgment, insight, experience, and available research evidence (Christiansen & Lou, 2001). *Evidence-based practice* is described as practice based on the investigation and appraisal of currently available research regarding intervention efficacy (Case-Smith & Arbesman, 2008; Christiansen & Lou, 2001). According to Christiansen and Lou (2001), practitioners also should consider relevant ethical principles such as patient benefit, truth, fairness, doing the right thing, avoiding harm, and respecting autonomy. Professional codes of ethics identify these principles to provide guidance for ethical practice and appropriate conduct. They also may be used to assist practitioners in making ethical decisions about less-traditional aspects of clinical practice.

In recent years, new technology-based interventions have appeared for children who have sensory processing difficulties. This Advisory Opinion summarizes several emerging technologies in this area and relevant ethical considerations.

EMERGING TECHNOLOGY-BASED INTERVENTIONS

A variety of specialized technology (from low to high) has emerged over the past few years to address the needs of children with diagnoses such as autism, attention deficit hyperactivity disorder, learning disabilities, and sensory modulation or sensory processing difficulties. One example of the application of specialized technology, the Sensory Learning Program, was developed in 1990 and is described as a multisensory approach that simultaneously stimulates the visual, auditory, and vestibular systems with light, sound, and motion to presumably assist with developmental learning (Bolles, 2004). On the basis of a specific protocol, a trochoidal motion table uses computerized positioning equipment that "slowly rises and descends in a circular pattern that can be rotated 90 degrees, providing vestibular stimulation while the client, who is supine, listens to gated or modulated music through headphones, and is exposed to combinations of diffuse color" (Bolles, 2004). The objective of the program is to allow the central nervous system to enhance sensory processing of information by facilitating the reorganization of the visual, vestibular, and auditory systems simultaneously. Allegedly, this is an "innovative, noncognitive approach" based on the concept of neuroplasticity that stimulates the senses, thereby enhancing "emergent faculties," and "is a therapy that accelerates sensory integration and develops learning abilities for individuals with acquired brain injury, learning/behavioral problems, ADD/ADHD, developmental delays, autism, and birth trauma" (Bolles, 2001). Unlike more traditional interventions, the cost of this modality can be several thousand dollars, which may not be covered by insurance and therefore is an out-of-pocket expense for the client and his or her family. However, there were no published articles found within the professional literature that described the Sensory Learning Program.

Another example of emerging technology-based intervention is sound-based therapy approaches that use the auditory system; these include auditory integration training (AIT) and other therapeutic listening programs (Baranek, 2002; Case-Smith & Arbesman, 2008; Sinha, Silove, Wheeler, & Williams, 2004; Tharpe, 1999). AIT (including the Tomatis and Berard methods) uses modulated music through headphones to remediate hypersensitivities and auditory processing abilities to decrease aberrant behaviors (Baranek, 2002; Case-Smith & Arbesman, 2008). This, too, has a specific protocol over several days (Dawson & Watling, 2000). Case-Smith and Arbesman (2008), however, indicated that evidence for the effectiveness of auditory or sound-based therapies was weak and inconclusive in promoting the integration and organization of the nervous system. Additional evidence-based reviews of this AIT intervention by Case-Smith and Arbesman (2008) and Sinha et al. (2004) came to the same conclusion related to efficacy for children with autism. In addition, the potential risks, adverse side effects, and lack of safeguards associated with hearing loss in some cases show that further studies are necessary (Baranek, 2002; Brown, 1999; Mudford et al., 2000; Sinha et al., 2004).

Additional technology interventions based on *syntonics,* or colored-light therapy, and ZYTO remote technology based on galvanic skin response also have emerged for potential use with these populations (B. T. Barrett, 2009; S. Barrett, 2009; Liberman, 1986, 1991; ZYTO Corporation, n.d.). However, as in the first two examples, limited research and questionable validity of studies preclude scientific support for the current application of these technologies to occupational therapy (B. T. Barrett, 2009; S. Barrett, 2009; Evans & Drasdo, 1991; Liberman, 1986).

ETHICAL CONSIDERATIONS RELEVANT TO EMERGING TECHNOLOGY-BASED INTERVENTIONS

Given the scarcity of conclusive evidence to validate the effectiveness and safety of these technologies, ethical principles must be considered in deciding whether to implement them. Practitioners need to carefully examine their own motivations, driving forces, and rationale (e.g., financial gain, innovative interventions) if they choose to use emerging technology-based interventions that appear to have little evidence for treatment efficacy.

Occupational therapy practitioners have an ethical obligation to be totally transparent in disclosing their ability to provide certain interventions and to avoid practice in areas of limited competence (i.e., professional limitations). They also have an ethical obligation to ensure that equipment is safe and effective for use with clients. The principle of nonmaleficence mandates that practitioners not inflict or cause harm to a client by using an intervention that does not have a reasonable expectation of benefit or that they are not competent to administer. In addition, practitioners must consider that, by virtue of their trust in the therapeutic relationship, consumers may be biased to accept recommendations about innovative technology to address their condition (balancing the probability or possibility of harm vs. benefit). Relevant ethical questions include the following:

- Does the client fully understand the risks and benefits, effectiveness, and safety factors associated with a new, nontraditional intervention when evidence is not available or is limited? Some risks may be unknown.
- Has existing, relevant literature been shared with the client regarding the proposed utility of an emerging technology-based treatment?
- What considerations should direct the ethical decision-making process when evidence is limited or the research does not demonstrate effectiveness?

Ethical reasoning and transparency can assist in communication and autonomous decision making with the client when there is minimal or no evidence. Specifically, the following principles from the American Occupational Therapy Association's (AOTA's) *Occupational Therapy Code of Ethics and Ethics Standards (2010)* (referred to as the "Code and Ethics Standards"; AOTA, 2010a) can assist practitioners in evaluating and making decisions about whether to incorporate emerging or nontraditional technologies in their practices. The following principles are applicable:

Beneficence: Principle 1. Occupational therapy personnel shall demonstrate a concern for the well-being and safety of the recipients of their services.

F. Occupational therapy personnel shall use, to the extent possible, evaluation, planning, intervention techniques, and therapeutic equipment that are evidence-based and within the recognized scope of occupational therapy practice.

G. Occupational therapy personnel shall take responsible steps (e.g., continuing education, research, supervision, training) and use careful judgment to ensure their own competence and weigh potential for client harm when generally recognized standards do not exist in emerging technology or areas of practice.

Principle 1 supports occupational therapy practitioners' obligation to provide interventions that they can reasonably expect to benefit clients; improve their quality of life; and have a safe, effective outcome.

Nonmaleficence: Principle 2. Occupational therapy personnel shall intentionally refrain from actions that cause harm.

C. Occupational therapy personnel shall avoid relationships that exploit the recipient of services . . . physically, emotionally, psychologically, financially, socially, or in any other manner that conflicts or interferes with professional judgment and objectivity.

G. Occupational therapy personnel shall avoid situations in which a practitioner, educator, researcher, or employer is unable to maintain clear professional boundaries or objectivity to ensure the safety and well-being of recipients of service. . . .

Principle 2 involves preventing any foreseeable harm caused by using an intervention for which safety or the potential for harm has not been determined. Similarly, a potential undue influence may pertain to financial incentives associated with providing these new technology-based interventions. For example, if a private practice owner has made a substantial investment in a particular piece of equipment, he or she may be inclined to promote or maximize its use for financial gain.

Autonomy, Confidentiality: Principle 3. Occupational therapy personnel shall respect the right of the individual to self-determination.

A. Occupational therapy personnel shall establish a collaborative relationship with recipients of service, including families, significant others, and caregivers in setting goals and priorities throughout the intervention process. This includes full disclosure of the benefits, risks, and potential outcomes of any intervention; the personnel who will be providing the intervention(s); and/or any reasonable alternatives to the proposed intervention.

C. Occupational therapy personnel shall respect the recipient of service's right to refuse occupational therapy services temporarily or permanently without negative consequences.

This principle is about respecting clients' values, interests, preferences, and privacy and their right to make their own decisions on the basis of those considerations, even if these decisions are not in agreement with practitioner recommendations.

It is important to distinguish between the concepts of informed consent and consent to treat. *Informed consent* is a client's right to full disclosure of what is to be expected in terms of objectives or goals, plan of care, and the known or unknown risks or benefits associated with therapy services and to make decisions on the basis of that information. *Consent to treat* refers to a client's autonomous decision to receive services by volitionally engaging in treatment. It is a professional and ethical mandate to obtain consent to treat from a client before the initiation of the evaluation and any subsequent services. If this is impossible, the practitioner must seek this consent from an individual with legal authority to make such decisions for the client (see Principle 3B of the Code and Ethics Standards). Respect for the patient rights of informed consent and consent to treat is the basis for the principle of autonomy and promotes free choice and trust in the therapist–client relationship. Because technology-based interventions may be at an experimental stage, they should be monitored until best practice, evidence-based, valid, and reliable outcome measures demonstrate definitive positive or negative results.

Procedural Justice: Principle 5. Occupational therapy personnel shall comply with institutional rules, local, state, federal, and international laws and AOTA documents applicable to the profession of occupational therapy.

E. Occupational therapy personnel shall hold appropriate national, state, or other requisite credentials for the occupational therapy services they provide.

F. Occupational therapy personnel shall take responsibility for maintaining high standards and continuing competence in practice, education, and research by participating in professional development and educational activities to improve and update knowledge and skills.

Ensuring competence is a professional responsibility, as is familiarity with applicable current research, to provide state-of-the-art intervention to the extent possible. However, if no evidence exists within the literature, additional professional resources should be sought and used (e.g., ethical reasoning, critical thinking skills, professional resources such as the *Occupational Therapy Practice Framework: Domain and Process;* AOTA, 2008). Maintaining current competency can be done through additional specialty training; certification, if available; or continuing education credits to competently and adequately deliver services.

Principle 5 also addresses occupational therapy practitioners' professional and ethical obligation to be familiar with and comply with state licensure laws (or applicable state regulations) that legally govern appropriate practice and conduct by a practitioner. In states with licensure, licensure laws legally define a profession's scope of practice or domain, and each state has jurisdiction, authority, and power to enforce the legally defined scope of occupational therapy practice in that state. However, language in state practice acts tends to be quite general, so practitioners may need to seek interpretation from the licensure board to assist in decisions about whether particular emerging technology interventions are within their scope of practice.

Veracity: Principle 6. Occupational therapy personnel shall provide comprehensive, accurate, and objective information when representing the profession.

A. Occupational therapy personnel shall represent the credentials, qualifications, education, experience, training, roles, duties, competence . . . accurately in all forms of communication about recipients of service, students, employees, research participants, and colleagues.

B. Occupational therapy personnel shall refrain from using or participating in the use of any form of communication that contains false, fraudulent, deceptive, misleading, or unfair statements or claims.

Principle 6 addresses two additional concepts that are relevant to ethical decision making: transparency and vulnerability. Regarding transparency, occupational therapy practitioners are mandated to provide full disclosure of the risks and benefits of emerging technology-based interventions, including lack of research if applicable or the rationale for why a practitioner is proposing to use a particular device or modality. The concept of vulnerability applies to clients with disabilities or their caregivers.

For example, parents of children with sensory processing disorders, like most parents, may be vulnerable because they are willing to seek and try any available intervention that they believe may help their child improve his or her functional and occupational performance skills. In some circumstances, all customary therapeutic options may have been exhausted, and when a new intervention becomes available, even if it is untried, parents may be in danger of being exploited as they seek positive outcomes. Consequently, parents may find themselves susceptible to costly interventions as they seek to leave no stone unturned to benefit the child, regardless of financial stress. Vulnerability involves issues of trust and the therapeutic relationship between practitioner and client—that is, the ethical principle of Veracity and the core value of truth. Clients in need of and receiving services are at a very vulnerable point in their life and must trust in the honesty of a therapist–client relationship in which their well-being is protected.

In some cases, emergent technology-based interventions have not demonstrated sufficient or conclusive evidence of effectiveness, and adequate evidence may never be obtained. What should the decision-making process be when evidence is limited or altogether absent? The following questions may facilitate the ethical and scope-of-practice reasoning process when limited evidence and guidelines are available for nontraditional interventions:

- Was this body of knowledge contained within the practitioner's core occupational therapy educational curriculum?
- Does the practitioner have adequate education and competence to provide this intervention on the basis of past education or current continuing education?
- "Is this intervention or practice usual and customary among occupational therapy practitioners, and would many of them agree? If not, is it defensible and consistent with the occupational therapy scope of

practice utilizing criteria previously outlined?" (Slater, 2004, p. 16)

- Has clarification from the state licensure board been sought in providing clarity to the less-defined emerging areas of practice within the scope of practice?
- Has the practitioner used AOTA's resources, such as position papers or official documents related to this practice area?
- "Is this occupational therapy?" Is occupation used to facilitate engagement in meaningful activities and engagement in life roles? (Slater, 2004, p. 16)

Practice must meet both ethical and legal criteria. The *Scope of Practice* (AOTA, 2010b) document is an excellent resource guide for reference when an emerging or nontraditional intervention is introduced to clinical practice. This document can provide practice domain guidance. However, AOTA official documents do not replace the legal language in state practice acts, which must be followed for compliance with state laws and regulatory board requirements.

CONCLUSION

Nontraditional technologies and interventions can have positive applications to occupational therapy clients but also can pose ethical challenges to occupational therapy practitioners seeking to integrate them into their practice. Clinicians must understand the level of education and training required to use these technologies and interventions competently from a legal and ethical perspective. Areas of emerging practice and specialization outside of traditional occupational therapy settings can raise similar issues. Practitioners have a professional responsibility to seek evidence and research related to these areas and interventions to assist in making appropriate clinical decisions in collaboration with clients. Furthermore, the principles of Beneficence, Nonmaleficence, Autonomy and Confidentiality, Procedural Justice, and Veracity, which form the basis of the therapeutic rela-

tionship, must be upheld to ensure that clients are protected in potentially ambiguous situations. Above all, occupational therapy practitioners have an obligation to promote benefit for the good of their clients.

REFERENCES

American Occupational Therapy Association. (2008). Occupational therapy practice framework: Domain and process (2nd ed.). *American Journal of Occupational Therapy, 62*, 625–683. doi:10.5014/ajot.62.6.625

American Occupational Therapy Association. (2010a). Occupational therapy code of ethics and ethics standards (2010). *American Journal of Occupational Therapy, 64*(6 Suppl.), S17–S26. doi:10.5014/ajot.2010.64S17

American Occupational Therapy Association. (2010b). Scope of practice. *American Journal of Occupational Therapy, 64*(6 Suppl.), S70–S77. doi:10.5014/ajot.2010.64S70

Baranek, G. T. (2002). Efficacy of sensory and motor interventions for children with autism. *Journal of Autism and Developmental Disorders, 32*, 397–422.

Barrett, B. T. (2009). A critical evaluation of the evidence supporting the practice of behavioural vision therapy. *Ophthalmic and Physiological Optics, 29*, 4–25.

Barrett, S. (2009). *ZYTO scanning: Another test to avoid.* Retrieved June 23, 2009, from Device Watch at http://www.devicewatch.org/reports/zyto/overview.shtml

Bolles, M. (2001). *Bolles Sensory Learning Program.* Retrieved June 1, 2009, from http://www.positivehealth.com/article-view.php?articleid=700

Bolles, M. (2004). *Sensory Learning Program.* Retrieved June 1, 2009, from www.sensorylearning.com

Brown, M. (1999). Auditory integration training and autism: Two case studies. *British Journal of Occupational Therapy, 62*, 13–18.

Case-Smith, J., & Arbesman, M. (2008). Evidence-based review of interventions for autism used in or of relevance to occupational therapy. *American Journal of Occupational Therapy, 62*, 416–429.

Christiansen, C., & Lou, J. (2001). Ethical considerations related to evidence-based practice. *American Journal of Occupational Therapy, 55,* 345–349. doi:10.5014/ajot.55.3.345

Dawson, G., & Watling, R. (2000). Interventions to facilitate auditory, visual, and motor integration in autism: A review of the evidence. *Journal of Autism and Developmental Disorders, 30,* 415–421.

Evans, B. J., & Drasdo, N. (1991). Tinted lenses and related therapies for learning disabilities: A review. *Ophthalmic and Physiological Optics, 11,* 206–217.

Liberman, J. (1986). The effect of syntonic (colored light) stimulation on certain visual and cognitive functions. *Journal of Optometric Vision Development, 17,* 133–144.

Liberman, J. (1991). *Light medicine of the future.* Santa Fe, NM: Bear & Co.

Mudford, O. C., Cross, B. A., Breen, S., Cullen, C., Reeves, D., Gould, J., et al. (2000). Auditory integration training for children with autism: No behavioral benefits detected. *American Journal on Mental Retardation, 105,* 118–129.

Sinha, Y., Silove, N., Wheeler, D., & Williams, K. (2004). Auditory integration training and other sound therapies for autism spectrum disorders (Art No. CD003681). *Cochrane Database of Systematic Reviews, 1.* doi:10.1002/14651858. CD003681.pub2

Slater, D. (2004, September 6). Legal and ethical practice: A professional responsibility. *OT Practice,* pp. 13–16.

Tharpe, A. (1999). Auditory integration training: The magical mystery cure. *Language, Speech, and Hearing Services in Schools, 30,* 378–382.

ZYTO Corporation. (n.d.). *16 commonly asked questions about ZYTO technology.* Retrieved June 3, 2009, from http://www.zyto.com/Documents/questions.pdf

Paige M. Johns, OTD, OTR/L
OTD Student, Creighton University

CHAPTER 28

Ethical Issues Around Payment for Services

The Issues

The current health care environment has created the potential for ethical issues regarding payment for occupational therapy services that may have appeared minimal or nonexistent to occupational therapy practitioners before the past 15 years. Central questions include, How do occupational therapy practitioners ethically apply rules for payment? provide quality care to achieve desired outcomes? manage resources? Additional concerns may arise from administrative decisions based on maximizing reimbursement (perhaps to offset escalating health care costs) rather than based on clinical judgment. These have the potential to erode trust and respect for the dignity of the client, both of which are the foundation of a therapeutic relationship, and to place clinicians in a quandary as they try to balance professional ethics with business ethics (Povar et al., 2004).

For example, in the clinical practice arena, payment for services is governed by a variety of federal and private payment guidelines. Clinicians may be confronted with providing treatment to several recipients of service with the same diagnosis but who are "entitled" by differing insurance plans to different levels of care (e.g., number of visits, coverage of equipment or splints, span of treatment) at different levels of reimbursement. For example, some plans provide for a 90% payment and 10% copay by the recipient of service, some plans provide for an 80%/20% split, and some have larger out-of-pocket costs. Different insurance plans provide certain levels and types of health care coverage, so in some instances, inevitable differences in care may result in the clinic.

Sometimes recipients of service are limited to designated facilities because of payer contract restrictions. In some cases, the facilities in the provider network may not necessarily be those best suited in terms of staff competence and equipment to address their specific medical needs. This raises ethical issues based on the concepts of beneficence, autonomy, and justice. Within the arena of payment for services are ethical concerns about who makes the decisions regarding length and duration of clinical services. Determination of approved services may be done by a third-party case manager without full regard for the complexity of the clinical aspects of a specific case. In the managed care model (including, in many cases, Medicare and Medicaid), the clinical decisions regarding treatment often are made by nonclinical personnel on what may appear to be arbitrary and rigid guidelines (Slater & Kyler, 1999).

For clinical practitioners whose altruism is usually the primary motivating force for seeking a career in occupational therapy and whose guiding principle of ethical practice is beneficence, or doing good for the recipient of service, these payment and clinical service issues can present frequent dilemmas. At the heart of these dilemmas may be the overriding question of professional autonomy based on who is most competent to direct medical care and the duty to advocate for the good of the patient within the system (Povar et al., 2004). The perception that conflicting motives (business vs. altruism) underlie this decision process has the inevitable potential to put the occupational therapy practitioner, the employer, and the insurance entity in conflict.

Ethical allocation of finite resources is yet another related and critical issue. Constraints have always existed in health care, as in other aspects of daily life. Material and human resources have never been unlimited. Yet the tremendous advances in medical technology and health care costs over the past few decades have brought the issue of allocating health care resources responsibility and fairly to the forefront (Povar et al., 2004). Managed care and other payer attempts to control spiraling health care costs have resulted in a swing of the pendulum to what many feel are excessive constraints on treatment that could potentially lead to blatant denial of care. Occupational therapists have faced arbitrary discharges or terminations of treatment because of limitations in health insurance coverage. Occupational therapy treatment may be cut short prematurely or never initiated because of policy limits or restrictions in services. However, occupational therapy practitioners have an ethical obligation to see that resources are most appropriately allocated according to the principle of distributive justice. The allocation of occupational therapy resources should weigh the skill level of the practitioner, the treatment intensity, the type of intervention needed, and the appropriate timing of that intervention so that consumers can achieve optimal outcome. It is unethical to waste resources.

The prevalence of capitated payment systems in skilled nursing facilities and most other traditional medical settings may promote efforts by management to dictate frequency and duration of therapy to ensure maximal reimbursement, resulting in pressure on clinicians to comply. If clinicians are not making these decisions according to their professional judgment, resources may be misallocated on the basis of payer source, with some patients getting unnecessary therapy and others receiving less benefit. Likewise, in these situations, practitioners may be tempted to modify their documentation of intervention needs to support increased reimbursement, which also is an ethical issue.

Finally, the growth in emerging or nontraditional practice areas (e.g., use of alternative or complementary interventions as an adjunct to more usual occupational therapy practice) presents its own potential ethical issues. In these cases, third-party payment is likely to be very limited or nonexistent. Practitioners need to be clear whether the services they provide fall within the scope of occupational therapy and legitimately can be billed as such. They also need to understand ethical considerations in developing fee schedules for a client group that may include private payment from individuals as well as reimbursement by third-party payers. In addition, they need to ensure that their provider contracts do not violate ethical or professional standards.

DISCUSSION

All these issues (e.g., payment rules that may present arbitrary limitations to care, quality of treatment to achieve outcomes, appropriate application of limited resources) can present awkward dilemmas for providers in their dealings with recipients of services. They also present ethical concerns for clinicians. In this environment, the concepts of beneficence, competence, informed consent, autonomy, and education are paramount. Familiarity with and reference to several documents from the American Occupational Therapy Association (AOTA) can provide a useful framework for making ethical decisions that are effective in daily practice. In addition, facility-based ethics committees, supervisors with ethics knowledge, and AOTA ethics staff and Ethics Commission (EC) members can assist practitioners in analyzing issues and identifying strategies to deal with ethical dilemmas. In many cases, these complex issues do not have clear-cut resolutions, so it is not in the client's best interest for clinicians to attempt to handle them on their own. As stated in Principle 5D of the *Occupational Therapy Code of Ethics and Ethics Standards (2010)* (referred to as the "Code and Ethics Standards; AOTA, 2010),

> Occupational therapy personnel shall be familiar with established policies and procedures for handling concerns about the Code and Ethics Standards, including familiarity with national, state, local, district, and territorial procedures for handling ethics complaints as well as policies and procedures created by AOTA and certification, licensing, and regulatory agencies.

LEVEL OF CARE AND INFORMED CONSENT

With respect to loss of autonomy in determining appropriate skill level, treatment intensity, and interventions needed to achieve optimal outcome or the greatest good for recipients of services, both managers and clinicians must rethink service delivery models and educate themselves about cost-effective methods of rendering care. A focus should be on increased collaboration when setting goals with recipients of services so that treatment time is used for the most direct benefit. This is consistent with a client-centered approach to care and with Principle 3A of the Code and Ethics Standards, which states that

> occupational therapy personnel shall establish a collaborative relationship with recipients of service, including families, significant others, and caregivers in setting goals and priorities throughout the intervention process. This includes full disclosure of the benefits, risks, and potential outcomes of any intervention; the personnel who will be providing the intervention(s); and/or any reasonable alternatives to the proposed intervention.

The concept of informed consent in any health care environment is particularly important. Clinicians must be able to discuss all treatment options with a patient and significant others so that they can be fully informed and make appropriate decisions about their care. Recommendations for care also must be free from influence by contractual or other arrangements the insurer may have with the provider (Povar et al., 2004). That does not, however, ensure that all interventions will be reimbursed. In some cases, providing services on a pro bono or private-pay basis may be an appropriate and viable option to improve access to care. Again, clients must be educated as to risks, benefits, and alternatives in an understandable manner (considering, e.g., language, culture, literacy) so that they can make an informed decision whether to consent to or refuse services (Povar et al., 2004).

Principle 4G of the Code and Ethics Standards supports this concept by providing an option for rendering pro bono services within certain parameters: "Occupational therapy personnel shall consider offering *pro bono* ("for the good") or reduced-fee occupational therapy services for selected individuals when consistent with guidelines of the employer, third-party payer, and/or government agency." Although it is not universally possible within the boundaries of employers' policy and financial resources, pro bono services can improve access to occupational therapy.

COMPETENCE

Practitioner competence is another way to help ensure that, irrespective of external payment limits, treatment sessions are focused on the goals established by the occupational therapy practitioner and the recipient of service. This issue is addressed directly in Principle 5F of the Code and Ethics Standards:

> Occupational therapy personnel shall take responsibility for maintaining high standards and continuing competence in

practice, education, and research by participating in professional development and educational activities to improve and update knowledge and skills.

Regardless of length of treatment, the recipient of service will gain the greatest good through clinicians who are highly competent to provide specific care, thus ensuring that the ethical concept of beneficence is central to the scope of occupational therapy services.

The concept of competence in today's health care environment is broad. Competence includes not only clinical competence but also knowledge and ongoing education about financial realities and compliance with reimbursement and regulatory guidelines. In addition, competence includes an occupational therapy practitioner's ability to advise recipients of alternative strategies to reach their goals of decreased impairment and increased occupational performance and participation. This is consistent with Principle 1E of the Code and Ethics Standards: "Occupational therapy personnel shall provide occupational therapy services that are within each practitioner's level of competence and scope of practice (e.g., qualifications, experience, the law)." Likewise, according to Principle 1F, "occupational therapy personnel shall use, to the extent possible, evaluation, planning, intervention techniques, and therapeutic equipment that are evidence-based and within the recognized scope of occupational therapy practice." Upholding this principle will assist occupational therapy practitioners in providing interventions that are most clinically appropriate and effective at the most appropriate point in the continuum of care.

EDUCATION AND ADVOCACY

Education and advocacy are additional realms of knowledge that aid occupational therapy practitioners in negotiating the potential minefield of payment guidelines. Principle 7H of the Code and Ethics Standards supports the development of skills to allow occupational therapy personnel

to "be diligent stewards of human, financial, and material resources of their employers." The trust so critical to the therapeutic relationship also includes "a responsibility to practice effective and efficient health care and to use . . . resources responsibly" (Povar et al., 2004, p. 133). Likewise, it also is a patient's responsibility to be knowledgeable about and share with his or her therapist the details about his or her insurance plan and reimbursement as related to occupational therapy services.

In cases in which there is lack of or limited coverage and the service is essential, there should be a clear and fair procedure for appeal. A clinician's ability to educate clients on advocacy strategies, rights, and options in the health care system is another way of doing good for recipients of services and resolving ethical dilemmas resulting from limitations to care. Advocacy on behalf of clients can include documentation of objective data and relevant evidence to support the positive outcomes of occupational therapy intervention.

It is not unusual for occupational therapy practitioners to treat several clients who have the same diagnosis but who, by virtue of different insurance plans, are entitled to different parameters of care. It is important to remember that recipients of services have chosen a health plan that entitles them to benefits that may not be the same across all payers (Kyler, 1996). It is also important to distinguish between recipients' perceived right to obtain services and the obligation of occupational therapy practitioners in their role as an employee of a health care facility to provide more services than are covered. According to Principle 4E, occupational therapy practitioners should "make efforts to advocate for recipients of occupational therapy services to obtain needed services through available means"; services do not need to be provided in the same way, only in a "goal-directed and objective" manner to the extent possible. This situation emphasizes the importance of occupational therapy practitioners' competence and presents an opportunity for clinicians to educate recipients of their services about advocacy skills in the greater health care system. It also facilitates a collaborative educational process as occupational therapy practitioners and clients may discuss treatment options, strategies, expected outcomes, and alternative methods of reaching goals.

This collaboration has the potential to make recipients of occupational therapy services more active participants in their own care, thereby increasing the likelihood of a positive outcome, and is consistent with the collaborative relationship called for in Principle 3A of the Code and Ethics Standards and within the core value of truth, which infers that prioritizing values is also done through thoughtful deliberation based on the given situation.

In sorting through any ethical dilemma presented in practice, the good of the recipient of services must always serve as the focal point from which intervention decisions are made, regardless of ongoing changes in the external environment. Payment regulations may present ethical dilemmas for occupational therapy practitioners. An important component of the occupational therapy professional role is knowledge about payment guidelines for services and strategies to assist clients in obtaining beneficial services. The ongoing knowledge base needed to maintain competence in the payment for services area includes financial information from federal and state laws, regulations, and guidelines that cover Medicare and Medicaid payment and private payer sources in both fee-for-service and managed care models. The occupational therapy role of educator and advocate also must be acknowledged. The concepts of informed decision making by both occupational therapy practitioner and client must be part of the service delivery process.

Conclusion

Guidelines and regulations for payment change. However, the need for current competency in this area does not change. The Code and Ethics Standards and other documents cited in this Advisory Opinion support the knowledge base to provide cost-effective services in an ethical manner. It is incumbent on occupational therapists and occupational therapy assistants to be familiar with these documents and use them in clinical practice.

References

American Occupational Therapy Association. (2010). Occupational therapy code of ethics and ethics standards (2010). *American Journal of Occupational Therapy, 64*(6 Suppl.), S17–S26. doi:10.5014/ajot.2010.64S17

Kyler, P. (1996). Ethics in managed care. *OT Week, 10,* 9.

Povar, G. J., Blumen, H., Daniel, J., Daub, S., Evans, L., Holm, R. P., et al. (2004). Ethics in practice: Managed care and the changing health care environment. *Annals of Internal Medicine, 141,* 131–136.

Slater, D. Y., & Kyler, P. L. (1999, June). Management strategies for ethical practice dilemmas. *Administration and Management Special Interest Section Quarterly,* pp. 1–2.

Deborah Y. Slater, MS, OTR/L, FAOTA
Chairperson, Commission on Standards and Ethics (2000–2001)

This chapter was originally published in the 2000 edition of the *Reference Guide to the Occupational Therapy Code of Ethics.* It has been revised to reflect updated AOTA official documents, Web sites, AOTA style, and additional resources.

CHAPTER 29

State Licensure, Professionalism, and the AOTA Occupational Therapy Code of Ethics and Ethics Standards

WHEN DOES YOUR STATE LICENSE EXPIRE?

If you are unable to answer this question, please read on to heighten your awareness regarding the importance of state licensure renewal. Although not all states and territories of the United States require licensure per se, they all require some form of regulation for those wishing to provide occupational therapy services. Depending on your location, except in a state with trademark law, all occupational therapists in the United States, District of Columbia, and Puerto Rico are required to be licensed, state certified, or registered or to hold a temporary license or permit in order to provide services to clients. The same is true for occupational therapy assistants except in states with trademark law and those that do not regulate occupational therapy assistants.

All occupational therapy practitioners are required to adhere to state occupational therapy statutes and regulations. States' statutes and regulations governing occupational therapy practice vary in their use of titles and initials. Occupational therapists and occupational therapy assistants need to be aware of the specific provisions in their states so that they and their practice are in compliance with the law. It is unlawful for an unlicensed occupational therapist or occupational therapy assistant to represent himself or herself as an occupational therapy practitioner unless he or she is licensed by the state. State licensees who practice occupational therapy without renewing their license may be subject to criminal prosecution depending on the regulations of the state, district, or province.

The American Occupational Therapy Association (AOTA) *Occupational Therapy Code of Ethics and Ethics Standards (2010)* (referred to as the "Code and Ethics Standards"; AOTA, 2010b) identifies standards that support regulatory bodies and licensing of occupational therapy practitioners. Licensure laws and the Code and Ethics Standards are requisite to protect recipients of services, the practitioner, and the profession. In other words, when practicing without a license, regardless of the reason, the offender not only is violating his or her licensing regulatory board laws but is also breaching the Code and Ethics Standards. Unfortunately, it is not uncommon for occupational therapy practitioners to have such hectic personal and professional lives that they may neglect to take the time to check when their state license requires renewal.

In today's busy world, a variety of life situations arise that may interfere with obtaining or renewing your license to practice occupational therapy. Relocating without leaving a forwarding address for your licensure board or moving to a new state may disrupt your typical pattern for licensure renewal. Having a baby, experiencing a serious personal illness, coping with the illness of a family member, or any other major life event is distracting and may leave practitioners forgetful about licensure renewal.

New practitioners may lack knowledge about how to obtain a license. Practitioners who change employment or work in more than one state may not be aware of each state's licensure requirements. Traveling and international practitioners face the challenge of keeping up with state licensing processes, which are contingent on their relocation, which can occur several times within a year.

These examples may sound familiar to you, and there can be understandable reasons for failing to apply for or renew one's license. However, regardless of the situation, each practitioner is ultimately responsible for ensuring that his or her license is current before practicing as an occupational therapist or occupational therapy assistant. AOTA's State Affairs Group maintains detailed information about state occupational therapy laws on the Association's Web site, including a directory of state occupational therapy regulatory authorities. Practitioners should contact individual state boards or agencies for specific questions about state regulatory requirements.

Licensure is not only a legal measure to protect consumers; it also serves as a safeguard for the profession, the practitioner, and the community at large by preventing nonqualified individuals from practicing occupational therapy. As a protective measure for recipients of service, licensure is a process that affords patient safety in that it prevents individuals who are not trained occupational therapists from assuming such a role and providing spurious intervention under false pretense. An employer, a client, the client's family members, an occupational therapy practitioner, a colleague of another discipline, licensing organizations, or a related professional organization may report practitioners who provide occupational therapy services without a license.

Practitioners reported to be providing occupational therapy services without a license may undergo a review and/or penalty from several professional oversight organizations such as the licensing state, district, or province; AOTA; and the National Board for Certification in Occupational Therapy (NBCOT). Unlicensed practitioners who are members of AOTA may be reported to the Association's Ethics Commission (EC) through a formal complaint process by one of the aforementioned groups or individuals. Depending on the nature of the violation as ascertained from thorough and objective information from relevant sources (e.g., the state regulatory board, NBCOT, the complainant, and/or the respondent), the EC determines the principles of the Code and Ethics Standards that have been violated. State and national regulatory boards and professional organizations such as NBCOT (*Certificant Code of Conduct;* NBCOT, 2010) may adopt AOTA's Code and Ethics Standards or similar ethical language. The following are examples of Code and Ethics Standards principles one would violate by practicing without a license or with an expired or lapsed license:

- Principle 5F: "Occupational therapy personnel shall take responsibility for maintaining high standards and continuing competence in practice, education, and research by participating in professional development and educational activities to improve and update knowledge and skills."
- Principle 5E: "Occupational therapy personnel shall hold appropriate national, state, or other requisite credentials for the occupational therapy services they provide."

All occupational therapy practitioners are ethically bound to adhere to and follow the credential requirements of their state, territory, or district in particular, maintaining the required credentials in a timely manner as required.

- Principle 5: "Occupational therapy personnel shall comply with institutional rules, local, state, federal, and international laws and AOTA documents applicable to the profession of occupational therapy." (Procedural Justice)

- Principle 5B: "Occupational therapy personnel shall be familiar with and seek to understand and abide by institutional rules, and when those rules conflict with ethical practice, take steps to resolve the conflict."

In the case of licensure and its legal ramifications, the understanding is that occupational therapy practitioners are ethically responsible for securing, reading, and understanding licensure rules and requirements for their state, territory, or district.

- Principle 5C: "Occupational therapy personnel shall be familiar with revisions in those laws and AOTA policies that apply to the profession of occupational therapy and inform employers, employees, colleagues, students, and researchers of those changes."

Occupational therapy practitioners are responsible for maintaining up-to-date knowledge about changes and additions to their state licensure requirements.

- Principle 5H: "Occupational therapy personnel shall provide appropriate supervision to individuals for whom they have supervisory responsibility in accordance with AOTA official documents and local, state, and federal or national laws, rules, regulations, policies, procedures, standards, and guidelines."

Occupational therapy practitioners who function in a leadership capacity are responsible for ensuring that occupational therapy professionals under their supervision have met all state requirements for licensure in the timely manner required by law.

- Principle 5L: "Occupational therapy personnel shall take reasonable steps to ensure that employers are aware of occupational therapy's ethical obligations as set forth in this Code and Ethics Standards and of the implications of those obligations for occupational therapy practice, education, and research.

All occupational therapy practitioners are responsible for communicating to their employer, supervisor, director, and so forth, up-to-date information regarding their licensure status.

- Principle 6: "Occupational therapy personnel shall provide comprehensive, accurate, and objective information when representing the profession." (Veracity)
- Principle 6A: "Occupational therapy personnel shall represent the credentials, qualifications, education, experience, training, roles, duties, competence, views, contributions, and findings accurately in all forms of communication about recipients of service, students, employees, research participants, and colleagues."

Any individual declaring himself or herself an occupational therapy practitioner and providing services to clients in that regard is required by the laws of his or her state, territory, or district and the AOTA to be credentialed according to the board regulations in their geographic area. This assures recipients of occupational therapy services that they are receiving care from individuals who are qualified to do so.

Three of the core values discussed in the Preamble of the Code and Ethics Standards reflect the commitment and responsibility of occupational therapy practitioners to maintain up-to-date practice credentials:

1. Justice—The concept of justice is most relevant, as it requires the practitioner to abide by laws and standards established by governing bodies:

   Occupational therapy practitioners, educators, and researchers relate in a fair and impartial manner to individuals with whom they interact and respect and adhere to the applicable laws and standards regarding their area of practice, be it direct care, education, or research (justice). (AOTA, 2010b, p. S17)

It is the responsibility of the occupational therapist and occupational therapy assistant to ensure that they are informed about regulatory requirements in their state, territory, or district to provide services they identify as occupational therapy.

2. Truth—The value of truth requires that "in all situations, occupational therapists, occupational therapy assistants, and students must provide accurate information, both in oral and written form" (AOTA, 2010b, p. S18). Further, veracity is shown by being accountable, honest, and authentic in both attitude and action. Occupational therapists and occupational therapy assistants should be accountable by acquiring their initial license and renewing it thereafter as required by their regulatory board. Practitioners are responsible for providing information to employers regarding their licensure status.

3. Prudence—The concept of prudence means that "occupational therapy personnel use their clinical and ethical reasoning skills, sound judgment, and reflection to make decisions to direct them in their area(s) of practice" (AOTA, 2010b, p. S18). Although regulatory boards may provide renewal information to practitioners, it is the sole responsibility of the professional to be self-disciplined in securing and maintaining the credentials required by their state, territory, or district.

When a credentialing violation has occurred, the EC applies the *Enforcement Procedures for the Occupational Therapy Code of Ethics and Ethics Standards* (AOTA, 2010a) as a disciplinary and protective measure on the basis of a range of circumstances. AOTA fully supports the legal and practice intent of credentialing out of concern for consumer and practitioner protection and enforces the Code and Ethics Standards in an effort to maintain the integrity of the profession. Examples of disciplinary actions that may be applied to cases involving the practice of occupational therapy without the appropriate credentials are as follows:

1.3.1. Reprimand—A formal expression of disapproval of conduct communicated privately by letter from the EC Chairperson that is nondisclosable and noncommunicative to other bodies (e.g., state regulatory boards, NBCOT).

1.3.2. Censure—A formal expression of disapproval that is public.

1.3.3. Probation of Membership Subject to Terms—Failure to meet terms will subject an AOTA member to any of the disciplinary actions or sanctions.

1.3.4. Suspension—Removal of AOTA membership for a specified period of time.

1.3.5. Revocation—Permanent denial of AOTA membership. (AOTA, 2010a, p. S5).

Case Scenario

You are an occupational therapy practitioner with 15 years of experience. You have been married for slightly over 2 years and have a 4-month-old baby. Your husband received a job transfer, and you have recently moved to a new state. Two months after relocating to your new state, you join the state occupational therapy association. Through the state association, you learn of a job opening; you apply and are hired. Although the state requires licensure, they provide you with a grace period of 3 months to get the process completed. You have worked in three other states, so you need to supply past licensure information from those states, as well as information about having successfully completed the National Certification Exam for occupational therapy practitioners.

You develop influenza and are very ill for at least 2 weeks. During this time, you are worried about your family and your new employment. Eventually you recover and return to work with a great deal to catch up on, both at work and at home. Along the way, you forget about the licensure requirement. It is now 15 months later, and you receive a notice from the state board stating that you are facing disciplinary action as a result of practicing without a license. Your initial response is that you actually completed the licensure process. You search for the information but are unable to locate any paperwork to verify that you actually completed the licensure process.

Even though your circumstances were challenging, the overriding issue is that you violated the law and practiced without a license for a significant period of time. Because of the collaborative professional relationship between organizations, state licensing boards routinely communicate information regarding lapsed licenses to the AOTA's EC. Referencing the aforementioned principles, the likelihood of disciplinary action from a variety of sources is probable. Regardless of your personal circumstances, the final determination will be influenced by the sum of information collected from all parties involved, including your supervisors from your place of employment.

CONCLUSION

In many states, achieving regulatory status required extensive lobbying and legislative efforts. The collaborative effort between AOTA and state associations has been instrumental in assisting states to achieve this professional status. This widespread, successful effort legally ensures the quality of occupational therapy service for consumers and prevents illegal behavior on the part of individuals without professional training and certification in occupational therapy who call themselves occupational therapists, thus aiding in the preservation of the integrity of the profession. Occupational therapy practitioners are legally bound by state requirements and are ethically responsible for compliance with them. This *Reference Guide to the Occupational Therapy Code of Ethics and Ethics Standards* serves as a helpful resource to understand the potential penalty for practicing as an unlicensed occupational therapy practitioner. An increased awareness and knowledge regarding the importance of state license renewal will protect occupational therapists, occupational therapy assistants, and students from unnecessary legal problems, work interruption, and professional and personal embarrassment.

REFERENCES

American Occupational Therapy Association. (2010a). Enforcement procedures for the *Occupational Therapy Code of Ethics and Ethics Standards*. *American Journal of Occupational Therapy, 64* (6 Suppl.), S4–S16. doi:10.5014/ajot.2010.64S4

American Occupational Therapy Association. (2010b). Occupational therapy code of ethics and ethics standards (2010). *American Journal of Occupational Therapy, 64*(6 Suppl.), S17–S26. doi:10.5014/ajot.2010.64S17

National Board for Certification in Occupational Therapy. (2010). *NBCOT candidate/certificant code of conduct.* Retrieved June 24, 2010, from http://www.nbcot.org/pdf/Candidate-Certifi cant-Code-of-Conduct.pdf

Melba J. Arnold, MS, OTR/L
Member, Commission on Standards and Ethics (1999–2005)

Diane Hill, COTA/L, AP, ROH
OTA Representative, Commission on Standards and Ethics (1999–2005)

This chapter was originally published in the 2006 edition of the *Reference Guide to the Occupational Therapy Code of Ethics*. It has been revised to reflect updated AOTA official documents, Web sites, AOTA style, and additional resources.

CHAPTER 30

Ethics in Governance

INTRODUCTION

Ethics in governance is about the qualities of leadership and the values expressed by the leaders themselves. Leaders set the tone and character of the organization of which they are stewards. *Values* are a core set of beliefs that guide actions. Ethics are derived from and based on a particular code of values (Campbell, 2003). Occupational therapy leaders are guided by the core values of the profession (American Occupational Therapy Association [AOTA], 2010).

THE ISSUES

Leaders in volunteer organizations, such as a professional association, are frequently faced with expectations by members to increase the performance of the organization but also are faced with limited resources and options. There are pressures to maintain or expand existing programs, membership benefits, and ideals while at the same time to change, be innovative, be creative, and be different (Merrill Associates, 2002). Leadership training to deal effectively with membership expectations often is learned in the course of performing the leadership role. The result may be ethical dilemmas and tough choices for the volunteers or elected leaders who challenge the profession's core values and beliefs. Dilemmas may evolve from conflicts of interest, conflict of commitment (i.e., accepting additional roles that have a negative impact on

the ability to meet current responsibilities), and/or a misunderstanding of one's fiduciary responsibility.

The values in leadership are similar to the values in practice. These values are trustworthiness, respect, responsibility, fairness, caring, and citizenship (Seel, 1996). The six values are based in part on the six pillars of character developed by the Josephson Institute for Ethics (2007). *Trustworthiness* includes "integrity, honesty, reliability, and loyalty" (Josephson Institute for Ethics, 2007, ¶ 7). *Respect* includes dignity, tolerance, acceptance, nonviolence, and courtesy. *Responsibility* includes duty, accountability, pursuit of excellence, and self-control. *Fairness* includes justice, impartiality, and openness. *Caring* includes concern for others and altruism. *Citizenship* includes doing your share and respecting authority. These six values are consistent with the core values of the American Occupational Therapy Association (AOTA, 2010): altruism, equality, freedom, justice, dignity, truth, and prudence.

DISCUSSION

These leadership values also are expressed and covered in the *Occupational Therapy Code of Ethics and Ethics Standards (2010)* (referred to as the "Code and Ethics Standards"; AOTA, 2010). They are illustrated in this document for clarity. *Trustworthiness* is part of Veracity (Principle 6) and is supported by

Fidelity (Principle 7). *Respect* is supported by Fidelity (Principle 7) and Autonomy, Confidentiality (Principle 3). *Fairness* is part of Procedural Justice (Principle 5). *Caring* is part of Beneficence (Principle 1) and Nonmaleficence (Principle 2). *Citizenship* and *responsibility* involve all seven principles. In addition, Principles 7E (conflict of interest) and 7D (resolving ethical issues in professional organizations) of the Code and Ethics Standards also are especially relevant.

Leaders need to constantly monitor their behavior to avoid the perception of seeking secondary gains from their position. For example, one situation in which the ethical conduct of leaders can be challenged is when they are called on to speak to members at local or state meetings and to represent AOTA at other organizational events. The content of their presentations and their conduct during their representations reflect directly on the reputation of the Association. Therefore, a volunteer who is in an AOTA leadership role must avoid projecting personal opinions or promoting his or her employer or policies that would benefit his or her employer. Following the principles of ethical conduct and good leadership provides sound guidance toward ensuring that AOTA will continue to be well respected and maintain its good reputation with both its members and outside groups.

Some examples of the ethical values in application may include the following statements adapted from the American Heart Association (AHA, 2006) and Josephson Institute for Ethics (2007):

- Be honest and truthful in personal conduct related to Association business, including the "handling of actual or apparent conflicts of interest between personal and professional relationships" (AHA, 2006, ¶ 11). (Trustworthiness)
- Be loyal to the Association and committed to maintaining its good reputation. (Trustworthiness)

- Treat members of the Association, fellow volunteers, and employees with good manners and with tolerance for differences. (Respect)
- Resolve disagreements without resorting to anger and insults. (Respect)
- "Comply with all applicable government laws, rules, and regulations" (AHA, 2006, ¶ 11). (Responsibility)
- "Protect and ensure the proper use of" (AHA, 2006, ¶ 11) Association assets. (Responsibility)
- Be open-minded and listen to what others (members, fellow volunteers, and employees) have to say. (Fairness)
- Do not take advantage of others or blame others carelessly. (Fairness)
- Provide Association members "with information that is accurate . . . objective, relevant, timely, and understandable" (AHA, 2006, ¶ 11). (Caring)
- "Proactively promote ethical behavior" (AHA, 2006, ¶ 11) among Association members, fellow volunteers, and employees. (Caring)
- Complete assigned tasks on time and perform to the best of personal ability. (Citizenship)
- Stay informed on topics of interest and concern to the Association and its members. (Citizenship)
- Cooperate with others to accomplish the goals and objectives of the Association and its members. (Citizenship)
- Be accountable for personal behavior and actions at all times. (Citizenship)

SUMMARY

Ethical behavior in governance is based on the same principles as the expected ethical conduct of all AOTA members. However, volunteer and elected leaders have accepted, by virtue of their position, additional responsibilities within the Association. These responsibilities include behaviors that require a higher level of ethical conduct than members without such responsibilities. The welfare and well-being of AOTA must remain the Number 1 concern of all leaders involved in Association governance. Adherence to the AOTA Code and Ethics Standards and the values on which they are based provides a sound approach to ensuring that AOTA will remain a vital force and voice in expressing the goals and objectives of the profession.

REFERENCES

American Heart Association. (2006). *Ethics policy*. Retrieved February 1, 2007, from http://www.americanheart.org/presenter.jhtml?identifier=3023721

American Occupational Therapy Association. (2010). Occupational therapy code of ethics and ethics standards (2010). *American Journal of Occupational Therapy, 64*(6 Suppl.), S17–S26. doi:10.5014/ajot.2010.64S17

Campbell, K. H. (2003, Fall/Winter). Ethics today: Personal, practical, and relevant. *The Connection.* Retrieved September 13, 2006, from www.casanet.org/

Josephson Institute for Ethics. (2007). *The six pillars of character*. Retrieved May 14, 2007, from http://www.josephsoninstitute.org/MED/MED-2sixpillars.htm

Merrill Associates. (2002). *Topic of the month: April 2002*. Retrieved September 13, 2006, from www.merrillassociates.net

Seel, K. (1996). The new AVA statement of professional ethics in volunteer administration. *Journal of Volunteer Administration, 14*(2), 33–38.

Kathlyn L. Reed, PhD, OTR, FAOTA, MLIS
Chairperson, Ethics Commission (2007–2010)

This chapter was originally published in the 2008 edition of the *Reference Guide to the Occupational Therapy Ethics Standards.* It has been revised to reflect updated AOTA official documents, Web sites, AOTA style, and additional resources.

CHAPTER 31

Organizational Ethics

INTRODUCTION

The health care system has changed in recent years from a model where health care relationships were defined primarily by the provider and patient to a more complex model where the organization in which the health care professional practices has a direct impact on the care provided to patients. The role of the organization in the delivery of care has introduced business, financial, and management pressures into the health care environment, often leading to ethical conflict among delivery, access, and reimbursement for service. As stated by the American Society for Bioethics and Humanities (1998), "Ethical issues in organizational behavior have become more evident in recent years with the emergence of a more explicit market approach to medicine" (p. 24). The market approach has resulted in the need for integrating organizational ethics into the health care environment. This integration has led to speculation regarding how business ethics and clinical ethics will coexist within the infrastructure of the health care institution. However, organizational ethics is more than clinical ethics and business ethics combined. Organizations must take into account values and moral positions that are defined both internally and externally (Spencer & Mills, 1999), including the professionals and the codes that shape their behavior and guide practice.

Strategies for shaping an ethical organization must include health care values and codes of ethics. Health care professionals have always been held to a high ethical standard; therefore, organizations that provide health care services also must be held to this standard. Ethics in organizations are often complicated by business pressures. Health care organizations have become more complex and more involved in managing care, especially in times of limited resources. There are ethical tensions resulting from pressures to do more with less. Health care organizations are expected to improve quality and expand access while reducing cost (Veterans Health Administration, National Center for Ethics, 2002). However, these pressures do not excuse organizations from their primary purpose of caring for people. In addition, if a health care professional works for an organization, ethical or otherwise, he or she cannot hide behind the policies or administration of the institution; his or her professional code and values must continue to guide practice. Ethical action requires the organization and the health care provider to demonstrate "integrity in the face of patients' exploitable vulnerability, [and] loyalty even to the point of personal sacrifice" (L. Emanuel, 2000, p. 155).

THE ISSUES

Occupational therapy practitioners are not immune to these market-based pressures. Most clinicians are familiar with the pressure to do more with less, whether manifested in lack of resources or increased productivity standards. Constraints in time and money will continue to exist in health care; therefore, occupational therapy practitioners must understand how to handle these problems ethically while addressing the needs of the patients and the communities they serve. Practitioners may work within an organization, but they also belong to a profession with core values based on concepts of altruism, equality, freedom, justice, dignity, truth, and prudence.

Health care providers are finding themselves enmeshed in relationships that extend beyond the provider and patient. These providers "interact on matters of accountability over many different domains and mechanisms [creating] what we might call a complex reciprocating matrix of accountability" (E. J. Emanuel & Emanuel, 1996, p. 231). The organization in which a health care professional practices often acts as a domain that influences the behavior of the practitioner. If the practitioner is an employee of the organization, then a level of accountability to that organization's culture, standards, and viability is subsumed. Although the focus of accountability is often limited to the dynamic of the provider–patient relationship, service delivery is influenced by relationships external to this dyad. The occupational therapy practitioner may be placed in situations where it is difficult to protect and maintain the provider–patient relationship. In some circumstances, occupational therapy practitioners will be pressured to provide services that conflict with their personal or professional code of ethics in order to support decisions made by individual physicians or made within the organization.

Ethics focuses on choices in at least three domains: (1) choices about what we ought to do or not do—that is, the actions we might undertake; (2) choices about the kind of persons we ought to be or not be—that is, the kind of character we ought to have or develop; and (3) more abstractly, choices about the conditions of doing and being, which are perhaps best illustrated in the context of the organizational cultures, structures, or policies that influence but do not determine what we do and who we are as persons (Heller, 1999, p. 346).

It is this influence of the organization that often leaves practitioners in the difficult position of attempting to respect the patient's rights while also attempting to support the organization's policies, procedures, and financial viability. Organizations are dominant moral actors in today's health arena, not only influencing policies within the hospital but also creating role expectations for health care providers that influence how they perform professionally within the organization (Goold, 2001).

In years past, relationships in health care were arguably less complicated. Practitioners' ethical obligations were primarily limited to the patient and acting within that patient's best interest (Gervais, 1998). Practitioners' roles and accountabilities were outlined by oaths and professional codes of ethics. These codes are designed to address conflict specific to the patient–provider relationship but are lacking when used to address more complex ethical dilemmas that extend beyond the bedside and encompass organizational ethics issues. With growing changes in health care, and with the shift in focus from health care providers to corporate institutions, "greater attention must be paid to the moral content or moral character of the actions of health care organizations" (Goold, Kamil, Cohan, & Sefansky, 2000, p. 69). In particular, one must be aware of the impact an organization's moral character has on its practitioners. Although organizations must consider the relationships between "institutions and patients, patient populations, professionals, and other institutions" (Khushf, 1998, p. 133), the organization cannot undermine the integrity of the provider–patient relationship:

[Organizations must take into] account interaction among individuals, health care workers, institutions, integrated delivery systems and the entire health care environment. Any account of organizational ethics that focuses only on one level of the environment, such as the team or the institution, without examining and accounting for interaction among the levels of the environment, is inadequate. (Boyle, DuBose, Ellingson, Guinn, & McCurdy, 2001, p. 8)

This goal of organizations to meet individual as well as comprehensive societal needs may at times seem to conflict with the provider's responsibility to the patient. When this conflict occurs, the provider is often presented with a dilemma to support either the organization's goals or the patient's rights. An ethical dilemma will be encountered when a morally correct course of action requires the therapist to support both the organization and the patient, but the supporting actions are mutually exclusive, meaning that the therapist cannot do both (Purtilo, 2005).

Although the organization is responsible for responding to all of these levels of the environment, the occupational therapy practitioner working within the organization cannot be accountable to all of these groups without risking an erosion of the provider–patient relationship. This dynamic appears to be a conflict between organizational ethics and those of the practitioner. A health care organization must be accountable to multiple parties and the community, but this extended accountability should not detract from the provider's relationship with the patient. The organization, therefore, cannot ethically require a practitioner to engage in decision making or actions that will undermine the provider–patient relationship: "Any social, organizational, administrative, and financial arrangement with practice settings that contribute to distancing [providers] from their patients will result in tendencies to dehumanize them and will ultimately diminish the [provider's] competence to heal" (Scott, Aiken, Mechanic, & Moravcsik, 1995, p. 81). There-

fore, although organizational and clinical ethics may seem to conflict initially, the care of the individual patient is the common tenet in both areas of ethics, and ultimately the destruction of the provider–patient relationship detracts from delivery of care and patients' outcomes (Mills, Spencer, Rorty, & Werhane, 2000). Unfortunately, not all health care organizations recognize the role the institution plays in sustaining the provider–patient relationship, and inevitably the provider encounters situations in which he or she must choose to act as directed by organizational administration or on behalf of the patient.

The conflict that arises from the health care professional's complex matrix of accountability often leads to lack of trust between patients and providers. These conflicts have resulted in eroded trust between health care provider and patient (Haskell, 2000). Trust is a necessary component of the health care relationship between therapist and patient: "The need for trust and the reliance on trust are especially important in health care because of the patient's acute vulnerability to suffering, lost opportunity, and lack of power" (Goold, 2001, p. 26). Within the provider–patient relationship, the occupational therapy practitioner has more power, and how he or she wishes to use that power can quickly degrade the trust of a patient. One potential abuse of that power presents itself in the form of paternalism. Practitioners who independently define the patient's best interest and provide care based on their assumptions of best interest—without the consent, or worse, against the will of the patient—are acting in a paternalistic manner. Health care in the United States has shifted away from a paternalistic manner that affords the professional the power to make decisions in the health care environment and has moved toward a focus on patient autonomy (Quill & Brody, 1996).

CASE SCENARIO AND DISCUSSION

An occupational therapist has received a referral to see a patient on the cardiac floor of a community hospital. When the therapist enters the room to complete her evaluation, the patient refuses occupational therapy services. The occupational therapist continues to see the patient over the course of the next week. On all occasions, the patient refuses to participate in therapy. During each visit the therapist explains to the patient and her family the importance of occupational therapy services, why her physician has referred her for treatment, and the risks of minimal activity after cardiac surgery. In addition, the occupational therapist speaks with nursing staff to determine whether the patient has been seen by a psychiatrist to rule out depression or any other emotional state that may be affecting participation. The nurse refers the occupational therapist to a report compiled by the psychiatrist indicating that the patient is slightly depressed but has full decision-making capacity and is therefore able to make health-care-related decisions. The occupational therapist decides to call the physician to tell her that she will be discharging the patient from services because of the patient's informed refusal of treatment. During this discussion, the physician states to the therapist that she will need to continue treatment and that she should "not allow the patient to refuse services" and then abruptly hangs up the phone.

When the occupational therapist arrives to work the next day, she has another written physician referral on her desk stating, "Evaluate and treat for occupational therapy services; do not allow the patient to refuse." This new order places the occupational therapist in a difficult position, and she does not know how to proceed. She wants to respect the patient's autonomy, and yet she feels a responsibility to maintain a positive working relationship with the physician. Her confusion is complicated by her obligation to the health care organization for which she is working, and she fears that aggravating the physician may result in a decrease in referrals for patients who may benefit from occupational therapy services and subsequent decreased revenue for the department.

Occupational therapists often work under the direction of a physician and within a health care organization. Organizations drive care because they have a vested interest in services provided and in ensuring continued physician referrals that support the financial solvency of the institution. This situation is especially true in communities where the physicians are not employed by the facility itself but also have privileges at competing hospitals within the same town. Of the three relationships—patient, physician, and organization—the patient relationship is often seen as the one to whom the occupational therapy practitioner is most responsible. There are serious questions about what accountability occupational therapy practitioners have to the organizations that employ them. Do employees have a fiduciary responsibility to support the organizations that employ them as well as other health care professionals within the organization, even if that relationship conflicts with their patient relationship?

Occupational therapy practitioners may perceive that the organization would support a team environment, which favors the physician, because there may be negative financial fallout if physician relationships are strained. However, it is in the organization's best interest to support provider–patient relationships that build trust, because these relationships make for better medical care (Goold, 2001). Ethical health care organizations should not require a practitioner to compromise standards in the delivery of care. Organizations that place providers in situations that jeopardize the patient–provider relationship are also jeopardizing the organization's relationship with the customer. In the case scenario above, if the occupational therapist were to violate the trust of the patient by forcing her to participate in therapy against her will, the therapist would inadvertently make the institution less trustworthy in the eyes of the patient. Because of this need to support individual provider–patient relationships, most organizations have policies and resources in place that can support the provider in making ethical choices.

In the case scenario, the occupational therapist should use her supervisor to help her in communicating with the physician. If a supervisor is not available, there is generally a medical director or administrator who can facilitate communication with the physician. Often organizational management can communicate with physicians in a way that minimizes power imbalances. In addition, a supervisor or administrator should be familiar with and able to locate patients' rights policies that objectively identify patient and provider roles and can assist the employee in identification of other organizational resources. The hospital ethics committee or consultation services may help resolve conflict between health care providers within the confines of the organization. In addition, organizational structures, such as incident reporting systems or safety hotlines, can be used to influence the behavior of providers in order to protect patient rights while keeping the reporting source anonymous so as to avoid strained relationships among team members. The occupational therapist walks a difficult line in balancing these team relationships with her responsibilities to the patient.

Helping patients exercise their autonomy effectively in today's health care environment has become more and more complicated. However, Principle 3 of the *Occupational Therapy Code of Ethics and Ethics Standards (2010)* (referred to as the "Code and Ethics Standards") requires occupational therapy personnel to respect their patients and assure that their rights are being upheld (American Occupational Therapy Association [AOTA], 2010). Because of the complex matrix of accountability faced when practicing in health care organizations, practitioners often find themselves not only in a relationship with the patient but also in collegial relationships with other health care providers and the institution. Although the provider–patient relationship is typically the theoretical focus for conflict resolution, other relationships also must be maintained by the provider to ensure safe, effective, and ethical delivery of health care services.

This concept of fidelity is also present in the Code and Ethics Standards under Principle 7: "Occupational therapy personnel shall treat colleagues and other professionals with respect, fairness, discretion, and integrity." However, an occupational therapist need not compromise a relationship with a patient in order to maintain other relationships. In fact, respecting the patient's right to refuse—thus maintaining the integrity of the provider–patient relationship—is ethically mandated in order to ensure ethical practices that support the moral structure of the health care environment.

In the case scenario above, the occupational therapist does have options for justifying a course of action. The therapist should pursue opportunities for communication with the physician; however, if the physician continues to rebuff the therapist's attempts at dialogue, the therapist should pursue another avenue for communication involving the administration. Depending on the organization's understanding of its role in fostering relationships between providers and patients, the therapist may or may not encounter a supportive advocate for resolution of the ethical dilemma. If this option does not resolve the conflict, the therapist may ultimately decide to transfer care of the patient to another therapist; refuse to treat the patient, which may result in termination of employment; or continue treating the patient. Continuing to treat a patient who is refusing services and has decision-making capacity would not be ethically justifiable. This option could lead to many adverse outcomes, including a decline in trust between patient and provider; the potential harm—both psychological and physical—imposed on the patient; the lack of benefit incurred when treating a patient against his or her will (also a legal issue because it can be construed as assault and battery); and, ultimately, a decline in trust between health care providers, organizations, and the individuals served.

Although the previously mentioned options are viable, it is important to actively advocate for the patient, but in a respectful manner that is least damaging to relationships between physician and therapist. Although patient trust is essential, one must also work to maintain trust between colleagues and team members.

CONCLUSION

Research demonstrates over and over again that patients most highly value having a strong relationship with their health care provider (Gervais, 1998). The humanistic characteristics of the occupational therapy profession, in which emphasis is placed on the patient's view of meaningful life, morally require respect for the patient's wishes, even when these wishes seem to conflict with clinical reasoning and their own benefit. It is not that autonomy-based obligations trump beneficence-based obligations; however, when there is no compelling beneficence-based obligation to consider, as demonstrated in the case study, a health care provider has no morally based option but to adhere to the patient's informed choice (Chervenak & McCullough, 1991). Although other health care professionals are often apprehensive about sharing decision-making powers with the patient (Henderson, 2003), occupational therapists rely on patient input to help identify the direction intervention should take. AOTA (2005) has acknowledged that "ethical decision making is a process that includes awareness of how the outcome will impact occupational therapy clients in all spheres" (p. S18) and encourages the implementation of core occupational therapy tenets that require the active participation of the client. Occupational therapy is a traditionally holistic profession with humanistic roots implying a "theoretical and practical commitment to treating patients in a caring, respectful and holistic manner that appreciates their dignity, individual needs and meaningful life circumstances" (Lohman & Brown, 1997, p. 11).

The occupational therapy practitioner has an ethical responsibility to maintain the integrity of the provider–patient relationship in the face of organizational pressures. Whether this relationship is maintained through respect for autonomy or advocating for patient rights and needs with regard to care, occupational therapists must be aware of their responsibilities to the well-being of the patient. Within the Code and Ethics Standards, the first principle calls on practitioners to act with beneficence. Although the therapist cannot disregard or neglect his or her relationships within an organization, a practitioner must remember that undermining the patient's trust promotes neither the integrity of the organization nor the integrity of the patient–provider relationship.

REFERENCES

American Occupational Therapy Association. (2010). Occupational therapy code of ethics and ethics standards (2010). *American Journal of Occupational Therapy, 64* (6 Suppl.), S17–S26. doi:10.5014/ajot.2010.64S17

American Society for Bioethics and Humanities. (1998). *Core competencies for health care ethics consultation: The report of the American Society for Bioethics and Humanities.* Glenview, IL: Author.

Boyle, P. J., DuBose, E. R., Ellingson, S. J., Guinn, D. E., & McCurdy, D. B. (2001). *Organizational ethics in health care: Principles, cases, and practical solutions.* San Francisco: Jossey-Bass.

Chervenak, F. A., & McCullough, L. B. (1991). Justified limits on refusing intervention. *Hastings Center Report, 21*(2), 7–12.

Emanuel, E. J., & Emanuel, L. L. (1996). What is accountability in health care? *Annals of Internal Medicine, 124,* 229–239.

Emanuel, L. (2000). Ethics and the structures of healthcare. *Cambridge Quarterly of Healthcare Ethics, 9,* 151–168.

Gervais, K. G. (1998). Changing society, changing medicine, changing bioethics. In R. DeVries & J. Subedi (Eds.), *Bioethics and society: Constructing the ethical enterprise* (pp. 216–232). Upper Saddle River, NJ: Prentice-Hall.

Goold, S. (2001). Trust and the ethics of health care institutions. *Hastings Center Report, 31*(6), 26–33.

Goold, S., Kamil, L., Cohan, N., & Sefansky, S. (2000). Outline of a process for organizational ethics consultation. *HEC Forum, 12*(1), 69–77.

Haskell, C. M. (2000, September/October). Healthcare ethics and integrity. *Veterans Health Systems Journal,* pp. 53–60.

Heller, J. C. (1999). Framing healthcare compliance in ethical terms: A taxonomy of moral choices. *HEC Forum, 11,* 345–357.

Henderson, S. (2003). Power imbalance between nurses and patients: A potential inhibitor of partnership in care. *Journal of Clinical Nursing, 12,* 501–508.

Khushf, G. (1998). The scope of organizational ethics. *HEC Forum, 10,* 127–135.

Lohman, H., & Brown, K. (1997). Ethical issues related to managed care: An in-depth discussion of an occupational therapy case study. *Occupational Therapy in Healthcare, 10*(4), 1–12.

Mills, A. E., Spencer, E. M., Rorty, M. V., & Werhane, P. H. (2000). *Organization ethics in health care.* New York: Oxford University Press.

Purtilo, R. (2005). *Ethical dimensions in the health professions* (4th ed.). Philadelphia: Elsevier/Saunders.

Quill, T. E., & Brody, H. (1996). Physician recommendations and patient autonomy. *Annals of Internal Medicine, 125,* 763–769.

Scott, R., Aiken, L., Mechanic, D., & Moravcsik, J. (1995). Organizational aspects of caring. *Milbank Quarterly, 73*(1), 77–95.

Spencer, E. M., & Mills, A. E. (1999). Ethics in health care organizations. *HEC Forum, 11,* 323–332.

Veterans Health Administration, National Center for Ethics. (2002, February). *Developing an integrated ethics program.* Presentation for Veterans Health Administration: Ethics Training, Detroit, MI.

Lea Cheyney Brandt, OTD, MA, OTR/L
Member at Large, Ethics Commission
(2005–2011)

CHAPTER 32

Occupational Therapist/Occupational Therapy Assistant Partnerships: Achieving High Ethical Standards in a Challenging Health Care Environment

INTRODUCTION

Health care reform, regardless of its design or policies, will likely influence the practice of occupational therapy in both traditional settings and emerging practice areas. Expected budget cuts in federal and state programs may affect occupational therapy in school systems, hospitals, community agencies, and skilled nursing facilities (SNFs) nationwide. There could be greater demand placed on occupational therapy assistants to fill positions for more direct delivery of occupational therapy services, freeing occupational therapists to focus on conducting evaluations and performing supervisory tasks. Managers with fiscal accountability may place higher productivity expectations on practitioners. In a field in which staffing shortages exist, practitioners need to stay focused on delivering high-quality care that meets ethical standards.

The American Occupational Therapy Association (AOTA) provides guidance to occupational therapy personnel regarding the ethical standards of the profession. Principle 5F of the *Occupational Therapy Code of Ethics and Ethics Standards (2010)* (referred to as the "Code and Ethics Standards"; AOTA, 2010) states that it is the duty of occupational therapy practitioners to "take responsibility for maintaining high standards and continuing competence in practice, education, and research by participating in professional development and educational

activities to improve and update knowledge and skills." Principle 5, Procedural Justice, guides occupational therapy personnel to "comply with institutional rules, local, state, federal, and international laws and AOTA documents applicable to the profession of occupational therapy." Occupational therapy assistants need to be supervised appropriately according to state practice acts, regulations, and organizational policies. Successful occupational therapy practitioners in an evolving health care delivery system must be familiar with and consider professional ethical standards as they confront potential new challenges of health care reform.

This advisory opinion addresses trends in the workforce, strategies for ensuring appropriate supervision of occupational therapy assistants, teamwork, and effective collaboration to provide high-quality occupational therapy services despite budgetary constraints. Case examples are included to illustrate ethical dilemmas and practical solutions in an occupational therapist/occupational therapy assistant partnership.

WORKFORCE TRENDS

As an occupational therapist working for a rehabilitation company that contracts with SNFs, Pat splits her day between two buildings. She is responsible for evaluating new patients and supervising the occupational therapy assistants in those facilities. The recruiter just hired a new occupational therapy assistant graduate who is working under a temporary license. The plan is that she will replace the occupational therapy assistant in one of Pat's facilities. The staffing coordinator says that Pat's working situation will remain the same. However, because of the restrictions placed on someone working with a temporary license, Pat knows that she, as the supervising occupational therapist, needs to be on site while the new occupational therapy assistant is working with clients.

Pat's strategy to address the ethical concern is to obtain a copy of the state licensure regulations and present them to the recruiter and staffing coordinator. She explains the restrictions for those working under a temporary license as well as the need for occupational therapy supervision and mentoring for new graduates and then discusses the importance of ensuring consistent service competency.

Jim works in a comprehensive outpatient rehabilitation facility (CORF) as an occupational therapy assistant. The rehab manager has asked Jim to do all the treatments so that the occupational therapist can spend more time on evaluations. Medicare guidelines state that in CORFs, the occupational therapy assistant cannot provide the final discharge treatment, because that visit is considered a reassessment. Jim's strategy is to explain to the rehab manager that even though the guideline on final discharge treatment is not specified in his state's practice act, Jim must comply with the more stringent Medicare policy.

Although the health care environment has been challenging in recent years, there is good news for the profession of occupational therapy. In part because of increasing numbers of aging baby boomers, the employment outlook for occupational therapy practitioners is bright. With increasing demand in the job market, it is critical that all parties adhere to rules and regulations related to supervision. As depicted in the case examples, there are times when department managers in other disciplines are not knowledgeable about regulations for delivering occupational therapy services. Principles 5 and 5C of the Code and Ethics Standards state that occupational therapy professionals must be familiar with rules and regulations that guide our practice and must inform those we work for and with of any changes to those laws and AOTA policies. With appropriate supervision to meet legal and ethical requirements, occupational therapy assistants can effectively deliver high-quality occupational therapy services in both traditional and emerging practice areas.

SUPERVISING OCCUPATIONAL THERAPY ASSISTANTS AND SHARING RESPONSIBILITIES

Kim is an occupational therapy assistant working on an inpatient rehabilitation unit. Her supervising occupational therapist has written a plan of care that includes the use of electrical stimulation with a patient who has had a stroke. Kim completed the required training and has documentation to support her competency in the use of physical agent modalities (PAMs). According to the state licensure law, Kim must be supervised by an occupational therapist who has also had the necessary training in PAMs. However, the supervising occupational therapist is not competent or qualified in the use of PAMs.

Kim's strategy is to show her supervisor a copy of the state licensure law's language regarding the use of PAMs and explain that she must be supervised by an occupational therapist who also has "verifiable competence" in the use of PAMs (AOTA, 2008). (If Kim's state did not specify requirements for the use of PAMs, then she should refer to the AOTA Position Paper on PAMs, which states, "Only occupational therapists with service competency in this area may supervise the use of PAMs by occupational therapy assistants" [AOTA, 2008].) Kim can request that another occupational therapist in the hospital who has competency in this area ascertain whether electrical stimulation is an appropriate intervention for this patient, and if so that occupational therapist should supervise its administration. In addition, Kim can suggest that the initial occupational therapy supervisor pursue training in PAMs if this is an intervention often required by patients in this facility.

Under Principle 1E of the Code and Ethics Standards, it is the duty of practitioners to ensure that they provide services "that are within each practitioner's level of competence and scope of practice (e.g., qualifications, experience, the law)" to benefit patients and avoid harm. As stated in Principle 2A, "occupational therapy personnel shall avoid inflicting harm or injury to recipients of occupational therapy services, students, research participants, or employees."

SUPERVISION AND THE COLLABORATIVE PROCESS

Scope of Practice

The manager of the rehabilitation department in an SNF, who is not an occupational therapist or occupational therapy assistant, asks Ari, the occupational therapy assistant, to evaluate a patient. The rehab manager says that the client's activities of daily living status needs to be established to determine if the patient's insurance will pay for her stay at the SNF. Ari is the only occupational therapy practitioner on site.

Ari's strategy is to provide the rehab manager with a copy of the state practice act and explain that, as per Medicare guidelines, AOTA documents, and state regulations, evaluation is not within the scope of practice of an occupational therapy assistant. Although the occupational therapy assistant may contribute to the evaluation process if he or she has been trained, competency has been documented, and tasks are delegated by the occupational therapist, the occupational therapist must first direct "all aspects of the initial contact during the occupational therapy evaluation" (AOTA, 2005). Only the occupational therapist is qualified to evaluate a patient's occupational performance deficits through standardized tests and other methods, identify deficits or barriers to performance that may be addressed by intervention,

interpret data, determine goals, and develop the plan of care.

The delivery of occupational therapy services should be a collaborative process between the occupational therapist and the occupational therapy assistant. Occupational therapy practitioners must familiarize themselves with their state practice act, licensure board regulations, and organizational policies. State regulatory language may include occupational therapy assistant scope of practice and specific supervision requirements. In addition, Medicare guidelines for rehabilitative services state that occupational therapy practitioners must provide services in accordance with state regulations. This practitioner role delineation is supported by Principle 5 of the Code and Ethics Standards, which states that it is the duty of occupational therapy personnel to "comply with . . . AOTA documents applicable to the profession of occupational therapy." The AOTA Web site has a link that lists each state or U.S. territory with occupational therapy regulations (AOTA, n.d.).

Supervision

The *Guidelines for Supervision, Roles, and Responsibilities During the Delivery of Occupational Therapy Services* (AOTA, 2009) provides guidance to those supervising occupational therapy assistants and occupational therapy aides. It is an excellent overview of occupational therapy assistant supervision and addresses the necessity for a "cooperative process" (p. 797). Occupational therapists are responsible and accountable for overseeing occupational therapy service delivery for consumers. Occupational therapy assistants work "under the supervision and in partnership with" occupational therapists (p. 797). For the benefit of consumers, the supervisory process promotes professional growth toward achieving competence. The guidelines for supervision place responsibility on both occupational therapists and occupational therapy assistants for devising a collaborative plan for the process.

According to Medicare guidelines, occupational therapy assistants must work under the supervision of a qualified occupational therapist. The occupational therapist must conduct the evaluation and establish the plan of care. The qualified occupational therapy assistant can then carry out delegated intervention (Centers for Medicare and Medicaid Services, 2009). Medicare guidelines do not define different levels of supervision that are necessary for less experienced assistants. However, state practice acts may contain more specific language about frequency and type of supervision as well as a definition of supervision levels.

Amount and type of supervision are dependent on several variables. State practice acts, Medicare, other payers, and institutional policies may differ in what is specified or required. Occupational therapy practitioners should adopt whichever regulation or policy is most stringent. However, occupational therapists need to use their judgment as to how much supervision is necessary beyond what is mandated by law. Variables such as the experience and competency skill level of the occupational therapy assistant, complexity and condition of clients, number of clients, and type of setting can determine the frequency and type of supervision. When working with clients who have more acute conditions that may require frequent care plan modifications, the occupational therapist should provide closer supervision of the occupational therapy assistant (AOTA, 2009; Ryan & Sladyk, 2005).

Ryan and Sladyk (2005) defined each level of occupational therapy assistant practice and the recommended amount of supervision that practitioners should receive based on AOTA guidelines. *Close supervision,* which should be provided to entry-level practitioners, is defined as providing "direct, on-site, daily contact" to practitioners who have less than 1 year of experience (Ryan & Sladyk, 2005, p. 512). Beyond the entry level and as the occupational therapy assistant develops greater competence, the amount and type of supervision change.

At that time, *general supervision* may be appropriate, which could consist of face-to-face meetings that occur at specific intervals, or a variety of supervision methods can be used, such as observation of treatment, documentation review, and written or electronic communication. However, because some state practice acts specify how frequently meetings should be held or what types of supervision are allowable, these regulations always take precedence.

Additionally, when feasible and appropriate for the situation, Ryan and Sladyk (2005) recommended minimum supervision times of 3 to 5 direct contact hours per week for full-time occupational therapy assistants and fewer hours for part-time occupational therapy assistants (e.g., 1.5–2.5 hours per week for half-time occupational therapy assistants). Occupational therapists who are supervisors need to use their discretion and consider their working partnerships with their supervisees when determining how much time should be devoted to supervision.

Getting to Know the Strengths and Weaknesses

Lee is an occupational therapy assistant who is a new employee in an acute care hospital. He is experienced in working with orthopedic patients; however, in this setting, he is being assigned to treat patients with neurological diagnoses. Lee realizes it is his duty to let his supervisor know that although he is licensed, and so technically qualified, he does not feel adequately competent to provide occupational therapy intervention to patients with complex neurological diagnoses. As stated in Principles 5F and 5G of the Code and Ethics Standards, Lee needs to have the experience, knowledge, and competence to meet the patient's occupational therapy needs. This could include continuing education courses to expand his knowledge of patients with neurological diagnoses and a mentor who can provide guidance to him.

The supervisory process is an interactive and dynamic relationship between the occupational therapist and the occupational therapy assistant. Both parties must make an effort to understand and communicate with each other so that their strengths and weaknesses can be identified. Above all, occupational therapy practitioners have a responsibility to the clients they serve, and by making the most of the supervisory relationship, they ensure that occupational therapy is delivered in a safe and competent manner. Service competency means that regardless whether it is the occupational therapist or the occupational therapy assistant who performs a task or test, the skill level is equivalent and the outcomes are the same. Competency should be documented and tested at appropriate intervals. As stated in the Code and Ethics Standards, Principle 6A, "Occupational therapy personnel shall represent the credentials, qualifications, education, experience, training, roles, duties, [and] competence . . . accurately in all forms of communication about recipients of service, students, employees, research participants, and colleagues." In addition, as previously stated, Principle 5F mandates maintaining high standards and continuing competence.

As Ryan and Sladyk (2005) noted, the occupational therapist is responsible for facilitating an atmosphere in which supervisees can increase their talents, knowledge, and skills to support professional development. Having the occupational therapy assistant complete a skills checklist is an excellent way to discover areas of competence and also the need for additional training and supervision. In addition, a critical component of supervision is to assess the supervisee's learning style to facilitate assimilation of new information. Does he or she learn best by observing? Does he or she need hands-on practice to grasp a concept and integrate technique?

Establishing clear guidelines and expectations to perform the job from the beginning can go a long way toward avoiding miscommunication and misunderstanding later. A job description should be provided, and the supervisor should make sure that the occupational

therapy assistant is informed of other expectations such as productivity and performance. The supervisee also should be made aware of any system of rewards for outstanding performance as well as consequences for unsatisfactory performance.

An effective supervisor is supportive, truthful, and fair when giving feedback; respects differences; gives credit where credit is due; is open to new ideas; and is a role model for high standards of occupational therapy practice. Principle 6H of the Code and Ethics Standards states, "Occupational therapy personnel shall be honest, fair, accurate, respectful, and timely in gathering and reporting fact-based information regarding employee job performance." The supervisee has a responsibility to readily accept feedback and modify behavior accordingly, be an active participant in the learning process, and seek additional support or clarification when needed. The supervisor also should be receptive to feedback to facilitate the process.

Ensuring Adequate Supervision: Communicate, Collaborate, Document

It is necessary for occupational therapist/occupational therapy assistant teams to determine the system they will use for the supervision process. State regulations may guide practitioners as to the minimum required supervision, frequency, and modes of acceptable communication. However, within any regulatory or guideline parameters, the team can determine what will work best for their supervisory process. Developing a supervisory plan that works for both parties is important for the process. Early in the relationship, the supervisor and supervisee should decide when, where, and how often supervision should occur.

Sufficient documentation of the supervisory process is the responsibility of both supervisor and supervisee and is good practice even if not required by state law. Developing a system for including evidence that discussions have taken place also is important. Cosignatures are not enough to prove that conversations have taken place. Although face-to-face supervision during client treatment may need to occur at certain intervals and may be dependent on variables, there are times throughout the duration of client treatment that supervision can be handled through other modes of communication as long as patient privacy is protected. When using voice mail or telephone systems, it is more difficult to protect patient confidentiality. Practitioners may benefit from certain technology that would allow more flexibility during collaborative delivery of occupational therapy, such as password-protected electronic medical records.

In all cases, communication must take place between the occupational therapist and occupational therapy assistant prior to initiating intervention or discontinuing services. During the course of intervention, it is important for both parties to collaborate and exchange ideas as issues come up or changes in the plan of care or goals are indicated.

CONCLUSION

Occupational therapists and occupational therapy assistants must practice due diligence in providing services to clients to deliver ethical, high-quality care. Both parties need to know the legal and ethical requirements for supervision. State practice acts, regulatory bodies, Medicare, and other sources of guidelines regarding supervision of occupational therapy assistants must be followed to ensure the delivery of occupational therapy services that meet the ethical standards of the profession.

REFERENCES

American Occupational Therapy Association. (2005). *Model state regulation for supervision, roles, and responsibilities during the delivery of occupational therapy services*. Retrieved May 25, 2010, from http://www.aota.org/Practitioners/Advocacy/State/Resources/Supervision/36447.aspx

American Occupational Therapy Association. (2008). Physical agent modalities [Position Paper]. *American Journal of Occupational Therapy, 62,* 343–354. doi:10.5014/ajot.62.6.691

American Occupational Therapy Association. (2009). Guidelines for supervision, roles, and responsibilities during the delivery of occupational therapy services. *American Journal of Occupational Therapy, 63,* 797–803. doi:10.5014/ajot.63.6.797

American Occupational Therapy Association. (2010). Occupational therapy code of ethics and ethics standards (2010). *American Journal of Occupational Therapy, 64*(6 Suppl.), S17–S26. doi:10.5014/ajot.2010.64S17

American Occupational Therapy Association. (n.d.). *Occupational therapy regulatory authority contact list.* Available online at http://www1.aota.org/state_law/reglist.asp

Centers for Medicare and Medicaid Services. (2009, September). *Medicare benefit policy manual* (rev. 111). Retrieved May 26, 2010, from http://www3.cms.gov/manuals/Downloads/bp102c12.pdf

Ryan, S., & Sladyk, K. (2005). *Ryan's occupational therapy assistant: Principles, practice issues, and techniques* (4th ed.). Thorofare, NJ: Slack.

Loretta Foster, MS, COTA/L
OTA Representative, Ethics Commission (2008–2011, 2011–2014)

Rae Ann Smith, OTD, OTR/L
Program Director, Allegany College of Maryland

CHAPTER 33

Outdated and Obsolete Tests and Assessment Instruments

INTRODUCTION

The evaluation process and use of test and assessment instruments in occupational therapy practice should be designed to benefit the client by accurately reporting the client's capabilities (strengths) and limitations (deficits and weaknesses). Occupational therapy practitioners have an ethical responsibility to provide proper individualized evaluation and a plan of intervention for all recipients of occupational therapy service (Principle 1B, *Occupational Therapy Code of Ethics and Ethics Standards (2010)* [referred to as the "Code and Ethics Standards"]; American Occupational Therapy Association [AOTA], 2010). In addition, occupational therapy practitioners have a responsibility to avoid the use of outdated or obsolete tests and assessments or data obtained from such tests in making intervention decisions or recommendations (Principle 1D, Code and Ethics Standards). Finally, occupational therapy practitioners are encouraged to provide evaluations that are evidence-based and within the recognized scope of occupational therapy practice (Principle 1F, Code and Ethics Standards). Therefore, occupational therapy practitioners also have a responsibility to determine when a test or assessment is considered outdated or obsolete and would not provide current and relevant data on which to develop an intervention plan and program.

THE ISSUES

Tests and assessment instruments most often become outdated and obsolete because of revisions. Occupational therapy practitioners should be aware of revisions and make an effort to determine if any of the reasons for revision are pertinent to the tests or assessments used in their practice areas. According to the *Standards for Educational and Psychological Testing* (American Educational Research Association, 1999),

> Tests and their supporting documents (e.g., test manuals, technical manuals, user's guides) are reviewed periodically to determine whether revisions are needed. Revisions or amendments are necessary when new research data, significant changes in the domain, or new conditions of test use and interpretation would either improve the validity of interpretations of the test scores or suggest that the test is no longer fully appropriate for its intended use. As an example, tests are revised if the test content or language has become outdated and, therefore, may subsequently affect the validity of the test score interpretations. (p. 42)

The problem of outdated and obsolete tests and assessment instruments is not unique to occupational therapy practice. Any discipline or profession that uses standardized tests and assessment instruments to gather client data has a similar concern and problem. However, certain types of data tend to require more frequent updating. Such data include developmental, cognitive, psychological, social and contextual, or environmental factors. Although knowledge about anatomical and physiological factors does change, the rate of change tends to be slower. Therefore, the normative data on range of motion tend to change less frequently than the normative data on child development. In addition, normative data appropriate for one segment of the population do not necessarily accurately measure another segment. Older tests and assessment instruments may have been based on normative data from a select group of subjects that does not include the characteristics of the client the occupational therapy practitioner is evaluating. Comparing a person to normative data that do not include a group of subjects similar to the client does not accurately indicate the client's capabilities and limitations.

Although there is no definitive checklist to determine if a test or an assessment is outdated or obsolete, some general guidelines can be stated. Any test or assessment instrument to be used with clients must meet the following criteria:

- The test or assessment instrument should be the most current edition or version available.
- The content of the test or assessment instrument should be based on currently accepted theory, frame of reference, or model of practice.
- The content of the test or assessment instrument should be recognized as within the scope of occupational therapy practice.
- If there is a similar test or assessment instrument with essentially the same content that was published more recently than the test or assessment being considered for use, consider using the more recent test or assessment instrument if feasible.
- Normative data should have been updated or reviewed for need to update within the past 20 years or other appropriate length of time.

- The sample on which the normative data are based should include subjects with the characteristics of the client being assessed (e.g., age, sex, ethnicity, symptoms, diagnosis).
- A literature search should be performed to ascertain that no statements in a recent publication have questioned the validity or reliability of the test or assessment instrument and provided evidence to substantiate the question(s) posed.
- The language of the test or assessment instrument should be consistent with current usage.
- The test items should be the same as or similar to those in daily use to measure functional ability, occupational performance, or participation.
- The test instrument should be in good condition (i.e., all parts available and in working order).

CASE ILLUSTRATIONS

Jamie, an occupational therapist, needs to evaluate Geoff, age 26 months. She chooses the Peabody Developmental Motor Scales (Folio & Fewell, 1992) and the Bayley Scales of Infant Development (Bayley, 1969) because both are recognized tests of infant development. She administers and scores each test according to the instructions but completes only the motor section of the Bayley. By previous arrangement, the psychologist completes the mental and behavioral sections of the Bayley. In the staff meeting, the psychologist tells team members that the test results Jamie provided in her report are meaningless and should be disregarded because the normative data for both tests are out of date. Jamie is asked to retest Geoff using current editions of the two tests. The Peabody Developmental Motor Scales was updated in 2000 (Folio & Fewell, 2000), and the Bayley Scales of Infant and Toddler Development, 3rd edition, was updated in 2005 (Bayley, 2005).

Sara is a pediatric occupational therapist who administers the Test of Visual–Motor

Skills—Revised (Gardner, 1995) and the Test of Visual Perceptual Skills, 3rd edition (Martin, 2006) to Laura, age 12, to assess her perceptual and perceptual–motor skills. Laura scores below her age level on both tests. At the guidance team meeting, the teacher asks Sara to explain the conceptual model or frame of reference on which the tests are based to help the teacher better understand Laura's perceptual problems. Sara is unable to find any information in the test manuals regarding a model or frame of reference. The guidance team requests that Sara retest Laura using perceptual and perceptual–motor instruments that provide a model to be used for understanding the test results and for supporting intervention in the classroom.

Ken, an occupational therapist working in a rehab hospital, administers the Cognitive Assessment of Minnesota (CAM; Rustad et al., 1993) to Mr. Clausen, age 57, who had a cerebral vascular accident 2 weeks ago. Ken skips the Money Skills section because he cannot find a 50-cent piece and the Visual Neglect section because the reproducible form is missing from the test manual. He summarizes the test results he has completed, but his supervisor refuses to allow them to be entered in Mr. Clausen's chart because the results are incomplete. The supervisor suggests looking for the missing pieces of the CAM or retesting Mr. Clausen with a similar assessment instrument.

DISCUSSION

As the cases illustrate, tests and assessment instruments that do not meet the bulleted criteria outlined in this article may not accurately report a client's capabilities and limitations. Such tests and assessment instruments may not benefit the client if one or more of the following are true: the normative data are out of date, the normative data sample did not include certain ethic or minority groups, the normative data sample did not include a range of ages from child to adult (if relevant), test item(s) have become dated and do not reflect current language

or life situations, errors in administrating and scoring have been observed and reported in published studies, validity or reliability have been questioned by researchers, or the conceptual model of the instrument is missing or may not be consistent with currently accepted theory (Adams, 2000; Butcher, 2000; Okazaki & Sue, 2000; Silverstein & Nelson, 2000; Strauss, Spreen, & Hunter, 2000). Inaccurate measurement during the evaluation process may result in intervention that is not needed or that does not address existing limitations. Sources of inaccurate measurement may include errors in administration and scoring or failure to administer some parts of the instrument altogether. The client may not receive the full benefit of occupational therapy services because important limitations or potential capabilities were not identified or were misidentified during the evaluation process. Planning and implementation for intervention may have been developed and carried out based on incomplete, inaccurate, or missing facts and data.

Occupational therapy practitioners have an ethical responsibility to select, administer, score, and interpret tests and assessment instruments that accurately reflect the client within the context of time and circumstances important to that client. Tests and assessment instruments that do not accurately measure the client should not be used unless the potential inaccuracies are noted within the assessment summary and allowances made for inaccurate interpretation. The occupational therapy practitioner should be knowledgeable about each assessment instrument used to measure client capacities and limitations. Any deficiencies in the application of the test or assessment instrument should be clearly stated in documentation reporting the data or summary.

For example, the dynamometer is basically a strain gauge that must be periodically recalibrated—like retuning a piano—to accurately measure grip strength. Arrangements and a maintenance schedule to have dynamometers recalibrated—or new ones purchased—are the responsibility of the occupational therapy practitioner.

A second example is perception tests, which were originally published with norms established primarily for children. In recent years, many of these perception instruments have been revised to include new norms for adults. Use of the newer instruments increases the potential for identifying perceptual dysfunction that may be interfering with the adult client's ability to perform daily living tasks and continues to be useful in assessing children. As tests and assessment instruments improve to measure more aspects of client capabilities and limitations, occupational therapy practitioners must be alert to the newer measurement tools and incorporate them into the evaluation process.

A third example is a developmental test that may become out of date because of changes in overall health, nutrition, and child-rearing practices. For example, the average age of walking has decreased from 18 months in the 1940s to under 1 year of age today. Using a development test that was standardized 40 or 50 years ago might not identify a performance deficit that should be addressed to improve the child's function in today's society.

A fourth example is a test without an identified conceptual model or theory or with a discarded model or theory. The conceptual model provides the basis for interpreting the significance or meaning for performance in everyday life. If knowledge of a foreign language is viewed as important for everyday functioning, then not knowing the language is important. However, if the ability to speak another language is not viewed as important, then a test result of ability that is three standard deviations below the mean may be an accurate measurement but probably is interpreted as insignificant to performing daily tasks.

A fifth example is test items that are out of date such as those that ask the client to identify a 50-cent piece. Because 50-cent pieces are not in common circulation today, such identification is not useful in interpreting the client's ability to handle coins or make change correctly.

Finally, tests and assessment instruments best provide useful information when the data are consistent with occupational therapy theory. Occupational therapy theories stress the importance of understanding and managing the process by which a task, activity, or occupation is performed. Some assessment instruments primarily measure the outcome or end result without providing a means of measuring the process (sequence or steps) by which the outcome or end result is obtained. Such assessment instruments may be useful for reporting to other professionals, families, or agencies about the results of therapy but are limited in assessing the need for occupational therapy intervention. Understanding the conceptual basis of an assessment can increase the chances that the information obtained will be useful in planning and implementing an occupational therapy service program.

SUMMARY

Occupational therapy practitioners use tests and assessment instruments as a means of gathering data about a client during the evaluation process. The tests and assessment instruments should provide accurate and up-to-date data about the client being evaluated. Occupational therapy practitioners must assume responsibility for selecting, administering, scoring, and interpreting tests and assessment instruments that are not outdated or obsolete. Although definitive guidelines for determining whether a test or instrument is outdated or obsolete do not exist, useful guidelines—like the criteria outlined in this chapter—can and should be observed by occupational therapy practitioners.

REFERENCES

Adams, K. M. (2000). Practical and ethical issues pertaining to test revisions. *Psychological Assessment, 12,* 281–286.

American Educational Research Association. (1999). *Standards for educational and psychological testing.* Washington, DC: Author.

American Occupational Therapy Association. (2010). Occupational therapy code of ethics and ethics standards (2010). *American Journal of Occupational Therapy, 64*(6 Suppl.), S17–S26. doi:10.5014/ajot.2010.64S17

Bayley, N. (1969). *Bayley Scales of Infant Development*. New York: Psychological Corporation.

Bayley, N. (2005). *Bayley Scales of Infant and Toddler Development* (3rd ed.). San Antonio, TX: PsychCorp.

Butcher, J. N. (2000). Revising psychological tests: Lessons learned from the revision of the MMPI. *Psychological Assessment, 12,* 263–271.

Folio, M. R., & Fewell, R. R. (1992). *Peabody Developmental Motor Scales*. Austin, TX: Pro-Ed.

Folio, M. R., & Fewell, R. R. (2000). *Peabody Developmental Motor Scales* (2nd ed.). Austin, TX: Pro-Ed.

Gardner, M. (1995). *Test of Visual–Motor Skills—Revised*. Hydesville, CA: Psychological and Educational Publications.

Martin, N. (2006). *Test of Visual Perceptual Skills* (3rd ed.). Hydesville, CA: Psychological and Educational Publications.

Okazaki, S., & Sue, S. (2000). Implications of test revisions for assessment with Asian Americans. *Psychological Assessment, 12,* 272–280.

Rustad, R. A., DeGroot, T. L., Jungkunz, M. L., Freeberg, K. S., Borowick, L. G., & Wanttie, A. M. (1993). *The Cognitive Assesment of Minnesota*. San Antonio, TX: Pearson.

Silverstein, M. L., & Nelson, L. D. (2000). Clinical and research implications of revising psychological tests. *Psychological Assessment, 12,* 298–303.

Strauss, E., Spreen, O., & Hunter, M. (2000). Implications of test revisions for research. *Psychological Assessment, 12,* 237–244.

Kathlyn L. Reed, PhD, OTR, FAOTA, MLIS
Chairperson, Ethics Commission (2007–2010)

CHAPTER 34

Patient Abandonment

INTRODUCTION

According to Dictionary.com (2011), *abandon* is defined as "to leave completely and finally." A legal definition clarifies what abandonment means in the health care setting: "withdrawal from treatment of a patient without giving reasonable notice or providing a competent replacement" (USLegal.com, n.d.).

One should note that according to this second definition, a health care professional can indeed "abandon" a patient appropriately, as long as some notice has been given. Tangential to withdrawing from a case in which treatment has already begun is the refusal to initiate treatment, which many patients also take as an act of abandonment. This "right" (as it is sometimes called) of health care professionals to withdraw from the treatment of a patient or to refuse to initiate treatment is supported by the American Medical Association's (AMA's) Principles of Medical Ethics, Principle VI: "A physician shall, in the provision of appropriate patient care, except in emergencies, be free to choose whom to serve, with whom to associate, and the environment in which to provide medical services" (AMA, 1994, p. 101). Similarly, the *Comprehensive Accreditation Manual for Hospitals* (Joint Committee on the Accreditation of Healthcare Organizations [JCAHO], 1998) calls for the development of policies and procedures within health care facilities governing "how staff may request to be excused from participating in an aspect of patient care on grounds of conflicting cultural values, ethics, or religious beliefs . . ." (p. HR-21).

Belief in this "right" of health care professionals to refuse to treat can be found throughout the health care system in this country, because it flows out of the strong value Americans place on freedom of choice. As biomedical ethicist Albert R. Jonsen (1995) explained,

> There has long been, in the United States, a reluctance to force one person to provide services to another against his or her will. . . . The right to refuse to care for a particular patient, either by not accepting that person as a patient or by discharging oneself from responsibility in a recognized way, is deeply embedded in the ethos of American medicine. (p. 100)

The issue of patient abandonment versus the health care professional's rights is one of several problems that contribute to the growing tension between patients and medical personnel. Finding and maintaining a balance between patient needs and the personal rights of those involved with health care delivery on this issue of abandonment would go far toward easing such tensions as we move into the next millennium.

CLARIFYING "PATIENT ABANDONMENT"

We must recognize that there are legitimate reasons across all fields of health care to cease providing treatment to a patient. Some of these are clear-cut. First, when treatment needs exceed the ability and expertise of a health care professional, the patient is best served by having care transferred to a more qualified practitioner. Because the goal of health care is the well-being of the patient, withdrawing from a case when one's skill can no longer be of benefit is justified, even though claims of abandonment may be raised by the patient. However, the manner in which one presents the need for a transfer of care and the degree to which the patient is made aware of this need and involved in the choice of a new practitioner are important factors in lessening the patient's perception of abandonment.

Second, it is commonly agreed that a health care practitioner may withdraw from the care of a patient who acts inappropriately within the health care setting. The most common situation discussed is when a patient becomes violent or acts in ways that endanger the practitioner, other patients, or staff. However, this would also include inappropriate sexual advances from a patient (or possibly from a patient's guardian, spouse, parent, and so forth). In such cases, a practitioner may, if necessary, withdraw from the treatment of the patient without abandoning the patient, as the health care relationship has already been severed and the bond of trust damaged.

A third area, but one that involves more difficulty, arises from issues regarding the cultural and religious values of health care practitioners. As noted in the *Comprehensive Accreditation Manual for Hospitals* (JCAHO, 1998), in the delivery of health care there should be respect for a health care practitioner's "cultural values, ethics, and religious beliefs and the impact these may have on patient care" (p. HR-21). The *Accreditation Manual* emphasizes that to respect all staff members, a health care institution (or practice) should establish policies for how staff members can make requests to discontinue care for ethical, religious, and cultural reasons, as well as policies for ensuring that patient care will not be negatively affected. It is further noted that addressing such issues in

advance, even at the time of hiring or contracting, will be the most helpful for maintaining an appropriate level of patient care.

What makes these issues difficult is the subjective nature of "personal values." Who is to say what represents a cultural value? What if one's culture is in the minority—do minority values still have weight? Religious values might also be difficult to determine, as not all members of the same religion hold the same values. Should those making the decisions recognize only mainstream values of the staff member's religion? And, of course, ethical values flow from the individual's own conscience. How should a manager or a supervisor regard a staff member's ethical claims? Should all expressed values carry the same weight, simply because someone claims they are important? The *Accreditation Manual* goes on to note that if an appropriate (in the judgment of the manager or supervisor) request has been made, accommodations should be made when possible and cites the following "Examples of Implementation" to support Standard HR.6:

> There will be an understanding that if events prevent the accommodation at a specific point because of an emergency situation, the employee will be expected to perform assigned duties so he or she does not negatively affect the delivery of care or services.
>
> If an employee does not agree to render appropriate care or services in an emergency situation because of personal beliefs, the employee will be placed on a leave of absence from his or her current position and the incident will be reviewed. (JCAHO, 1998, p. HR-21)

Such cases will surely be difficult for all involved, especially if they have not been addressed prior to the emergent situation. The issue here is further complicated by the fact that even though health care is becoming more diverse, when we work with each other we are not always aware of each other's diverse beliefs, nor are we always open and understanding about such differences. Supervisors and employers need to become more aware of their staff's values, and staff need to continue to keep patient care at the focus of their work during times of personal conflict.

Beyond the above reasons for discontinuing patient care, disagreement begins to arise. What about refusing to treat a noncompliant patient? What if that patient is extremely noncompliant, rather than only occasionally noncompliant? In another vein, what about the patient who does not pay his or her bills? Is refusing to treat such a patient justifiable? What if the patient is unable to pay the bills? Would this make a difference? Or one might consider an especially demanding patient. If a patient takes time away from the care of others and continually calls the practitioner beyond normal care hours, is withdrawal from the care of such a patient acceptable? Yet another problematic case might involve a patient whose appearance or manners disgust a practitioner. If a practitioner is so put off by a patient that it impedes his or her ability to be an effective therapist, would withdrawing from the case be an act of abandonment or patient benefit? Finally, perhaps the most addressed cases involve persons with AIDS. Does the fear of contagion validate withdrawal from treating such a patient? Across the literature, there is little agreement as to what constitutes abandonment in such situations. Legal cases have not added much clarity (Southwick, 1988, pp. 37–41).

THE DUTY TO TREAT

Although there is disagreement about the issue of abandonment and the duty of health care professionals to treat patients, even in the face of personal inconvenience or risk, some helpful insights can be gained from the thought of bioethicist Edmund D. Pellegrino. In his chapter "Altruism, Self-Interest, and Medical Ethics," Pellegrino (1991) addressed the particular case of physicians and the treatment of persons with AIDS. To begin, the author questioned the notion that "medicine is an occupation like any

other, and the physician has the same 'rights' as the businessman or the craftsman" (Pellegrino, 1991, p. 114). As a counter to this notion, Pellegrino drew out three things specific to the nature of medicine that he argued establish a duty of physicians to treat the sick, even in the face of personal risk. Pellegrino first pointed out the uniqueness of the medical relationship, in that it involves a vulnerable and dependent person who is at risk of exploitation who must trust another to be restored to health. As Pellegrino explained, "Physicians invite that trust when offering to put knowledge at the service of the sick. A medical need in itself constitutes a moral claim on those equipped to help." Next, the author points out that, in short, medical education is a privilege. Societies make special allowances for people to study medicine for the good of the society, thereby establishing a covenant with future health care professionals. Based on this, Pellegrino concluded, "The physician's knowledge, therefore, is not individually owned and ought not be used primarily for personal gain, prestige, or power. Rather, the profession holds this knowledge in trust for the good of the sick." Finally, Pellegrino pointed to the oath that physicians take before practicing medicine: "That oath—whichever one is taken—is a public promise that the new physician understands the gravity of this calling and promises to be competent and to use that competence in the interests of the sick." Although the debate continues, several have asserted that Pellegrino made a strong case for the duty to treat (Arras, 1991; Jonsen, 1995). And although Pellegrino's comments were directed toward physicians, his reasoning cuts across all fields of medical practice.

THE DUTY TO TREAT, PATIENT ABANDONMENT, AND OCCUPATIONAL THERAPY

The points presented by Pellegrino (1991) have direct bearing on the profession of occupational therapy. The Preamble to the *Occupational Therapy Code of Ethics and Ethics Standards (2010)* (referred to as the "Code and Ethics

Standards"; American Occupational Therapy Association [AOTA], 2010) recognizes the vulnerability of the people who seek their services and are aware of the trust that is required in the healing relationship. Even though the recipient of treatment depends on the occupational therapist, the core value of equality "refers to the desire to promote fairness in interactions with others" (AOTA, 2010, p. S17). The core value of dignity emphasizes "the promotion and preservation of the individuality . . . of the client, by assisting him or her to engage in occupations that are meaningful to him or her regardless of level of disability" (AOTA, 2010, p. S18). The need to respect the vulnerability of patients and build trust is also expressed in the Code and Ethics Standards in Principle 1, which states, "Occupational therapy personnel shall demonstrate a concern for the well-being and safety of the recipients of their services." Principle 2 adds, "Occupational therapy personnel shall intentionally refrain from actions that cause harm." Principle 2C also explicitly states that "Occupational therapy personnel shall avoid relationships that exploit the recipient of services . . . physically, emotionally, psychologically, financially, socially, or in any other manner that conflicts or interferes with professional judgment and objectivity." Principle 3 further demonstrates the concern of occupational therapists for building trust between practitioners and the persons in their care: "Occupational therapy personnel shall respect the right of the individual to self-determination." Under this principle, the importance of collaborating with, gaining informed consent from, and respecting the confidentiality of service recipients is recognized.

As to the second point raised by Pellegrino, occupational therapists do indeed recognize the importance of their training and education. This is emphasized in Principle 5F of the Code and Ethics Standards: "Occupational therapy personnel shall take responsibility for maintaining high standards and continuing competence in practice, education, and research. . . ."

The impact of this principle goes beyond just receiving specialized training; occupational therapists seek to maintain competence "by participating in professional development and educational activities." Principle 5G also directs occupational therapists to protect service recipients in the discharge of their knowledge and skill by ensuring that "duties assumed by or assigned to other occupational therapy personnel match credentials, qualifications, experience, and scope of practice." Through these actions, occupational therapists can truly demonstrate that they do not acquire their knowledge for "personal gain, prestige, or power. Rather, the profession holds this knowledge in trust for the good of the sick" (Pellegrino, 1991, p. 114).

Finally, occupational therapists also make a public pledge to promote the well-being of others through the Code and Ethics Standards. The Preamble to the Code and Ethics Standards states, "Members of AOTA are committed to promoting inclusion, diversity, independence, and safety for all recipients in various stages of life, health, and illness and to empower all beneficiaries of occupational therapy" (AOTA, 2010, p. S17). Principle 1 of the Code and Ethics Standards further supports this pledge for the well-being of the recipients of occupational therapy. Finally, the dedication of occupational therapists to the well-being of those they treat is echoed in the core value of altruism: "the individual's ability to place the needs of others before their own" (AOTA, 2010, p. S17).

This understanding of the duty of health care professionals to treat patients as drawn from the perspective of occupational therapy can provide some guidance for the initial concern of patient abandonment. There is, indeed, a strong claim here to treat all patients to the fullest of one's ability as an occupational therapist. The two limiting factors to this are when a more competent therapist is needed and when the patient's actions make further treatment imprudent. But aside from such cases, the Code and Ethics Standards challenge occupational therapists to act from a higher level of responsibility than the general norms of society. Thus, even though it may be standard practice to refuse to serve customers and clients at one's discretion in business, occupational therapists have a higher standard to follow. Prudential decisions will need to be made about initiating or ceasing treatment when such actions are valid and necessary. However, to avoid the genuine abandonment of patients, occupational therapists must act according to both the letter and the spirit of the Code and Ethics Standards. Kyler (1995) summed up these points well when she wrote,

> As ethical health care practitioners, we are guided by the fundamental belief in the worth of our clients. This belief is based on our social responsibility, as stated in the AOTA Code of Ethics and in the Standards of Practice. An ethical practitioner treats clients and delivers services not simply because of a contractual agreement, but because of a social responsibility to do so. (p. 176)

CONCLUSION: ABIDE, NOT ABANDON

As Purtilo (1993) noted, the actual physical abandonment of patients by health care professionals is no longer as prevalent as it had once been. However, she added that "psychological abandonment often replaces what used to be experienced as the more obvious bodily abandonment of the patient" (p. 156). Psychological abandonment still involves treating a patient, but in such a manner "that the patient becomes a total non-person to the health professional." One of the dangers here is that physical abandonment is rather obvious and can be empirically validated. Psychological abandonment is far more subtle and may even occur without the practitioner's conscious knowledge—for example, as a type of defense mechanism in a difficult case. Nonetheless, even this form of abandonment must be guarded against. But how?

Purtilo (1993) offered a simple but thought-provoking suggestion. She explained that the "opposite of abandonment is to stay with or abide with the patient." Learning to abide with those in need, those who are difficult, those whose actions appear immoral to us, and those whom we fear because of their specific health problems will certainly not be easy. However, as Purtilo noted, health care professionals "can overcome their tendency to flee (physically or psychologically) only when the attitude of compassion is combined with an understanding of how much harm is induced by abandonment" (p. 157). Learning to abide with the recipients of occupational therapy may be one of the most important ways to safeguard against patient abandonment.

REFERENCES

American Medical Association. (1994). American Medical Association's principles of medical ethics. In G. R. Beabout & D. J. Wennemann (Eds.), *Applied professional ethics* (p. 101). New York: University Press of America.

American Occupational Therapy Association. (2010). Occupational therapy code of ethics and ethics standards (2010). *American Journal of Occupational Therapy, 64*(6 Suppl.), S17–S26. doi:10.5014/ajot.2010.64S17

Arras, J. D. (1991). AIDS and the duty to treat. In T. A. Mappes & J. S. Zembaty (Eds.), *Biomedical ethics* (3rd ed., pp. 115–121). St. Louis, MO: McGraw-Hill.

Dictionary.com. (2011). *Abandon.* Retrieved February 2, 2011, from http://dictionary.reference.com/browse/abandon

Joint Commission on the Accreditation of Healthcare Organizations. (1998, January). *Comprehensive accreditation manual for hospitals* (pp. HR-21–HR-22). Washington, DC: Author.

Jonsen, A. R. (1995). The duty to treat patients with AIDS and HIV infection. In J. D. Arras & B. Steinbock (Eds.), *Ethical issues in modern medicine* (4th ed., pp. 97–106). Mountain View, CA: Mayfield.

Kyler, P. (1995). Ethical Commentary—Commentary on Chapter 10, "Contracts and Referrals to Private Practice." In D. B. Bailey & S. L. Schwartzberg (Eds.), *Ethical and legal dilemmas in occupational therapy* (pp. 174–176). Philadelphia: F. A. Davis.

Pellegrino, E. D. (1991). Altruism, self-interest, and medical ethics. In T. A. Mappes & J. S. Zembaty (Eds.), *Biomedical ethics* (3rd ed., pp. 113–114). St. Louis, MO: McGraw-Hill.

Purtilo, R. (1993). *Ethical dimensions in the health professions* (2nd ed.) Philadelphia: W. B. Saunders.

Southwick, A. F. (1988). *The law of hospital and health care administration* (2nd ed.). Ann Arbor, MI: Health Administration Press.

USLegal.com. (n.d.). *Patient abandonment law and legal definition*. Retrieved February 2, 2011, from http://definitions.uslegal.com/p/patient-abandonment/

John F. Morris, PhD
Public Member, Commission on Standards and Ethics (1998–2001, 2001–2004)

This chapter was originally published in the 2000 edition of the *Reference Guide to the Occupational Therapy Code of Ethics*. It has been revised to reflect updated AOTA official documents, Web sites, AOTA style, and additional resources.

CHAPTER 35

Plagiarism

What Is Plagiarism?

The *Oxford Desk Dictionary and Thesaurus* defines *plagiarize* as taking and using "the thoughts, writings, inventions, etc. of another" as one's own or "passing off thoughts, etc. (of another) as one's own" (Abate, 1997). Among its word alternatives to plagiarism, the thesaurus lists *piracy, theft, stealing, appropriation,* and *thievery.*

These definitions remind readers that plagiarism's scope extends beyond the failure to reference a published quote. Plagiarism involves the taking of another's ideas, thoughts, and concepts from any source. The sources can include printed or formally published works, electronic media, presentations or workshops, videotaped or audiotaped materials, and information obtained from the Internet.

Plagiarism can occur in several contexts. Individuals can take someone else's complete work and represent an identical work as their own (University of Victoria Libraries, 2009). One can omit references to borrowed phrases or sentences incorporated into one's work. Authors can paraphrase statements from other sources and fail to cite the source. And finally, writers can represent another's ideas or concepts as their own without including a reference to the creator or source.

Plagiarism can take several forms. One can actively or intentionally use the words, ideas, or concepts of another without citing the author as the source (Duke University, Office of the Dean of Academic Affairs, Trinity College, 2009). Examples are as follows:

- Copying entire documents and presenting them as your own
- Cutting and pasting from the work of others without properly citing the authors
- Stringing together the quotes and ideas of others without connecting their work to your own original work
- Asserting ideas without acknowledging their sources, reproducing sentences written verbatim by others without properly quoting and attributing the work to them
- Making only minor changes to the words or phrasing of another's work without properly citing the authors. (Washington State University, 2009).

Unintentional plagiarism occurs as well:

Unintentional plagiarism, or the misuse of sources, is the accidental appropriation of the ideas and materials of others due to a lack of understanding of the conventions of citation and documentation. Misuse of sources might include a lack of understanding of paraphrasing, not being clear about the parameters of common knowledge, and/or the statute of limitations on the attribution of ideas (Washington State University, 2009, italics added).

Sometimes after dedicating long hours to research on a specific topic, one may find it difficult to discern one's own ideas from the ideas of the many readings one has undertaken. Unintentional confusion of another's ideas with one's own still constitutes plagiarism (Skandalakis & Mirilas, 2004).

Increased use of online sources allows individuals to cut and paste content from a variety of Internet sources into a "new" document—a form of passive or unintentional "electronic plagiarism" (Sinha, Singh, & Kumar, 2009). One should understand that a paper comprising "patchwork" or "pastiche" taken from various Internet sources fails to rise to the level of an original work (Blum, 2009, quoted in Rosen, 2009). One also may commit unintentional plagiarism when one fails to cite another's ideas or concepts—even if they are paraphrased—because of ignorance of how or when to use citations (University of Victoria Libraries, 2009).

HOW DOES THE OCCUPATIONAL THERAPY PROFESSION VIEW PLAGIARISM?

As a profession, occupational therapy embraces a set of basic beliefs as put forth in the *Occupational Therapy Code of Ethics and Ethics Standards (2010)* (referred to as the "Code and Ethics Standards"; American Occupational Therapy Association [AOTA], 2010). As stated in the Preamble of the Code and Ethics Standards, the core value of truth requires that "in all situations, occupational therapists, occupational therapy assistants, and students must provide accurate information, both in oral and written form" (AOTA, 2010, p. S18). Truthfulness or veracity also is demonstrated by being accountable, honest, and authentic in both attitude and actions.

AOTA's Code and Ethics Standards expand on the concept of truth in Principle 6, Veracity, and Principle 7, Fidelity. Principle 6B states that "occupational therapy personnel shall refrain from using or participating in the use of any form of communication that contains false, fraudulent, deceptive, misleading, or unfair statements or claims." Principle 7 states that "occupational therapy personnel shall treat colleagues and other professionals with respect, fairness, discretion, and integrity." Principle 6I elaborates further on Veracity: "Occupational therapy personnel shall give credit and recognition when using the work of others in written, oral, or electronic media." The Code and Ethics Standards also remind us that we need to comply with laws and policies relevant to plagiarism, such as federal copyright laws. Principle 5 explicitly states, "Occupational therapy personnel shall comply with institutional rules, local, state, federal, and international laws and AOTA documents applicable to the profession of occupational therapy." Principle 6J states specifically the prohibition against plagiarism: "Occupational therapy personnel shall not plagiarize the work of others."

EXAMPLES OF PLAGIARISM IN OCCUPATIONAL THERAPY

- A local charity asks an occupational therapy practitioner to write an article for its newsletter explaining how occupational therapy can help the charity's constituents. The practitioner reads all of the major occupational therapy literature on the subject and surfs the Internet. She paraphrases the materials as she goes, collecting several pages of notes. At the end of her search, she puts her notes together in a coherent manner and submits her article. If the occupational therapy practitioner omits references to the ideas she paraphrased from the work of others, she commits plagiarism. *(intentional plagiarism)*
- Before writing a paper, a graduate student reads another student's paper. Two days later, she sits down and writes her own paper. Upon review of the paper, many ideas sound strikingly similar to the other student's paper. Although the student never intended to copy her fellow student's ideas, her conduct falls under the umbrella of plagiarism. *(confusion of one's own ideas with another's ideas)*
- An occupational therapy practitioner accepts a position to open a new, community-based

occupational therapy program. As she develops her evaluation forms and policies and procedures, she reviews a collection of material she has gathered from previous employers and others. She cuts and pastes pieces from the various sources and cuts and pastes content from her Google search results to compose her "new" forms and policies and procedures. She includes no references in her documents. Because the practitioner took materials written by others and failed to give them credit, this constitutes plagiarism. *(cutting and pasting ideas of others)*

- An occupational therapy practitioner attends a workshop. On her return, her employer requests that she present the material to the other occupational therapy practitioners. The occupational therapy practitioner copies and distributes to her colleagues the handout given out at the workshop. She reproduces the slide handout onto overheads and presents the material to the staff. Although everyone knows this material came from a workshop presented by a world-renowned occupational therapy practitioner, none of the materials or slides contain a reference. If the occupational therapy practitioner uses the materials without referencing their source, she plagiarizes the materials. This also may violate copyright laws. *(unintentional plagiarism due to ignorance)*

How Can Occupational Therapy Practitioners and Students Avoid Plagiarism?

Occupational therapists, occupational therapy assistants, and occupational therapy students may take several steps to avoid committing plagiarism. One must always put direct quotes in quotation marks and include the appropriately cited source (Stolley & Brizee, 2010). If authors borrow significant words from the work of another, they must quote those words and give credit to the author who coined them. When paraphrasing statements or borrowing concepts or ideas from another's work, one must include a reference to the source following the adopted information. One should consider introducing the quote or paraphrased language by crediting the author by name in an introductory statement, such as "According to Reilly . . ." (Stolley & Brizee, 2010).

As members of AOTA, we respect a standard of professionalism. Professionalism requires occupational therapists, occupational therapy assistants, and students of occupational therapy at all levels to treat the works of others as an extension of respect for the author. When in doubt, one should cite the source of words, thoughts, and ideas that may have originated from others. Writers must never represent someone else's words, thoughts, or ideas as their own. Plagiarism is not acceptable in any form.

References

Abate, F. R. (1997). *Oxford desk dictionary and thesaurus.* New York: Berkley Books.

American Occupational Therapy Association. (2010). Occupational therapy code of ethics and ethics standards (2010). *American Journal of Occupational Therapy, 64*(6 Suppl.), S17–S26. doi:10.5014/ajot.2010.64S17

Blum, S. D. (2009). *My word! Plagiarism and college culture.* Ithaca, NY: Cornell University.

Duke University, Office of the Dean of Academic Affairs, Trinity College. (2009). *Plagiarism tutorial at Duke University.* Durham, NC: Author. Retrieved July 30, 2010, from https://plagiarism.duke.edu/intent/

Rosen, C. (2009, April 16). It's not theft, it's pastiche. *Wall Street Journal,* p. A13. Retrieved July 30, 2010, from http://online.wsj.com/article/NA_WSJ_PUB:SB123984974506823779.html

Sinha, R., Singh, G., & Kumar, C. (2009). Plagiarism and unethical practices in literature. *Indian Journal of Ophthalmology, 57,* 481–485. Retrieved July 30, 2010, from http://www.ncbi.nlm.nih.gov/pmc/articles/PMC2812776/

Skandalakis, J. E., & Mirilas, P. (2004). Plagiarism. *Archives of Surgery, 139,* 1022–1024. Retrieved January 20, 2011, from http://archsurg.ama-assn.org/cgi/reprint/139/9/1022.pdf

Stolley, K., & Brizee, A. (2010, April 21). *Safe practices*. West Lafayette, IN: OWL, Purdue Online Writing Lab, Purdue University. Retrieved July 30, 2010, from http://owl.english.purdue.edu/owl/resource/589/03/

University of Victoria Libraries. (2009). *Plagiarism*. Victoria, BC, Canada: Author. Retrieved July 30, 2010, from http://library.uvic.ca/site/lib/instruction/cite/plagiarism.html#top

Washington State University. (2009). *Plagiarism: What is it?* Retrieved January 19, 2011, from http://www.wsulibs.wsu.edu/plagiarism/what.html

OTHER HELPFUL RESOURCES

College Board. (2008, September 29). *How to avoid plagiarism*. Retrieved July 30, 2010, from http://www.collegeboard.com/student/plan/college-success/10314.html

Office of the Faculty, Cornell University. (2006). *Acknowledging the work of others*. Ithaca, NY: Author. Retrieved July 30, 2010, from http://theuniversityfaculty.cornell.edu/pdfs/AIAckWorkRev90620.pdf

Pennsylvania State University. (2010, March 24). *Plagiarism tutorials for students*. Retrieved July 30, 2010, from http://tlt.its.psu.edu/plagiarism/tutorial

Plagiarism.org. (n.d.). *Educational tips on plagiarism prevention*. Retrieved July 30, 2010, from http://www.plagiarism.org/plag_article_educational_tips_on_plagiarism_prevention.html

Rutgers, The State University of New Jersey. (n.d.). [Paul Robeson Library: Video on plagiarism.] Retrieved July 30, 2010, from http://library.camden.rutgers.edu/EducationalModule/Plagiarism/

University of Wisconsin—Madison Writing Center. (2009). *How to avoid plagiarism*. Madison, WI: University of Wisconsin—Madison. Retrieved July 30, 2010, from http://writing.wisc.edu/Handbook/QPA_plagiarism.html

Writing Resource Center. (2006). *Avoiding plagiarism*. Bemidji, MN: Bemidji State University. Retrieved July 7, 2010, from http://www.bemidjistate.edu/students/wrc/sources.html

Barbara L. Kornblau, JD, OT/L, FAOTA, AAPM, ABDA, CCM, CDMS
Chairperson, Commission on Standards and Ethics (1998–2000)

This chapter was originally published in the 2000 edition of the *Reference Guide to the Occupational Therapy Code of Ethics*. It has been revised to reflect updated AOTA official documents, Web sites, AOTA style, and additional resources.

CHAPTER 36

Social Justice and Meeting the Needs of Clients

INTRODUCTION

Social justice is an ethical concept related to the equitable division of assets among members of society. In the area of health care, it addresses the importance of ensuring access to care to all persons in need of it (Beauchamp & Childress, 2009). In an environment of health care disparities and limited resources, occupational therapy practitioners can find themselves in ethical dilemmas related to providing appropriate levels of care. Some clients may use their extensive insurance coverage to pressure practitioners into providing more therapy than is needed to meet their occupational performance deficits. Yet others may have considerable needs but little or no coverage to pay for services. Further, employers may pressure practitioners to provide those services based on the reimbursement potential. This advisory opinion discusses the ethical standards that should guide decision making in these challenging situations.

THE ISSUES

Occupational therapy practitioners often face ethical issues involving service delivery because of a complex system of insurance rules and regulations. Practitioners must balance the needs of the individual client, the financial survival of the institution, and the laws regarding appropriate care. In general, clients should get the therapy they need, no more and no less. However, "need" cannot always be clearly defined and may differ in the opinion of different practitioners.

In addition, should clients who are motivated and engaged be presumed to derive more benefit and therefore to be more deserving of services than those who are not?

A reality of health care organizations is that they need to be paid for providing services, and health care is a labor-intensive "business." If organizations do not remain financially viable, they will not be available to provide any services, thereby further limiting access to resources. Are clients who pay for insurance coverage entitled to receive services based on that coverage even if they can no longer continue to benefit from therapy services? If so, how does that affect the resources (e.g., staff, time) that are then available to those with lesser financial means? Three case studies are presented to illustrate the issues.

Case Scenario 1

Jackie was a 39-year-old woman who sustained a right cerebral vascular accident (CVA) due to a previously undiagnosed pancreatic growth that caused severe hypertension. Prior to the CVA, she had been employed in sales at a large home repair chain. She was single, lived alone, and was thus responsible for all home management tasks. Jackie received comprehensive inpatient rehabilitation, including occupational, physical, and speech therapy, and was referred for further outpatient services after her discharge from the hospital. Jackie received services for approximately 1 month, at which time her former employer notified her by mail that they were cancelling her insurance. Although

209

she had applied for disability and Medicaid, she had not yet been approved. Jackie did not have the financial resources to self-pay for her therapies, and as a result, she discharged herself from outpatient physical therapy, occupational therapy, and speech therapy.

Case Scenario 2

Bob was a 62-year-old Vietnam War veteran who had had multiple CVAs and a history of hypertension and diabetes. After his CVAs, he spent a few years in several nursing homes receiving rehabilitation therapies. He was then referred to a day rehabilitation program for 6 weeks of intensive outpatient therapy. After discharge from day rehabilitation, he was referred to the outpatient clinic for continued occupational and physical therapy. Bob lived alone in an accessible apartment and had an aide who assisted him in all his activities of daily living (ADLs) and home management tasks. Bob's stated goal for occupational therapy was to "do more for himself."

Over the course of several months of occupational therapy, it became apparent that Bob was not using the skills he attained in therapy in his home environment. He was continuing to rely on his aide for dressing, bathing, toileting, and cooking, even though he required only setup or minimal assistance with these tasks. When confronted with the discrepancy between his abilities and his actual performance, Bob admitted that he enjoyed having the aide do these things for him and did not want to do them himself at this time. The occupational therapist reviewed Bob's goals and progress with him and stated her intention to discharge him from occupational therapy. Bob became irate, stating that he had multiple funding sources, including Medicare, Medicaid, and the Veterans Administration, and that if he wanted to have therapy, then he could have it as long as he wanted.

Case Scenario 3

Ashley was a 12-year-old girl who had cerebral palsy resulting in left hemiplegia. She had been receiving occupational therapy three times a week since a routine screening at age 2 identified her as eligible for related services because of an orthopedic impairment. Ashley was in a regular classroom and was currently on the honor roll. Her occupational therapist determined that direct services were no longer necessary and placed her on consult status for occupational therapy. Ashley's mother was fighting this change as she believed that her child still needed occupational therapy to "fix her left arm." The occupational therapy report stated, "Ashley has met her goals and gained maximum benefit from occupational therapy in the school environment. Ashley no longer requires the direct support of occupational therapy to benefit from her current educational placement."

Practitioners working in a school setting often encounter difficulty in clarifying the role of occupational therapy in an educational setting versus a rehabilitation or medical setting. Parents, hoping to maximize their child's function, may see services provided in the school as a way to ensure that their child continues to progress when health insurance for therapy is nonexistent or exhausted. The occupational therapy practitioner working in the schools has the responsibility to help the parent understand the role of the Individuals With Disabilities Education Act and occupational therapy as a related service as well as to direct them to other resources in the community that may be helpful to their child (e.g., United Cerebral Palsy, therapeutic recreation). Individualized education program meetings should be conducted in such a manner as to ensure that all parties understand the rationale for changes in the service plan and have opportunities for discussion and clarification.

DISCUSSION

These case studies provide examples of occupational therapy practitioners who found themselves in a quandary when making decisions regarding service provision or confronting inequities in allocation of available resources. Principle 1 of the *Occupational Therapy Code of Ethics and Ethics Standards (2010)* (referred to as the "Code and Ethics Standards"; American Occupational Therapy Association [AOTA], 2010) calls on occupational therapy practitioners to "demonstrate a concern for the well-being and safety of the recipients of their services," whereas Principle 5 calls on them to "comply with . . . laws and AOTA documents applicable to the profession of occupational therapy"; balancing these two imperatives can sometimes be difficult. Most insurance carriers reimburse for occupational therapy services only when those services are deemed medically necessary, are part of a plan of care that has been developed to improve functional performance, and require skilled intervention. If individuals like Bob are no longer progressing toward the stated goals, they must be reassessed to determine whether the goals were unrealistic and need modification or whether they have maximized their functional performance at this time and reached a plateau. Principle 1C of the Code and Ethics Standards states, "Occupational therapy personnel shall reevaluate and reassess recipients of service in a timely manner to determine if goals are being achieved and whether intervention plans should be revised."

Principle 1H of the Code and Ethics Standards further instructs the practitioner to "terminate occupational therapy services in collaboration with the service recipient or responsible party when the needs and goals of the recipient have been met or when services no longer produce a measurable change or outcome." The occupational therapy practitioner is ethically bound to be truthful in documentation (Principle 6C) and to not use language in such a way as to deceive the insurance carrier or agency into approving additional resources for persons when they are not meeting standards for reimbursement of care. Thus, the occupational therapy practitioner could not ethically revise Bob's notes to give the appearance that he was progressing toward his goals when he was not, and she could not omit his conflicting subjective statements regarding his interest in performing his ADLs

more independently. Billing codes and documentation must accurately reflect the procedures that were performed and the outcomes that resulted; they should never be modified based on the potential for maximizing reimbursement (see Principles 6B, 6C, and 6D).

Practitioners should "be diligent stewards of human, financial, and material resources of their employers" (Principle 7H). Facilities and agencies have limited staffing and financial resources and must allocate those resources carefully to remain viable. Therefore, they may face ethical challenges in prioritizing how therapy is provided. Facilities and agencies must balance the needs of the public with their ability to provide services that are likely to have the greatest positive effect on the lives of service recipients. Although Principle 4G holds that occupational therapy practitioners may "consider offering *pro bono* ('for the good') or reduced-fee occupational therapy services for selected individuals," this can be done only "when consistent with guidelines of the employer, third-party payer, and/or government agency." Thus, the occupational therapy practitioner treating Jackie would need to be sure that continuing to treat her for free or at a reduced rate would not be against department policy or law. In fact, because practitioners also have an obligation to "make efforts to advocate for recipients of occupational therapy services to obtain needed services through available means" (Principle 4E), they should also be aware of sliding scale fees or other assistance that may be available through the facility for clients in need.

The level of reimbursement for services, as in Bob's situation, should not dictate the plan of care. The ethical practitioner does not allow himself or herself to be coerced by administrators or clients or their families into keeping someone on the caseload who is no longer progressing toward a functional outcome or who does not have measurable goals. Clients without reimbursement, and those whose reimbursement has been discontinued or "maxed out," as in Jackie's situation, should be directed to community resources. Such resources can include indigent care and crime victims' funds, Medicaid, and other resources if financial assistance is not available within the facility. Clients should also be given the option to self-pay for services if their insurance has been exhausted but they are continuing to benefit from services. In addition to an ethical obligation to advocate for clients to receive needed services (Principle 4E), practitioners should educate clients on options other than skilled occupational therapy when their goals have been met or further progress is unlikely. Transition services to ensure continuity of care are the responsibility of the practitioner. These services may include support groups or community programs such as city therapeutic recreation programs to maintain or advance motor skills, improve endurance, or provide socialization.

Home programs, although generally part of most rehabilitation, can also be an important strategy to continue the client's progress when further in-clinic therapy is no longer possible or appropriate. These programs should be developed with the needs of the client and their available support network in mind. It is occupational therapy practitioners' responsibility to familiarize themselves with the community resources available to their clients and to help them make a smooth transition to the next phase of their rehabilitation or to independent resumption of daily life activities.

It is critical to recognize the social and emotional ties that are created in the therapeutic relationship, which is based on trust and developed during a vulnerable period in a client's life. Therefore, the practitioner may expect and should acknowledge the client's feeling of loss when therapy is terminated. The ethical practitioner espouses a "no surprises" approach to discharge and continuously lays the groundwork for the eventual release from skilled care.

Summary

The increasing number of individuals in need of occupational therapy services and the expanded awareness of the benefits offered by occupational therapy can result in a shortage of practitioners to meet the needs of the population. Skyrocketing medical costs have led insurance carriers and agencies to limit services for their participants on the basis of strict dollar amounts, number of visits, or progress made. Occupational therapy practitioners often find it difficult to ethically and comfortably balance the needs of the client, the facility or agency, and the payer source. Application of the *Occupational Therapy Code of Ethics and Ethics Standards (2010)* (AOTA, 2010) can assist in managing these challenging situations, permitting this battle between seemingly opposing forces to be resolved in a way that is mutually beneficial and meets the needs of all involved.

References

American Occupational Therapy Association. (2010). Occupational therapy code of ethics and ethics standards (2010). *American Journal of Occupational Therapy, 64*(6 Suppl.), S17–S26. doi:10.5014/ajot.2010.64S17

Beauchamp, T., & Childress, J. (2009). *Principles of biomedical ethics* (6th ed.). New York: Oxford University Press.

Individuals With Disabilities Education Act of 1990, Pub. L. 101–476, 20 U.S.C., Ch. 33.

Ann Moodey Ashe, MHS, OTR/L
Practice Representative, Ethics Commission (2008–2011)

CHAPTER 37

Online Social Networking

INTRODUCTION

Over the past several years, social activity has intersected with the Internet to popularize *online social networking (OSN)*. OSN is the sharing of user-generated information and media with friends, families, professional colleagues, and even strangers via designated Web sites (Terry, 2009). Millions of teenagers and adults worldwide access such popular OSN sites as Facebook, MySpace, Friendster.com, LinkedIn, and Xanga.com (Barnes, 2006). Facebook is the most popular site (Bemis-Dougherty, 2010), boasting more than 500 million members worldwide (Facebook, 2010). Users create and post profiles that may include such personal information as "name, age, sex, contact information, photographs, areas of interest, educational background, employment, hobbies, and relationship status" (Bemis-Dougherty, 2010, p. 42). Using Facebook and similar sites allows people to communicate and connect with hundreds of others by posting information about their lives via instant messaging, chat rooms, file sharing, and blogging (Klich-Heartt & Prion, 2010), as well as photos, videos, and links to other sites (Bemis-Dougherty, 2010).

Use of social networking sites offers many benefits in terms of staying connected with family, friends, acquaintances, and others, but the type and amount of information shared may result in ethical conflict related to one's professional roles. Persons who are friends within social networking sites have no legal obligation to protect confidential information. In addition, due to the often unclear personal relationships associated with social networking friendships, those individuals accessing shared information may feel no moral obligation to refrain from disclosing information posted by others.

INAPPROPRIATE USE

The potential exists for OSN users to post insensitive, inflammatory, offensive, or illegal content. Sites attempt to prevent this through expectations for responsible use as delineated in user terms and conditions. Facebook's *Statement of Rights and Responsibilities* (Facebook, 2010) and MySpace's *Terms of Use Agreement* (MySpace, 2009) prohibit inappropriate postings including, but not limited to, those that are offensive, harassing, exploitative, illegal, defamatory, or libelous or that violate the privacy rights of others. Despite these terms of agreement, the popular media continue to report incidents of inappropriate use. For example, a management company sued a tenant for libel after she used electronic social networking to broadcast that her apartment was moldy (Heussner, 2009). In another instance, a political aide resigned after posting an offensive remark about President Obama on her Facebook page (Gentile, 2009). Social networking sites are also being accessed by employers who are making decisions not to hire people (Clark & Roberts,

2010) or to fire employees (Greenhouse, 2010) on the basis of inappropriate postings about colleagues and supervisors.

Although privacy filters are available, people may not use them. There is also the chance that someone may post publicly accessible inappropriate information about other people. That is, if you "friend" someone on your OSN page, in essence you are agreeing that anything you post on your page can be made public by that friend. Other people have no legal obligation to keep confidential information that you have posted. Once you post information, you lose control of who may view it. Furthermore, once information is posted online, a visitor to the site or third-party storage program can save it; for this reason, posted information should be considered permanent, even after it has been deleted (Bemis-Dougherty, 2010).

ISSUES FOR OCCUPATIONAL THERAPY EDUCATORS, PRACTITIONERS, AND STUDENTS

Use of OSN sites by health care providers presents unique concerns due to the blurring of the line between one's personal and professional lives (McBride & Cohen, 2009). In most settings, a health care professional's behavior during personal time (i.e., away from the health care setting) does not intersect with his or her professional behavior (Thompson et al., 2008). The exception to this may be active participation in OSN sites. Although posting information on an OSN site is not inherently unprofessional, health care providers need to be cognizant of their responsibility to carefully select the content and amount of information they post. As health care providers, occupational therapy practitioners, educators, and students should ensure that their postings are consistent with professional legal and ethical standards, behavior the term *e-professionalism* was coined to describe (Jannsen, 2009).

Unprofessional postings can have unintended and far-reaching consequences. Posting negative information about one's employer or colleagues can diminish one's credibility in the eyes of the community and result in legal action against the person who posted the information (McBride & Cohen, 2009). Equally important are ramifications related to the recipient–health care provider relationship. Of utmost concern are the legal and ethical mandates to keep protected health information confidential and thus avoid posting identifying information about clients. Another concern involves the posting of inappropriate or inflammatory (but not identifiable) information about colleagues, which can result in a negative impact on relationships with other health care providers and/or clients.

Information shared by health care providers whose sites are public or who engage in online friendships with clients can jeopardize professional boundaries by involvement in a dual relationship with service recipients (Guseh, Brendel, & Brendel, 2009). Health care providers must weigh the risks and benefits of self-disclosure and the potential for a client's knowledge of the provider's personal information to lead to an erosion of trust between client and provider (McBride & Cohen, 2009). Similarly, providers may learn information about service recipients that places the provider in the awkward position of deciding if or how to use the information and whether or not to document the information in the client's medical records (Guseh et al., 2009). The same principles that apply to health care providers also apply to educators, researchers, and students.

Occupational therapy students may be especially vulnerable to issues related to e-professionalism. Students are in the process of learning to incorporate high standards of professional behavior. As such, they may not understand the ramifications of unprofessional, unethical, or illegal postings on social networking sites. Popular media reports include multiple incidents of college students who experienced negative consequences related to online postings (Cain, 2008), including a nursing student who was expelled from a university because of her inappropriate postings about a patient on a social networking site (Lipka, 2009).

Although there is no research about occupational therapy students' online posting habits, results of studies with medical students document the prevalence of unprofessional postings (Chretien, Greysen, Chretien, & Kind, 2009; Thompson et al., 2008). These included violations of patient confidentiality, use of profanity, discriminatory language, depiction of intoxication, and use of sexually suggestive language (Chretien et al., 2009). Postings that students perceive as harmless or normal may actually be deemed unprofessional, unethical, or illegal by faculty, administrators, or potential employers (Cain, 2008).

CASE SCENARIO

Sara was a 27-year-old occupational therapy student who had completed half of her second Level II fieldwork placement in adult physical disabilities at a local general hospital. Her performance at this point was below passing level. Jessica, Sara's supervisor, gave Sara the feedback that she was taking too long to complete patient documentation, was having difficulty establishing rapport and interacting with patients, and could not be left alone with patients because of her lack of consistency in following safety precautions.

Sara was an avid user of Facebook, checking her page and posting information 5 to 6 times each day. Thinking it would help Jessica get to know and understand her better, Sara decided to invite Jessica to be her Facebook friend. Jessica declined and provided verbal feedback to Sara concerning the inappropriateness of being her Facebook friend. Throughout that day, Sara was impatient with her patients and became easily frustrated when they couldn't complete the activities she had planned for them. Around 1:30 p.m., Sara decided she needed a break, so she returned to the occupational therapy department, logged on to a computer, and accessed Facebook. Sara began to vent on her page. She wrote,

I can't believe how unprofessional my supervisor J is! What a witch! How she ever

got to be an OT is beyond me! Believe it or not, she REFUSED to be my Facebook friend. . . . This hospital stinks . . . you don't EVER want to be a patient here, let alone work here! The patients are crazy. . . . I just saw Mabel—Miss "I don't care what you want me to do, I just had a total hip replacement, and I'm going to rest." . . . All she does is make me look bad—and J blames ME! Only three more hours . . . I CAN'T WAIT to go home, kick back, and drink a bottle (or two ☺) of wine!!!!!!

Several aspects of Sara's behavior in the case scenario are in direct violation of the *Occupational Therapy Code of Ethics and Ethics Standards (2010)* (referred to as the "Code and Ethics Standards"; American Occupational Therapy Association [AOTA], 2010). Her behavior violates Principle 5, Procedural Justice, which states, "Occupational therapy personnel shall comply with institutional rules, local, state, federal, and international laws and AOTA documents applicable to the profession of occupational therapy." Occupational therapists have an ethical obligation to adhere to legal regulations. Sara's posting violated a federal statute, the Health Insurance Portability and Accountability Act of 1996 (HIPAA). HIPAA is a confidentiality and privacy statute that requires individually identifiable health information to be held confidential in all forms of communication (e.g., verbal, written, electronic) unless explicitly permitted by an individual (U.S. Department of Health and Human Services, 2010). The Department of Health and Human Services holds enforcement powers and may seek civil penalties and criminal punishments against people who violate HIPAA standards (Allen, 2004). Although Sara did not divulge her patient's full name, identifying her by her first name and diagnosis may well provide enough information for the patient, her family members, or others in the community to identify her as Sara's patient.

Sara also violated Principle 3, Autonomy and Confidentiality, which states, "Occupational therapy personnel shall respect the right of the individual to self-determination." Specifically, Principle 3G requires occupational therapy personnel to respect recipients' confidentiality and right to privacy. Principle 3H explicitly requires "all verbal, written, electronic, augmentative, and nonverbal communications" to be held confidential, "including compliance with HIPAA regulations." As noted above, Sara divulged personal information about her patient Mabel without Mabel's permission.

Sara's negative postings about Jessica also directly violate Principle 7 (Fidelity) of the Code and Ethics Standards, which states, "Occupational therapy personnel shall treat colleagues and other professionals with respect, fairness, discretion, and integrity." Information about their supervisory relationship should be considered private and should be preserved and respected as such (Principle 7B).

In contrast, Jessica's decisions were consistent with expected behaviors as outlined in the Code and Ethics Standards. Jessica's decision not to accept Sara's invitation to be her friend on Facebook was in adherence with Principle 2 (Nonmaleficence) and Principle 7 (Fidelity). By not accepting a friend invitation from Sara on Facebook, Jessica avoided a situation that could potentially have exploited Sara socially or that could have compromised Jessica's own professional judgment and objectivity as Sara's supervisor (Principle 2C). Additionally, Jessica's refusal allowed her to maintain clear professional boundaries and thus ensure Sara's well-being (Principle 2G). With regard to Principle 7, by not engaging in a personal relationship with a student outside of the workplace, Jessica avoided potential conflicts of interest as Sara's fieldwork educator (Principle 7E).

Sara's posting also included several elements of questionable professional behavior. Speaking negatively about the facility and her patients not only cast Sara in a negative light but also may have diminished the facility's reputation in the community. The reference to drinking up to two bottles of wine may have been exaggerated or said in jest. Nevertheless, these comments also cast Sara in a negative light. Colleagues, patients, administrators, or faculty who read these comments may pass judgment on Sara and question her judgment and professionalism or may even suspect that she may be impaired by the influence of alcohol. Although alcohol-related postings may be acceptable on a personal level, this incident shows them to be problematic on a professional level.

SUMMARY AND CONCLUSIONS

The advent of OSN sites offers millions of people worldwide opportunities to easily stay connected with friends and loved ones. Many may feel that their postings are personal in nature and as such are not subject to review by or judgment of others. However, the personal–professional boundary lines may blur when considering the appropriateness of content posted on personal social networking sites. This issue is of particular concern to health care providers.

Health care practitioners need to be aware that there may be an unintended audience viewing material posted on social networking sites (Jannsen, 2009). Personal information is readily available and may include content that should not be disclosed in provider–patient relationships (Thompson et al., 2008). As noted in the case scenario, professional relationships with coworkers may be compromised when using this arena for communication. Although in many instances these sites are seen as a means to facilitate communication, when used inappropriately they may lead to a breach of ethics standards set forth by the health professions, including occupational therapy.

Inappropriate postings by health care providers have ethical and potentially legal ramifications that may not be applicable to laypeople. As health care providers, occupational therapy personnel need to be cognizant of ethical boundaries related to content posted on personal social networking sites and should carefully consider whether or not the information they post is consistent with ethical standards as outlined in the *Occupational Therapy Code of Ethics and Ethics Standards (2010)*. If one doubts whether information to be posted is appropriate, one should err on the side of being conservative and avoid sharing the content on social networking sites.

REFERENCES

Allen, A. L. (2004). Privacy in healthcare. In S. Post (Ed.), *Encyclopedia of bioethics* (3rd ed., pp. 2120–2128). New York: Thomson Gale.

American Occupational Therapy Association. (2010). Occupational therapy code of ethics and ethics standards (2010). *American Journal of Occupational Therapy, 64*(6 Suppl.), S17–S26. doi:10.5014/ajot.2010.64S17

Barnes, S. (2006). A privacy paradox: Social networking in the United States. *First Monday, 11*(9). Retrieved February 5, 2011, from http://firstmonday.org/htbin/cgiwrap/bin/ojs/index.php/fm/article/view/1394/1312

Bemis-Dougherty, A. (2010, June). Professionalism and social networking. *PT in Motion,* pp. 40–47. Retrieved February 5, 2011, from http://web.ebscohost.com.ezproxy.uky.edu/ehost/pdfviewer/pdfviewer?vid=3&hid=22&sid=ea7bcf36-851b-4475-b254-3cffe7026deb%40sessionmgr10

Cain, J. (2008). Online social networking issues within academia and pharmacy education. *American Journal of Pharmaceutical Education, 72,* 1–7. Retrieved February 5, 2011, from https://www.ncbi.nlm.nih.gov/pmc/articles/PMC2254235/pdf/ajpe10.pdf

Chretien, K. C., Greysen, S. R., Chretien, J., & Kind, T. (2009). Online posting of unprofessional content by medical students. *JAMA, 302,* 1309–1315. doi:10.1001/jama.2009.1387

Clark, L. A., & Roberts, S. J. (2010). Employer's use of social networking sites: A socially irresponsible practice. *Journal of Business Ethics, 95,* 507–525. doi: 10.1007/s10551-010-0436-y

Facebook. (2010, October 4). *Statement of rights and responsibilities.* Retrieved February 5, 2011, from http://www.facebook.com/terms/#!/terms.php

Gentile, S. (2009, July 26). Stringer deputy press sec slams O-dumb-a. *City Hall.* Retrieved February 5, 2011, from http://www.cityhallnews.com/newyork/print-article-817-print.html.

Greenhouse, S. (2010, November 8). Company accused of firing over Facebook post. *New York Times.* Retrieved February 5, 2011, from http://www.nytimes.com/2010/11/09/business/09facebook.html?sq=socialnetworking.

Guseh, J. S., Brendel, R. W., & Brendel, D. H. (2009). Medical professionalism in the age of online social networking. *Journal of Medical Ethics, 35,* 584–586. doi:10.1136/ jme.2009.029231

Health Insurance Portability and Accountability Act of 1996 (HIPAA), Pub. L. 104–191.

Heussner, K. (2009, July 29). *Top 10 social media gaffes.* Retrieved February 9, 2011, from http://abcnews.go.com/Technology/AheadoftheCurve/story?id=8201190&page=1

Jannsen, M. (2009). Social networking and e-professionalism. *American Journal of Health System Pharmacy, 66,* 1672. Retrieved from http://web.ebscohost.com.ezproxy.uky.edu/ehost/pdfviewer/pdfviewer?vid=3&hid=110&sid=03767a2b-8f0a-46fa-bfd8-2173d07e0265%40sessionmgr115

Klich-Heartt, E. I., & Prion, S. (2010). Social networking and HIPAA: Ethical concerns for nurses. *Nurse Leader, 8*(2), 56–58. doi:10.1016/j.mnl.2010.01.007

Lipka, S. (2009, March 13). Nursing student sues after U. of Louisville expels her for online posts about patients. *Chronicle of Higher Education.* Retrieved February 5, 2011, from http://chronicle.com/article/Nursing-Student-Sues-After-U/42558

McBride, D., & Cohen, E. (2009, July). Misuse of social networking may have ethical implications for nurses. *ONS Connect,* 17. Retrieved from http://web.ebscohost.com.ezproxy.uky.edu/ehost/pdfviewer/pdfviewer?vid=4&hid=110&sid=6c9dcac8-ce38-4d9d-ad33-2c3c449444fe%40sessionmgr115

MySpace. (2009, June 25). *MySpace.com terms of use agreement.* Retrieved February 5, 2011, from http://www.myspace.com/help/terms

Terry, M. (2009). Twittering healthcare: Social media and medicine. *Telemedicine and e-Health, 15,* 507–511. doi:10.1089/tmj.2009.9955

Thompson, L., Dawson, K., Ferdig, R., Black, E., Boyer, J., Coutts, J., et al. (2008). The intersection of online social networking with medical professionalism. *Journal of General Internal Medicine, 23,* 954–957.

U.S. Department of Health and Human Services. (2010). *Health information privacy.* Retrieved February 5, 2011, from http://www.hhs.gov/ocr/privacy/

Joanne Estes, MS, OTR/L
Education Representative, Ethics Commission (2009–2012)

Lea Cheyney Brandt, OTD, MA, OTR/L
Member at Large, Ethics Commission (2005–2008, 2008–2011)

Copyright © 2011, by the American Occupational Therapy Association. The authors acknowledge the contribution of Katilyn Elrod, OTA, to the literature reviewed in this article.

CHAPTER 38

Avoiding Plagiarism in the Electronic Age

INTRODUCTION

Plagiarism is the "act of using another person's words or ideas without giving credit to that person" (Merriam-Webster, 2011a). The concept of plagiarism encompasses not only material that has been copyrighted and published but also unpublished works, speeches, tweets, blogs, photographs, drawings, and the like. With the increasing use of electronic media as resources, occupational therapists, occupational therapy assistants, and students face additional challenges in appropriately citing sources when they write a paper or article for the classroom or for publication.

Although the Internet has certainly simplified the process of research for the practitioner, researcher, educator, and student by making information readily available, it has resulted in confusion regarding the issues of defining intellectual property and public domain. The *public domain* is defined as "the realm embracing property rights that belong to the community at large, are unprotected by copyright or patent and are subject to appropriation by anyone" (Merriam-Webster, 2011b). Guidelines for what is considered to be in the public domain include work that was never copyrighted (e.g., work done before copyright law was established), those works for which the copyright has expired, the work of government agencies, and facts such as census information (University of Maryland University College, 2010).

Information available to all on the Internet is not necessarily in the public domain. When in doubt as to whether information is in the public domain, look for guidance on the bottom of the Web page as to the author's willingness to freely disseminate the information. Proper citation is important even when the information is in the public domain; this is an important way for others to locate further information on a topic. Experienced practitioners who might have a great deal of clinical knowledge but who have been out of their academic training for some time may find themselves entering a new world of documentation that requires that they cite less traditional sources such as Web sites and unpublished works.

ISSUES

Importance of Proper Citation

The *Occupational Therapy Code of Ethics and Ethics Standards (2010)* (referred to as the "Code and Ethics Standards"; American Occupational Therapy Association [AOTA], 2010) establishes that "occupational therapy personnel shall give credit and recognition when using the work of others in written, oral, or electronic media" (Principle 6I), thereby documenting their sources, whether they be books, journals, or Web sites. More importantly, copyright law requires that we either present only our own ideas or accurately cite those of others, making plagiarism both a legal and an ethical issue (U.S. Copyright Office, n.d.). Copyright law applies not just to literary works

(§102.a.1) but to pictorial and graphic works (among others) as well (§102.a.5). It gives the holder of the copyright the exclusive right to reproduce copyrighted works (§106.1). Under the fair use section of the copyright law (§107), one may reproduce copyrighted material for teaching, scholarship, or research as long as it is cited, is used for nonprofit educational purposes, and does not affect "the potential market for or value of copyrighted work" (§107.4). Lack of awareness about correct citation of information acquired through electronic media or other sources does not excuse the writer from the obligation to provide accurate documentation of those sources.

Guidance for Citation of Electronic Sources

The prevalence of online journals and the Internet in disseminating knowledge has led to new protocols that delineate the proper way to identify online sources of information, including blogs, conference abstracts, or online books. Those unfamiliar with the standards for citing references should consult such resources as the *Publication Manual of the American Psychological Association* (American Psychological Association, 2010). In addition, writers should seek out those with more experience in publishing to mentor them in the process of preparing an article or paper correctly. Additionally, many universities offer Web-based resources for preparing citations correctly (see list of resources at the end of this advisory opinion). Students may be able to use tools such as Safe Assign (www.safeassign.com), a plagiarism prevention service available on Blackboard, to determine if their papers could be construed as plagiarized. Safe Assign assists students by teaching them proper citation and educators by providing a mechanism to identify plagiarism by their students (www.blackboard.com).

Rules and Ethics Standards Regarding Plagiarism

All educational institutions have rules against plagiarism reflected in their student guides, and many have honor codes as well. Some universities have useful guides for students that help them avoid the pitfalls of plagiarism when preparing papers (see, e.g., Princeton University, 2008). In many universities, plagiarism is grounds for academic suspension or probation and may even lead to expulsion. It is crucial that students preparing everything from papers for the classroom to doctoral dissertations learn how to avoid plagiarism.

The Code and Ethics Standards address the concept of plagiarism both directly and indirectly, primarily within Principle 6 (Veracity) and its subprinciples. For example, Principle 6J directs occupational therapy personnel to "not plagiarize the work of others." This directive could not be clearer. Principle 6I states that "occupational therapy personnel shall give credit and recognition when using the work of others in written, oral, or electronic media." This principle highlights the ethical obligation to represent and document the contributions of others accurately in all forms of communication. Principle 6B additionally reminds occupational therapy personnel to "refrain from using or participating in the use of any form of communication that contains false, fraudulent, deceptive, misleading, or unfair statements or claims." Failing to cite a source appropriately can deceive the reader into believing that the thoughts contained in the document are those of the author. Any reader who then cites that author further diminishes the credit due the original source.

CASE SCENARIOS

Case Scenario 1. Tiffany

Tiffany recently started work at an outpatient clinic in town. She did her internship at a different hospital, where they had a well-developed arthritis program. Tiffany went online to the Web site of the hospital where she did her fieldwork, downloaded their handouts on joint protection, and reprinted them with the logo of her current employer's clinic.

Tiffany's actions constituted several breaches of the Code and Ethics Standards. By substituting the logo of her new facility, she was deceiving the public into believing that the handouts were created at that facility. This is an act of plagiarism, violating Principles 6J and 6I. Tiffany's actions could also be considered a breach of Principle 7, Fidelity, as she used her position as a student to gather information from another organization to provide a benefit to her new facility, thus creating a conflict of interest (Principle 7F). Tiffany must first ask permission to use the handouts from the facility that developed them. If granted, she must then acknowledge the facility that developed the handouts if she is going to use them and state that they are reprinted or used with permission, even if she paraphrases language or changes the order of the instruction sheets.

Case Scenario 2. Bob

Bob was a newly hired instructor in the occupational therapy assistant program at a local community college. His teaching course load included a class on physical disabilities. Bob prepared his lecture on stroke and included information on neurodevelopmental treatment (NDT) and proprioceptive neuromuscular facilitation that he received while in occupational therapy school and at continuing education courses. He long since sold the reference books that he had in school, but he assumed that the NDT principles were now "general knowledge" and in the public domain in the rehabilitation sciences and that specific citations were not necessary.

Although Bob may have felt that the information is general knowledge in the field, it is still mandatory that he cite references for his information, and adequate documentation will help students locate further information on the topic. A reference librarian or medical library may be helpful in locating the original source. Information gained from continuing education courses, although often not copyrighted, must still be referenced when preparing a lecture.

Case Scenario 3. Carlotta

Carlotta was required to do an in-service as part of her clinical affiliation. She gathered information from Web-based sources about her topic. She did not know how to format citations for the Web sites she used, so she left those sources off her reference list.

Carlotta failed to prepare her in-service properly. It is imperative that all information be referenced appropriately. Because information from the Web varies significantly in its reliability, it is especially important that the person receiving the information knows the source so that he or she can weigh its usefulness and quality. Providing the URL of a document helps readers locate the material on the Internet, and retrieval dates are necessary if the information is time sensitive or likely to change. In addition, providing a document's digital object identifier (DOI) helps readers locate the source (American Psychological Association, 2010). It is important that students and practitioners carefully document all of their sources when preparing in-services, as these are an excellent avenue for clinicians to update their knowledge.

SUMMARY AND CONCLUSION

Clinicians, researchers, educators, and students in the field of occupational therapy must be vigilant about avoiding plagiarism. Accurate citations and references to electronic sources when preparing in-services, continuing education presentations, or facility handouts or when authoring research or other articles are crucial to maintaining professional integrity and supporting appropriate ethical conduct as delineated in the Code and Ethics Standards.

REFERENCES

American Occupational Therapy Association. (2010). Occupational therapy code of ethics and ethics standards (2010). *American Journal of*

Occupational Therapy, 64(6 Suppl.), S17–S26. doi:10.5014/ajot.2010.64S17

American Psychological Association. (2010). *Publication manual of the American Psychological Association* (6th ed.). Washington, DC: Author.

Merriam-Webster. (2011a). *Plagiarism.* Retrieved February 5, 2011, from http://www.learners dictionary.com/search/plagiarism

Merriam-Webster. (2011b). *Public domain.* Retrieved February 9, 2011, from http://www. merriam-webster.com/dictionary/public%20 domain

Princeton University. (2008). *Examples of plagiarism.* Retrieved February 5, 2011, from http://www. princeton.edu/pr/pub/integrity/08/plagiarism/

U.S. Copyright Office. (n.d.). *Copyright law of the United States of America.* Retrieved February 5, 2011, from http://www.copyright.gov/title17/ 92chap1.html

University of Maryland University College. (2010). *Copyright and fair use in the classroom, on the Internet, and the World Wide Web.* Retrieved February 9, 2011, from http://umuc.edu/library/ copy.shtml

RESOURCES

Blackboard's plagiarism prevention service: www.safeassign.com/

Copyright law: http://www.copyright.gov/title17/ 92chap1.html

OWL Purdue Online Writing Lab: http://owl. english.purdue.edu/owl/

Princeton University Academic Integrity Web site: www.princeton.edu/pr/pub/integrity/08/ plagiarism

Ann Moodey Ashe, MHS, OTR/L
Practice Representative, Ethics Commission (2008–2011, 2011–2014)

APPENDIXES

Glossary of Ethics Terms

altruism The promotion of good for others and the consideration of the consequences of the action for everyone except oneself.

autonomy (*auto* = self, *nomos* = law) The right of an individual to self-determination; "self-rule that is free from both controlling interference by others and from certain limitations . . . that prevent meaningful choice" (Beauchamp & Childress, 2009, p. 58).

beneficence (*bene faceae* = to do well) Doing good for others or bringing about good for them; the duty to confer benefits on others.

bioethics A type of *normative ethics* involving the application of ethical principles in health care delivery, medical treatment, and research.

care ethics An ethical concept found primarily in nursing and feminist literature that states that the attitude of being a moral person is based on the concepts of receptivity, relatedness, and responsiveness by the caregiver to the one being cared for.

casuistry Ethical decision making based on the understanding of a specific situation in relation to past events and historical records of similar cases; particular features of a case versus the broad overarching principles are studied.

categorical imperative A maxim described by philosopher Immanuel Kant as a "command" that has three components: universality, respect, and autonomy. Together, they establish that an action is properly called "morally good" only if we can will all persons to do it, if it enables us to treat other persons as ends and not merely as the means to our own selfish ends, and if it allows us to see other persons as mutual lawmakers. Arguments are grounded in reason as opposed to tradition, emotion, or intuition.

confidentiality Nondisclosure of data or information that should be kept private to prevent harm and to abide by policies, regulations, and laws.

deontology (*deon* = duty) A classical ethical theory that states that the concept of *duty* is independent of the concept of good or the consequences of the action. People's actions are assessed by their ability to follow such things as religious codes, laws, and professional codes of ethics.

dilemma A situation in which one moral conviction or right action conflicts with another; exists because there is no one, clear-cut, right answer.

duty Actions required of professionals by society or actions that are self-imposed.

ethical relativism Moral judgments that depend on subjective criteria or cultural acceptance.

ethics A systematic view of rules of conduct that is grounded in philosophical principles and theory; character and customs of societal values and norms that are assumed in a given cultural, professional, or institutional setting as ways of determining right and wrong.

fidelity Faithful fulfillment of vows, promises, and agreements and discharge of fiduciary responsibilities.

fiduciary A person, often in a position of authority, who obligates himself or herself to act on behalf of another (as in managing money or property) and assumes a duty to act in good faith and with care, candor, and loyalty in fulfilling the obligation; one (as an agent) having a fiduciary duty to another.

impairment Problem in body function or structure as a significant deviation or loss (World Health Organization, 2001, p. 12).

justice The act of distributing goods and burdens among members of society. Three types include
- **compensatory justice** The making of reparations for wrongs that have been done.
- **distributive justice** "Fair, equitable, and appropriate distribution determined by justified norms that structure the terms of social cooperation. *Distributive justice* refers broadly to the distribution of all rights and responsibilities in society" (Beauchamp & Childress, 2009, p. 226).
- **procedural justice** The assurance that processes are organized in a fair manner.

law A body or system of rules used by an authority to impose control over a system or humans.

metaethics A branch of philosophy that studies the underlying reasons for setting and making moral judgments.

morality Personal beliefs regarding values, rules, and principles of what is right or wrong; may be culture based or culture driven.

morals Personal beliefs regarding values, rules, and principles of what is right or wrong;

may be culture based or culture driven (see *ethical relativism*).

nonmaleficence Not harming or causing harm to be done to oneself or others; the duty to ensure that no harm is done.

normative ethics The study of right and wrong from a societal perspective; the goal is the harmonious function of society and the welfare of the individual member of society.

paternalism An action taken by one person in the best interests of another without his or her consent.
- **strong paternalism** Action taken that is exercised against the competent wishes of another.
- **weak paternalism** Action taken that is presumed to be according to the wishes of the person, usually done because of the individual's age or mental status.

rights Specific legal, moral, and social claims humans possess that require others to act in specific ways toward us. With all rights is the implied obligation or duty on the part of each of us.

situational ethics The consideration of circumstances and situations used along with ethical principles and rules in the decision-making process.

social contract ethics An ethical theory that promotes the concept that each individual as a member of society adheres to moral norms in his or her relationships with others and that the larger community has special responsibilities to protect the more vulnerable members of society.

teleology (*telos* = end) An ethics theory that focuses on outcomes or consequences. This classical theory states that the morally right action is determined by the outcome it produces; frequently stated as "the ends justify the means."

utilitarianism An ethical theory that states that right actions are those that maximize utility (the greatest good for the greatest number) and result in the best consequences for all involved.

veracity A duty to tell the truth.

virtue ethics A form of philosophy that emphasizes character and personal integrity; involves deliberation, the quality of choice, and one's responses to one's poor choices.

REFERENCES

Beauchamp, T. L., & Childress, J. F. (2009). *Principles of biomedical ethics.* New York: Oxford University Press.

World Health Organization. (2001). *International classification of functioning, disability and health.* Geneva, Switzerland: Author.

Ethics Resources

ASSOCIATIONS, ORGANIZATIONS, AND ETHICS CENTERS

American Occupational Therapy Association
4720 Montgomery Lane
P.O. Box 31220
Bethesda, MD 20824-1220
301-652-2682
TDD: 1-800-377-8555
Fax: 301-652-7711
http://www.aota.org/Consumers/ Ethics.aspx
    (consumers and nonmembers)
http://www.aota.org/Practitioners/
    Ethics.aspx (additional resources for
    members)
ethics@aota.org

American Physical Therapy Association
1111 North Fairfax Street
Alexandria, VA 22314-1488
800-999-APTA (2782)
703-684-APTA (2782)
TDD: 703-683-6748
Fax: 703-684-7343
http://www.apta.org/AM/ Template.cfm?
    Section=Ethics_and_Legal_Issues1&
    Template=/TaggedPage/
    TaggedPageDisplay.cfm&TPLID=48&
    ContentID=63612

American Society for Bioethics and Humanities
(formerly Society for Health and Human Values)
4700 West Lake Avenue
Glenview, IL 60025-1485
847-375-4745
Fax: 847-375-6482
http://www.asbh.org
info@asbh.org

American Society of Law, Medicine & Ethics
765 Commonwealth Avenue, Suite 1634
Boston, MA 02215
617-262-4990
Fax: 617-437-7596
http://www.aslme.org
info@aslme.org

American Speech–Language–Hearing Association
2200 Research Boulevard
Rockville, MD 20850-3289
301-296-5700
Phone Members: 800-498-2071
Phone Nonmembers: 800-638-8255
TTY: 301-296-5650
Fax: 301-296-8580
http://www.asha.org/practice/ethics/
    roundtable/default.htm
actioncenter@asha.org

Association for Practical and Professional Ethics
Indiana University
618 East Third Street
Bloomington, IN 47405-3602
812-855-6450
Fax: 812-855-4969
http://www.indiana.edu/~appe/
appe@indiana.edu

Bioethics on the Web
National Institutes of Health
9000 Rockville Pike
Bethesda, MD 20892
301-496-4000
http://bioethics.od.nih.gov/
BioethicsResources@mail.nih.gov

Bioethics Research Library
Georgetown University
Kennedy Institute on Bioethics
Box 571212
Washington, DC 20057-1212
202-687-3885
Fax: 202-687-8089
http://bioethics.georgetown.edu/nrc/

Center for Academic Integrity
Clemson University
Clemson, SC 29634
864-656-3311
http://www.academicintegrity.org

Center for Bioethics
University of Pennsylvania
3401 Market Street, Suite 320
Philadelphia, PA 19104-3308
215-898-7136
Fax: 215-573-3036
http://www.bioethics.upenn.edu/

Center for Practical Bioethics
Harzfeld Building
1111 Main Street, Suite 500
Kansas City, MO 64105-2116
800-344-3829
816-221-1100
Fax: 816-221-2002
http://www.practicalbioethics.org/
bioethic@practicalbioethics.org

Center for the Study of Ethics in the Professions
Illinois Institute of Technology
Hermann Hall, Room 204
3241 South Federal Street
Chicago, IL 60616
312-567-3017
Fax: 312-567-3016
http://www.iit.edu/departments/csep/
csep@iit.edu

Consortium Ethics Program
University of Pittsburgh
Center for Bioethics and Health Law
3708 Fifth Avenue, Suite 300
Pittsburgh, PA 15213
412-647-5834
Fax: 412-647-5877
http://www.pitt.edu/~cep/
cep@pitt.edu

Ethics Updates
The Values Institute
University of San Diego
5998 Alcalá Park
San Diego, CA 92110-2492
619-260-4787
Fax: 619-260-5950
http://ethics.sandiego.edu/
hinman@sandiego.edu

Hastings Center
21 Malcolm Gordon Drive
Garrison, NY 10524-4125
845-424-4040
Fax: 845-424-4545
http://www.thehastingscenter.org/
mail@thehastingscenter.org

Hoffberger Center for Professional Ethics
University of Baltimore
1420 North Charles Street
Baltimore, MD 21201
410-837-4200
http://www.ubalt.edu/template.cfm?page=1882

Institute for Global Ethics
91 Camden Street, Suite 403
Rockland, ME 04841
207-594-6658
800-729-2615 (U.S. only)
Fax: 207-594-6648
http://www.globalethics.org/
ethics@globalethics.org

Kennedy Institute of Ethics
Georgetown University
Healy Hall, 4th Floor
Washington, DC 20057
202-687-8099
Fax: 202-687-8089
http://kennedyinstitute.georgetown.edu/
kicourse@georgetown.edu

Legal Information Institute
American Legal Ethics Library
Cornell University Law School
Myron Taylor Hall
Ithaca, NY 14853-4901
607-255-1221
http://www.law.cornell.edu/ethics/

Markkula Center for Applied Ethics
Santa Clara University
500 El Camino Real
Santa Clara, CA 95053-0633
408-554-5319
Fax: 408-554-2373
http://www.scu.edu/ethics/
ethics@scu.edu

National Board for Certification in Occupational Therapy (NBCOT)
12 South Summit Avenue, Suite 100
Gaithersburg, MD 20877-4150
301-990-7979
Fax: 301-869-8492
http://www.nbcot.org/
info@nbcot.org

National Center for Ethics in Health Care
U.S. Department of Veterans Affairs
810 Vermont Avenue, NW
Washington, DC 20420
202-501-0364
Fax: 202-501-2238
http://www.ethics.va.gov/
vhaethics@va.gov

Neiswanger Institute for Bioethics and Health Policy
(formerly Center for Ethics and Social Justice)
Loyola University Stritch School of Medicine
2160 South First Avenue, Building 120, Room 280
Maywood, IL 60153
708-327-9200
Fax: 708-327-9209
http://bioethics.lumc.edu/
bioethics@lumc.edu

Presidential Commission for the Study of Bioethical Issues
1425 New York Avenue, NW, Suite C-100
Washington, DC 20005
202-233-3960
Fax: 202-233-3990
www.bioethics.gov/
info@bioethics.gov

Werner Institute for Negotiation and Dispute Resolution
Creighton University School of Law
2500 California Plaza
Omaha, NE 68178
402-280-2700
http://www.creighton.edu/werner/

ETHICS JOURNALS

American Journal of Bioethics:
http://www.bioethics.net/journal/

Cambridge Quarterly of Healthcare Ethics:
http://journals.cambridge.org/action/
    displayJournal?jid=CQH

Canadian Medical Association Journal:
http://www.cmaj.ca/misc/bioethics_e.shtml

Hastings Center Report:
http://www.thehastingscenter.org/
    Publications/HCR/Default.aspx

HEC Forum:
http://www.springer.com/philosophy/ethics/
    journal/10730

Journal of Clinical Ethics:
http://www.clinicalethics.com/

Journal of Medical Ethics:
http://jme.bmj.com/

Kennedy Institute of Ethics Journal:
http://muse.jhu.edu/journals/ken/

INTERNET RESOURCES

The following Internet sites have been selected to inform readers rather than to persuade or advertise. These sites offer multiple links to other information sites and are updated frequently.

Bioethics Discussion Pages:
http://www-hsc.usc.edu/~mbernste/

Bioethicsline, Kennedy Institute of Ethics, Georgetown University:
http://wings.buffalo.edu/faculty/research/
    bioethics/bio-line.html

Bioethics.net:
http://www.bioethics.net/beta.php

Complete Guide to Ethics Management: An Ethics Toolkit for Managers:
www.mapnp.org/library/ethics/ethxgde.htm

Health Insurance Portability and Accountability Act of 1996 (HIPAA):
http://www.hipaa.org/

U.S. Office of Government Ethics:
http://www.usoge.gov

Women's Bioethics Project:
http://womensbioethics.blogspot.com/

ONLINE ETHICS CERTIFICATE, MASTER'S, AND UNIVERSITY-BASED PROGRAMS

Albany Medical College, Alden March Bioethics Institute:
http://aldenmarch.org/education/graduate/
    index.php?page_id=3

College of St. Rose, Ethics Minor:
http://www.strose.edu/academics/
    schoolofartsandhumanities/philosophy_
    and_religiousstudies/ethics_minor

Loyola University Chicago, Neiswanger Institute for Bioethics & Health Policy:
http://bioethics.lumc.edu/

St. Joseph's University, Online Master's Degree in Health Administration, Health Care Ethics Specialization:
http://www.sju-online.com/programs/masters-health-administration-ethics.asp

Union Graduate College, Mount Sinai School of Medicine, Bioethics Program:
http://www.bioethics.union.edu/acacertif-certificate_in_bioethics_health_policy_law_clinical_ethics.html

University of Missouri, Center for Health Ethics:
http://ethics.missouri.edu/

University of Pennsylvania, Center for Bioethics:
http://www.bioethics.upenn.edu/

University of Washington School of Medicine, Ethics in Medicine:
http://depts.washington.edu/bioethx/tools/index.html

ANNOTATED BIBLIOGRAPHY

Beauchamp, T. L., & Childress, J. F. (2009). *Principles of biomedical ethics* (6th ed.). New York: Oxford University Press.
Beauchamp, the author or coauthor of many books over 40 years, is with the Kennedy Institute of Ethics and the Department of Philosophy at Georgetown University, a major center for bioethics nationally. Childress is with the Department of Religious Studies at the University of Virginia and also is a well-known author. This book was first published in 1977 and is one of the earliest texts to focus on bioethics. Each of the subsequent revisions (the 6th edition was published in 2009) has been well researched and expanded. This book is considered by many to be a standard for the field. It describes traditional bioethics theory and application.

According to the authors, "*Ethics* is a generic term for various ways of understanding and examining the moral life" (p. 1). The book starts with chapters on moral norms and character (including a revision in ethics of care as a form of virtue ethics), followed by a new third chapter on moral status. It then devotes a chapter to each of four basic groups of principles: respect for autonomy, nonmaleficence, beneficence, and justice. The chapter on justice has expanded treatment of "obligations of justice at the international level, based on globalization and new philosophical thinking about the global order" (p. vii). The next chapter discusses the moral rules of veracity, privacy, confidentiality, and fidelity in the context of professional–patient relationships. The remaining two chapters examine moral theories such as utilitarianism and duty-based theory and models of theory and application.

The book assumes that readers have some knowledge of philosophy, and it may be a somewhat difficult read as a first book in bioethics. However, *Principles of Biomedical Ethics* is one of the most often referred to and cited texts by major authors in bioethics and is considered a standard and authoritative text in the field.

Beauchamp, T. L., & Walters, L. (2003). *Contemporary issues in bioethics* (6th ed.). Belmont, CA: Thomson/Wadsworth.
This collection of essays and court opinions on ethical issues in medicine includes information on ethical theories and ethics in relation to the law and public policy. Appropriate for graduate students.

Boss, J. A. (2008). *Ethics for life: A text with readings* (4th ed.). Boston: McGraw-Hill.
This volume covers a variety of ethnic and religious groups' ethical philosophies. Cases and personal reflection exercises appear throughout the chapters. Appropriate for all levels of students.

Bowie, G. L., Higgins, K. M., & Michaels, M. W. (1998). *Thirteen questions in ethics and social philosophy* (2nd ed.). New York: Harcourt Brace Jovanovich.

Ideal for introductory courses in ethics, applied ethics, or moral problems, this book responds to rising student interest in multiculturalism and reflects the current issues of today. This edition has been updated with new articles and discussions on a variety of topics from sexual harassment to medical ethics. Appropriate for graduate students.

Jonsen, A. R., Siegler, M., & Winslade, W. J. (2006). *Clinical ethics: A practical approach to ethical decisions in clinical medicine* (6th ed.). New York: McGraw-Hill.

This volume offers advice about the often-difficult decisions health professionals encounter daily concerning ethics and medical issues and provides a broad knowledge base as well as different perspectives so the best solution can emerge. A physician, lawyer, and ethicist combine their expertise and supply invaluable insight on AIDS, economics of care, and more. Clinical cases coupled with counseling instruction highlight the material. Appropriate for graduate students.

Monagle, J. F., & Thomasma, D. C. (2005). *Health care ethics: Critical issues for the 21st century.* Sudbury, MA: Jones & Bartlett.

Readers encounter an array of ethical dilemmas that they may see professionally and personally. Chapters focus on the plight of reinstitutionalized persons with chronic mental disorders, domestic violence, genetics, elderly persons living in nursing homes, HIV/AIDS, the business of health care, and advance directives.

Percesepe, G. (1995). *Introduction to ethics: Personal and social responsibility in a diverse world.* Englewood Cliffs, NJ: Prentice Hall.

This comprehensive overview of ethics includes discussion of theory and reading groups, as well as chapters related to race and power, sex and power, community, and more. Each chapter includes additional readings. Appropriate for all levels.

Purtilo, R. (2004). *Ethical dimensions in the health professions* (4th ed.). Philadelphia: W. B. Saunders.

This introductory textbook for students in the health care professions provides sets of learning objectives at the beginning of each chapter and questions interspersed in the text to allow readers time to reflect on particular issues or points. It includes new chapters on organizational ethics, diversity, and assisted suicide. Each chapter uses case examples to illustrate and explain key points. Appropriate for all levels.

Purtilo, R. B., Jensen, G. M., & Royeen, C. B. (Eds.). (2005). *Educating for moral action: A sourcebook in health and rehabilitation ethics.* Philadelphia: F. A. Davis.

The book, the result of a 3-day conference on Leadership in Ethics Education for Physical Therapy and Occupational Therapy at the Center for Health Policy and Ethics at Creighton University in September 2003, is divided into three major sections. Section 1, "Broadening Our Worldview of Ethics," includes chapters on topics such as respect, empathy, competence (client-centered and cultural), ethics of social responsibility and leadership, and the ethic of care as illustrated in the moral dimensions of a chronic illness. Section 2 centers on the health care environment, with chapters discussing moral agency, neuroethics, the impact of institutional practices and policies, roles of professional organization ethics committees, a process model for ethical decision making, and a discussion of what chapter author John Glaser refers to as the three realms of ethics: (1) individual, (2) organizational, and (3) societal. The editors note that "currently the individual realm has a hold on our moral thinking and action" (p. x), and Glaser and other authors in this text argue convincingly that occupational and physical therapists must broaden their view of what is right, moral, and ethical beyond the individual patient. Section 3 is devoted specifically to ethics education in physical and occupational therapy. Topics include mindfulness, the link between spiritual self-awareness and ethical behavior, adult education models and ethics curricula, clinical education, research ethics, ethics of teaching, and the application of the scholarship of teaching and learning to critical inquiry about ethics education in the health professions.

Although the book will be of interest to ethics educators, it is not intended to be used as another ethics textbook for the classroom. Rather, it is intended to be both a resource and a springboard for further discussion and comment.

Scott, R. (1998). *Professional ethics: A guide for rehabilitation professionals.* Philadelphia: Mosby.
This book uses a multidisciplinary focus to address issues of informed consent, professional business arrangements, and more. Appropriate for all levels of occupational and physical therapy students and clinical educators.

Sieber, J. E. (1992). *Planning ethically responsible research: A guide for students and internal review boards.* Newbury Park, CA: Sage.

This excellent small text addresses practical issues and concerns for those doing research in an academic or clinical environment. Appropriate for graduate students.

Veatch, R. M., & Flack, H. E. (1997). *Case studies in allied health ethics.* Upper Saddle River, NJ: Brady/Prentice Hall.
More than 80 cases from the areas of occupational therapy, physical therapy, clinical laboratory sciences, dietetics, and other allied health professions help answer the question, "Do all allied health professions impose ethical standards and obligations on their practitioners?" Appropriate for all levels of students.

Weiss, J. W. (2006). *Business ethics: A stakeholder and issues management approach.* Mason, OH: Thomson South-Western.
Integrating current and emerging issues from today's complex workplace, this comprehensive text spotlights major contemporary and international topics in business ethics. Following the premise that, although ethical issues change, ethical principles remain constant, the text equips readers with practical guidelines to apply to the ethical dilemmas they will ultimately face in their world of work.

Index

Medicare and Medicaid, 119, 136, 138, 142, 143, 163, 167, 188–190, 210

mercy, kindness, and charity (Principle 1), 125, 130, 142, 144, 150, 151, 157, 166, 176, 189, 193, 202, 210, 211

nonmaleficence (Principle 2), 136–138, 145, 157, 176, 189, 202, 216

normative data for tests, accuracy of, 193–197

organizational (health care system) ethics, 179–185

OT assistants, partnerships with, 187–192

outdated and obsolete tests and assessment instruments, 193–197

payment for OT services. *See* insurance and payment for OT services, *above, under this heading*

plagiarism, 205–208, 219–222

practicing without license, 169–173

private practice, 141–146

procedural justice (Principle 5), 130, 145, 150, 151, 158, 165, 170, 171, 176, 187, 189, 191, 202, 206, 211, 215

products, sales to recipients of OT services, 135–139

professional education of OT students with disabilities, 147–154

professional organization governance and leadership, 175–177

refusal of treatment by patients, 181–184

Rehabilitation Act of 1973, 147–149

risks and benefits of technology-based interventions, 155–161

safety of technology-based interventions, 155–161

self-determination (Principle 3), 124, 130, 137, 150, 157, 158, 165, 167, 176, 183, 202, 216

selling products to recipients of OT services, 135–139

social justice (Principle 4), 125, 130, 142, 144, 165, 166, 209–212

social networking, 213–218

state licensure and regulation of OT services, 169–173

students with disabilities, professional education of, 147–154

supervision of OT assistants, 187–192

technology-based interventions, 155–161

tests, outdated and obsolete, 193–197

veracity (Principle 6), 136, 138, 151, 159, 171, 175, 191, 206, 211, 219

withdrawal from patient treatment, 199–204

alternative healing, 127

altruism, defined, 225

Americans With Disabilities Act (ADA), 147–149

annotated bibliographies of ethics resources, 115, 116, 233–235

AOTA Ethics Commission (EC), 3, 26–28, 55, 56

    correspondence related to EC complaints, 24

    investigations, 25, 26

    jurisdiction, 37–39

    members, 56

    refuting decisions of, 20, 31

    See also enforcement procedures

appeals process, 20, 31

arbitration clauses in contracts, 118

Arts and Crafts movement, 59, 60, 65, 66, 69

aspirational ethics codes, 50

assessment and testing, outdated and obsolete instruments, 193–197

assistants. *See* occupational therapy assistants

associations and organizations, ethics resources, 229, 230

attorneys' assistance in enforcement procedures, 30

autonomy and confidentiality (Principle 3)

    advisory opinions regarding, 124, 130, 137, 150, 157, 158, 165, 167, 176, 183, 202, 216

    explanation of, 10, 11, 225

B

baccalaureate degree requirement, history of OT as profession, 69

balancing patients' rights and practitioners' values, 123–126 beneficence (Principle 1)

    advisory opinions regarding, 125, 130, 142, 144, 150, 151, 157, 166, 176, 189, 193, 202, 210, 211

    explanation of, 9, 49, 225

best practices, 95, 96

    Association on Higher Education and Disability, 148

    organizational support for, 111

    Standards of Practice for Occupational Therapy, 95

    technology-based interventions at experimental stage, 158

biases, cultural, 131

bibliography of ethics resources, 233–235

billing practices, 86

    advisory opinion regarding payment for OT services, 163–167

    maximizing billable hours and extending staff, 94

        moral distress resulting from. *See* moral distress

        unrealistic productivity requirements, 96

    record keeping and documentation, 52, 143, 144

bioethics, defined, 225

business transactions with clients

    advisory opinion regarding, 135–139

    See also billing practices

C

calibration of instruments, accuracy, 195

capitated payment systems, 118, 164

care ethics, defined, 225

casuistry, defined, 225

categorical imperative, defined, 225

CE. *See* continuing education

censure, 22, 39–41, 56, 81, 91, 172

certificate programs in ethics, 232, 233

certification and other regulation of OT services, 169–173

charges in enforcement procedures, 26, 29, 52

    See also complaints

charity. *See* beneficence (Principle 1)

choice of law clauses in contracts, 118

citation of work of others, advisory opinions regarding, 205–207, 219–221

Code and Ethics Standards, 3, 4, 21

    See also Occupational Therapy Code of Ethics and Ethics Standards (2010)

colleagues, defined, 9

college programs in ethics, 232, 233

commission, acts of, vs. acts of omission, 101

compensation

    advisory opinion regarding payment for OT services, 163–167

    capitated payment systems, 118, 164

    contracting with managed care companies and vendors, 118, 119

    See also billing practices; payment for services

compensatory justice, defined, 226

complainant, defined, 23

complaints, 19, 23, 24, 26

    conflicts of interest, 25, 28, 29, 31

    de jure complaints, 19, 24, 27

comprehensive client safety programs, 104

concurrent and group therapy, 93–95

    defined, 93

    Medicare and Medicaid requirements, 93, 95

confidentiality

    defined, 225

    HIPAA (Health Insurance Portability and Accountability Act of 1996), 215

    investigation and enforcement process, 23

    patient confidentiality. *See* autonomy and confidentiality (Principle 3)

conflict of values between patient and practitioner, advisory opinion regarding, 124

conflicts of interest, 10, 15, 115

    advisory opinions regarding, 135, 144, 175, 216, 221

    between investigators, complainants, and respondents, 25, 28, 29, 31

    full and open disclosure of competing businesses and potential financial gain, 84

conscience, matters of, 73, 75, 123, 125, 200

consensus in therapeutic relationships
explanation of, 73–79
patients' rights vs. practitioner values, 123
consent. *See* informed consent
contesting charge of ethics violation, 27
continuation of complaint process, 24
continuing education (CE), 9, 39, 82, 85, 102
    advisory opinions regarding, 144, 150,
        157–159, 190, 221
    Everyday Ethics: Core Knowledge for
      Occupational Therapy Practitioners
      and Educators, continuing education
      course on, 108
continuing to treat patients who have refused
    services, 183
contracting with managed care companies
    and vendors, 117–119
    choice of law clauses, 118
    compensation, 118, 119
    disputes between contracting parties, 118
    indemnification and hold-harmless clauses,
      118
    integration clauses, 119
correspondence related to EC complaint, 24
costs, containing. *See* productivity
credentialing. *See* state licensure and other
    regulation of OT services
criminal violations, 53, 81, 82, 119, 143
    HIPAA violations, 215
    jurisdiction, 41
    practicing without license, 169
cultural competency, advisory opinion
    regarding, 127–133, 200
customary practices, 85, 86

D
decision-making process for ethical dilemmas,
    73–80
definitions, 9, 225–227
    colleagues, 9
    complainant, 23
    concurrent therapy, 93
    dovetailing, 93
    employees, 9
    ethical dilemmas, 225
    glossary of ethics terms, 225–227

moral distress, 107
occupational therapy, formal definition of,
    66
public, 9
public domain, 219
recipients of service, 9
research participants, 9
respondent, 23
scope of practice, 84
service recipients, 9
students, 9
de jure complaints, 19, 24, 27
deontology, defined, 225
development of OT as profession. *See* history
    of OT as profession
dialogue in ethical decision making, 74
disabled OT students, professional education
    of, 147–154
disciplinary actions. *See* enforcement
    procedures
Disciplinary Council, 28–31
disclosure of information
    in ethics complaint process, 23
    practitioners' financial holdings in
      equipment company, 137
    See also confidentiality
discontinuing patient care, 200
discounted fees for services, 118
dismissal of complaints, 25
distributive justice (Principle 4)
    advisory opinions regarding, 125, 130,
      142, 144, 165, 166, 211, 212
    explanation of, 11, 12, 226
documentation in billing practices, 52, 143,
    144
domestic violence, suspected, 124
dovetailing, defined, 93
due care, 10
duty, defined, 225
duty to treat patients, 199–204

E
EC. *See* AOTA Ethics Commission (EC)
educational ethics codes, 50
education and training, 43–119
    OT students. *See* students

practitioners' education of patients on advocacy strategies, rights, and options, 166

proactive vs. reactive approach to reducing errors, 102

See also continuing education (CE)

educative letters, 22

electronic media, plagiarism, 206, 219–221

emerging technology-based interventions, 155–161

employees

defined, 9

employment contracts and position descriptions, 51

fiduciary responsibility of OTs to organizations vs. patients, 182

ends justifying means, 226

enforcement procedures, 4, 17–33

acceptance of charge of ethics violation, 27

AOTA Ethics Commission (EC), review and decision, 26–28

appeals process, 31

assistance of counsel, 30

censure, 22

complaints. *See* complaints

confidentiality throughout investigation and enforcement process, 23

conflicts of interest between investigators, complainants, and respondents, 25

contesting charge of ethics violation, 27

continuation of complaint process, 24

correspondence, 24

de jure complaints, 19, 24, 27

Disciplinary Council, 28–31

disclosure of information in ethics complaint process, 23

dismissal of complaints, 25

educative letters, 22

Enforcement Procedures for the Occupational Therapy Code of Ethics and Ethics Standards, 19, 21, 55

ethical issues to inform and educate AOTA membership, 22

evidence, 22, 23, 29

fairness to parties in ethics complaints, 21

hearing, 29, 30

interested party complaints, 23, 24

investigations by EC, 25, 26

jurisdiction, 22

modification of time periods, procedures, or application of enforcement procedures for good cause, 32

notice, enforcement procedures, 24, 29, 30, 32

objectivity and fundamental fairness to parties in ethics complaints, 21

preliminary review and investigation by EC, 25, 26

probation of AOTA membership, 22

professional responsibility, 21

publication of decision after appeals process, 32

records and reports on completion of enforcement process, 32

reprimands, 22

respondent

defined, 23

response of, 27

revocation of AOTA membership, 22

sanctions, 22

sua sponte complaints, 24

time limits. *See* time limits

witnesses, 29

Enforcement Procedures for the Occupational Therapy Code of Ethics and Ethics Standards, 19, 21, 55

environmental factors, controllable or uncontrollable, 101

equipment, as cause of error, 101

equitable and appropriate distribution of resources, 11

errors, common practice errors and preventive strategies, 99–104

ethical decision-making process, 73–80

ethical dilemmas, 74, 75

decision-making process for resolving, 73–80

defined, 225

ethical leadership, 112

ethical relativism, defined, 225

ethics, defined, 225

ethics centers as resources, 229, 230

Ethics Commission. *See* AOTA Ethics Commission (EC)

ethics complaint process. *See* enforcement procedures

Ethics Office at AOTA, availability for assistance, 20

ethics resources, 233–235

evidence at hearings, 22, 23, 29

F

faculty and fieldwork educators of students with disabilities, 147–154

fair, equitable, and appropriate distribution of resources, 11

fairness to parties in ethics complaints, 21

fair treatment, 12

Family Educational Rights and Privacy Act (FERPA), 147–149

fees for services, 118

See also compensation

FERPA (Family Educational Rights and Privacy Act), 147–149

fidelity (Principle 7)

advisory opinions regarding, 131, 145, 150, 166, 176, 183, 206, 211, 216, 221

explanation of, 14, 15, 50, 226

fiduciary, defined, 226

fiduciary responsibility of OTs to organizations vs. patients, 182

financial goals of organizations, pressure to use as basis for action, 91

forum selection, contracts, 118

fraud, 52, 89

free or reduced-rate services, 211

G

glossary of ethics terms, 225–227

governance of professional organization, advisory opinion regarding, 175–177

grading procedures, unfair, 52

graduate education, history of OT as profession, 69

group therapy. *See* concurrent and group therapy

H

harm. *See* nonmaleficence (Principle 2)

health care industry

advisory opinions regarding, 166, 179–185, 187

business practices and profits, 89

education of patients on advocacy strategies, rights, and options, 166

fiduciary responsibility of employees to organizations vs. patients, 182

financial goals, pressure to use as basis for action, 91

health care reform and demands on OT assistants, 187

interdisciplinary research, 110, 111

moral distress in. *See* moral distress

multidimensional causes of errors, including poorly structured organizations, 101

health insurance. *See* insurance benefits

Health Insurance Portability and Accountability Act of 1996, 215

hearings, 29, 30

evidence at hearings, 22, 23, 29

See also enforcement procedures

highest level of moral reasoning, 78

HIPAA (Health Insurance Portability and Accountability Act of 1996), 215

history of OT as profession, 57–64

activities of daily living, focus for OT, 68

adoption of formal definition of OT, 66

Arts and Crafts movement, 59, 60, 65, 66, 69

baccalaureate degree requirement, 69

basic principles of early OT, 59, 60

graduate education, 69

neuropsychiatry, 65

prescription vs. referral, 68

principles drawn from values and beliefs from 1904 to 1929, 61–63

registration vs. licensure, 69

research covering 1930 to 1949, 63

science-based profession, evolution as, 65

state licensure, 69

subject areas influencing development or application of OT, 60

war, treatment of returning soldiers, 59, 68

I

impairment, defined, 226

indemnification and hold-harmless clauses, contracts, 118

independent practice, advisory opinion regarding, 141–146

informed consent, 158, 165

    vs. consent to treat, 158

insurance benefits

    advisory opinions regarding, 138, 141, 142, 145, 156, 163–167, 189, 209–212, 215

    fraud, 52

    HIPAA (Health Insurance Portability and Accountability Act of 1996), 215

    indemnification and hold-harmless clauses, contracts, 118

    productivity requirements, illegal or unethical, 96

    reimbursement environments, 96

    social justice issues, 209–212

    See also Medicare and Medicaid

integration clauses, contracts, 119

integrity. *See* veracity (Principle 6)

interdisciplinary research, 110, 111

interested party complaints, 23, 24

Internet

    ethics resources online, 232

    plagiarism of online information, 206, 219–221

    social networking, advisory opinion regarding, 213–218

intervention phase, practice errors occurring during, 101

investigations, 19, 25, 26

    conflicts of interest, 25, 28, 29, 31

J

jurisdiction, 19, 22, 35–42, 51

    AOTA Ethics Commission (EC), 37–39

    chart of responsibility, NBCOT vs. SRBs vs. AOTA, 38

contracting with managed care companies and vendors, 118

criminal violations, 41

National Board for Certification in Occupational Therapy (NBCOT), 37–40

state regulatory boards (SRBs), 37, 38, 40, 41

justice, defined, 226

K

kindness. *See* beneficence (Principle 1)

L

law, defined, 226

leadership and governance of professional organization, 175–177

legal matters, 83–87

    distinguished from ethical dilemmas, 75, 81, 82

    law, defined, 226

    payer policies, 86

    reasoning in legal and ethical practice challenges, 87

    scope of practice, 83, 84

    state licensure laws, 85, 86

    usual and customary practices, 85, 86

    See also criminal violations

M

mail related to EC complaint, certified, return receipt requested, 24

master's programs in ethics, 232, 233

Medicare and Medicaid

    advisory opinions regarding, 119, 136, 138, 142, 143, 163, 167, 188–190, 210

    concurrent and group therapy, 93, 95

    fraud, 89

    payer policies, 85, 86, 90, 91

mercy, kindness, and charity. *See* beneficence (Principle 1)

metaethics, defined, 226

mistakes and preventive strategies, 99–104

model for ethical decision making, 74–78

moral distress, 107–112
  appropriate staffing, 112
  communication, 112
  defined, 107
  ethical leadership, 112
  patients' inability to pay, 111
morality, defined, 226
moral reasoning, 76–78
morals, defined, 226
moral vs. technical errors, 99
multidimensional causes of practice error, 101
multiple clients, provision of care at one time, 93–95

N

National Board for Certification in Occupational Therapy (NBCOT), 53
  chart of responsibility, NBCOT vs. SRBs vs. AOTA, 38
  jurisdiction, 37–40
neuropsychiatry, 65
nonmaleficence (Principle 2)
  advisory opinions regarding, 136–138, 145, 157, 176, 189, 202, 216
  explanation of, 9, 10, 49, 226
nontraditional treatment
  alternative healing, 127
  technology-based interventions, 155–161
normative data for tests, accuracy of, 193–197
normative ethics, defined, 226
notice, 29, 30, 32
  correspondence related to EC complaint, 24

O

objectivity and fundamental fairness in ethics complaints, 21
occupational therapy assistants, 89, 90
  Code and Ethics Standards, use in guidance of, 21
  many roles of, 3, 7, 39
  partnerships between OTs and OT assistants, 187–192

professional responsibility to know and understand regulations governing practice, 86, 90
roles and responsibilities, 83
supervision of, 83, 187–192
Occupational Therapy Code of Ethics and Ethics Standards (2010), 3, 7–15, 55
  Principle 1. *See* beneficence
  Principle 2. *See* nonmaleficence
  Principle 3. *See* autonomy and confidentiality; self-determination
  Principle 4. *See* distributive justice; social justice
  Principle 5. *See* procedural justice
  Principle 6. *See* veracity
  Principle 7. *See* fidelity
  replacement of 2005 Code, 4
occupational therapy students. *See* students
omission, acts of, vs. acts of commission, 101
one-on-one direct service, 94, 95
online ethics educational programs, 232, 233
online resources. *See* Internet
organizational (health care system) ethics, 108
  advisory opinion regarding, 179–185
  See also health care industry
OT assistants. *See* occupational therapy assistants
OT students. *See* students
outdated and obsolete tests and assessment instruments, 193–197
ownership of practice, 142, 143

P

partnerships between OTs and OT assistants, 187–192
paternalism, defined, 226
patients' rights vs. practitioner values, 123
payment for services, 86
  billing practices. *See* billing practices
  insurance. *See* insurance benefits
  moral distress, patients' inability to pay, 111
  See also compensation
per diem compensation, 118

personal integrity in ethical decision making, 74, 75

plagiarism, 205–208, 219–222

position descriptions and employment contracts, 51

power in relationship between patient and practitioner, unequal distribution of, 129

practice errors and preventive strategies
approaches to reducing errors, proactive vs. reactive, 102
multidimensional causes of error, 101

practicing without license, 169–173

preliminary review and investigation by EC, 25, 26

prescription vs. referral, history of OT as profession, 68

preventive strategies for common practice errors, 99–104

principles of conduct within OT profession
historical information, 59–63
Principle 1. *See* beneficence
Principle 2. *See* nonmaleficence
Principle 3. *See* autonomy and confidentiality; self-determination
Principle 4. *See* distributive justice; social justice
Principle 5. *See* procedural justice
Principle 6. *See* veracity
Principle 7. *See* fidelity

private practice, advisory opinion regarding, 141–146

proactive vs. reactive approach to reducing practice errors, 102, 104

probation, AOTA membership, 22, 24

pro bono OT services, 165, 211

procedural justice (Principle 5)
advisory opinions regarding, 130, 145, 150, 151, 158, 165, 170, 171, 176, 187, 189, 191, 202, 206, 211, 215
explanation of, 12, 13, 49, 226

procedural matters in enforcement of ethics code and standards, 19, 20
See also enforcement procedures

process for ethical decision making, 73–80

productivity, 93–97
maximizing billable hours and extending staff, 94
moral distress resulting from. *See* moral distress
unrealistic productivity requirements, 96
See also best practices

products, sales to recipients of OT services, 135–139

professional organization governance and leadership, 175–177

professional responsibility, 21
knowing and understanding regulations governing practice, 86, 90

psychological abandonment of patients, 203

psychological disequilibrium of OTs. *See* moral distress

publication of decisions after appeals process, 32

public, defined, 9

public domain, defined, 219

purposes of *Occupational Therapy Code of Ethics and Ethics Standards*, 8

R

recalibration of instruments, 195

recipients of service, defined, 9

record keeping and documentation, 52, 143, 144

records and reports, completion of enforcement process, 32

reduced-fee and pro bono OT services, 165, 211

reductionist therapy interventions, 94

referrals, advisory opinion regarding, 141, 142

reflection in ethical decision making, 74

refusal of treatment
by patients, 181–184
by practitioners, 199

registration vs. licensure
history of OT as profession, 69
See also state licensure and other regulation of OT services

regulatory ethics codes, 50

About the Editor

Deborah Yarett Slater, MS, OT/L, FAOTA, is the staff liaison to the Ethics Commission and the Special Interest Sections at the American Occupational Therapy Association (AOTA). She has over 35 years of experience in administration and management within diverse health care organizations, including oversight of large single and multidisciplinary departments in both inpatient and outpatient settings. She has developed startup off-site satellite clinics for several organizations, including new program development, and has extensive experience in financial management and reimbursement. Ms. Slater has also been active in a variety of volunteer leadership positions for her state occupational therapy association, and before working at AOTA, she served as committee member and chair of the Administration and Management Special Interest Section, chair of the Special Interest Section Council, practice representative to the Ethics Commission (EC), and chair of the EC from 2000 to 2001. She also has been a member of the AOTA Board of Directors and chair of the ad hoc committee on Scope of Practice.

Ms. Slater has done numerous presentations on ethical issues and their application to clinical practice at state and national conferences. She has also published articles and advisory opinions on topics related to ethics. Most recently, she coauthored a chapter "Ethical Reasoning" in the text *Clinical and Professional Reasoning in Occupational Therapy* (Lippincott Williams & Wilkins, 2008) and a chapter "Ethical Dimensions of Occupational Therapy" for the 5th edition of *The Occupational Therapy Manager* (AOTA Press, 2011). In addition, she coedits the AOTA *Scope of Practice Issues Update* newsletter and has done conference workshops and an AudioInsight Continuing Education presentation on "Understanding and Asserting the Occupational Therapy Scope of Practice" with AOTA colleagues.

Ms. Slater is an AOTA fellow and has received numerous Service Awards for her volunteer leadership positions. In 2002, she received the Herbert J. Hall Award from the Massachusetts Association for Occupational Therapy, and in May 2005, she received the Distinguished Alumna Award from Columbia University in New York City.